Prototype of a Biomimetic Multi-Spiked Connecting Scaffold
for a New Generation
of Resurfacing Endoprostheses

The monograph comprehensively presents the research on the prototype of the biomimetic Multi-Spiked Connecting Scaffold (MSC-Scaffold) for cementless fixation of the components of a new generation of resurfacing arthroplasty (RA) endoprostheses. This research, carried out by a bioengineering-surgical team from three Polish universities, includes bioengineering design, rapid prototyping, manufacturing in selective laser melting, functionalization, surface modification, numerical studies, experimental *in vitro* studies, and pilot surgical experiments in an animal model.

Features:

- Presents the prototype of the multi-spiked connecting scaffold for a new generation of resurfacing endoprostheses of the knee and the hip.
- Explains this prototype scaffold as the first worldwide design of the biomimetic fixation of components of diarthrodial joints resurfacing endoprostheses.
- Insights into the entire process of bioengineering design and research on this novel way of resurfacing endoprostheses fixation.
- Reviews main results of the scaffold prototyping and SLM manufacturing, structural and osteoconductive functionalization, and surface modification.
- Reports experimental and numerical investigations of mechanical behaviour of the scaffold-bone system, cell culture studies, and pilot surgical experiments in animal models.

This book is aimed at professionals and graduate students in biomedical engineering, biomaterials engineering, and bone & joint surgery.

Prototype of a Biomimetic
Multi-Spiked Connecting Scaffold
for a New Generation
of Resurfacing Endoprostheses

Ryszard Uklejewski, Piotr Rogala,
and Mariusz Winiecki

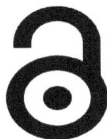

CRC Press
Taylor & Francis Group
Boca Raton London New York

CRC Press is an imprint of the
Taylor & Francis Group, an **informa** business

Designed cover image: Jan Rogala and Ryszard Uklejewski

First published in English 2024
by CRC Press
6000 Broken Sound Parkway NW, Suite 300, Boca Raton, FL 33487-2742

and by CRC Press
4 Park Square, Milton Park, Abingdon, Oxon, OX14 4RN

CRC Press is an imprint of Taylor & Francis Group, LLC

Funded by the Polish Ministry of Education and Science from funds awarded to the Kazimierz Wielki University in Bydgoszcz (Poland), and by the Endomedic Sp. z o.o., Poznan (Poland).

The precursory text (version) of this monograph was published in Polish by Academic Publishing House „EXIT", Warsaw 2021 (ISBN: 9788378371151); APH „EXIT" has waived to CRC Press all copyright claims to the text and of the monograph.

ISBN: 9781032418445 (hbk)
ISBN: 9781032428260 (pbk)
ISBN: 9781003364498 (ebk)

DOI: 10.1201/9781003364498

Typeset in Times
by codeMantra

Publication co-financed by the state budget (Poland) under the program of the Minister of Education and Science under the name "Excellent Science – Support for scientific monographs", project number DNM/SP/548211/2022, co-financing amount 66,962.50 PLN, total project value 74,412.50 PLN.

To our Friends and Colleagues from the Polish Society for Biomaterials,

affiliated Member of the European Society for Biomaterials

Contents

Forewords

Hip joint arthroplasty is one of the most widely performed orthopaedic surgeries in the world. There are many types of endoprostheses available on the medical market that, depending on the method of fixation in the bone, are divided into cemented and uncemented. Both solutions, however, require the excision of the femoral head and neck, as well as the preparation of the femoral medullary canal into which the endoprosthesis stem is inserted. In addition, the use of bone cement exposes the patient's tissues to the local increase in temperature from the cement setting, resulting in tissue necrosis. Furthermore, in the case of uncemented prostheses, patient rehabilitation and convalescence are relatively long, due to the highly traumatic surgery and the time needed for the biological fixation of the stem in the bone canal.

In many cases, patients can be offered resurfacing joint endoprostheses that are less traumatic and allow to save joint tissues to a greater extent than in the case of typical long-stem endoprostheses implantation. However, their fixation with bony structures with the use of cement is not optimal and may result in postoperative complications such as local blood circulation deficiency, stress shielding, aseptic loosening, and even hip fracture.

Therefore, taking into account the obstacles of contemporary solutions, an interdisciplinary team led by Prof. Uklejewski, Prof. Rogala, and Dr. Winiecki has been working for several years on new-generation uncemented resurfacing arthroplasty prostheses for the hip and other joints.

In nine chapters of this monograph, the reader can find a brief review of currently used cement-based hip joint resurfacing arthroplasty endoprostheses, followed by the presentation of the author's original, internationally patented concept of the multi-spiked connecting scaffold (MSC-Scaffold) for entirely uncemented fixation of resurfacing endoprostheses components in the periarticular bone. The MSC-Scaffold, through its structural and biomechanical biomimetism, preservation of bone tissue, and blood supply, may be regarded as a breakthrough approach to fixation of such endoprostheses. Presented are the results of the comprehensive bioengineering research programme on the MSC-Scaffold, which include the design, prototyping, manufacturing, surface modification, and *in vitro*, *in vivo*, and *ex vivo* studies. These results demonstrate the great potential of biomimetic fixation of resurfacing endoprostheses components via the MSC-Scaffold. The results have been partly published and have also been presented, e.g., during the annual conferences of the Polish Society for Biomaterials in Rytro and during the 27th European Conference on Biomaterials ESB 2015 in Kraków, Poland.

The monograph will be appreciated by all those who are interested in biomaterials design and modelling, biomedical engineering, biomechanics, cell/tissue-material interaction, and the development of innovative implants. I personally believe that this monograph will serve as a valuable reading for academics, physicians, researchers, and students. I highly recommend this book to these groups of people.

Prof. Dr. Elżbieta Pamuła, PhD, DSc, Eng.
Fellow Biomaterials Science and Engineering
President of the Polish Society for Biomaterials
AGH University of Science and Technology in Kraków, Poland

Foreword to the First Edition of the book published in Polish language
The monograph presents the overall course of the research tasks and the fundamental scientific results obtained within the frames of two Research Projects of the Polish Ministry of Science and Higher Education (No. 4T07C05629) and the National Science Centre Poland (No. NN518412638) and their continuation, accomplished at the Poznan University of Technology in cooperation with research teams from the Poznan University of Medical Sciences (from the Wiktor Dega Orthopaedic and Rehabilitation Clinical Hospital of the Poznan University of Medical Sciences) and from the Kazimierz Wielki University in Bydgoszcz (from the Department of Fundamentals of Medical Bioengineering at the Institute of Technology at the Faculty of Mathematics, Physics and Technology).

The most important of these results have been partially published in good and very good international and national scientific journals, mentioned by the authors in the Introduction to this monograph. The author of the concept of a new generation of hip resurfacing arthroplasty endoprosthesis and other joints is Professor Piotr Rogala, Ph.D., MD, an orthopaedic surgeon from the Poznan University of Medical Sciences. The bioengineering research on the prototype of the above-mentioned endoprosthesis with the multi-spiked connecting scaffold was headed by Professor Ryszard Uklejewski, Ph.D., Eng., Ph.D., MD – an expert from the National Centre for Research and Development, while Dr. Mariusz Winiecki, Ph.D., Eng., cooperates within the above-mentioned bioengineering research team as key co-investigator from its beginning.

The reader of this monograph – whether a bioengineer or an orthopaedist – can receive an almost direct insight into the entirety of bioengineering research works necessary to develop a functional prototype of an orthopaedic implant, prepared for the next stage of experimental surgical treatment using an innovative, entirely cementless hip joint resurfacing arthroplasty endoprosthesis, which shall be carried out at the university orthopaedic clinic, with the consent of the Bioethics Committee.

The developed prototype of innovative hip resurfacing arthroplasty endoprosthesis, the components of which are entirely embedded in the periarticular bone by means of the biomimetic multi-spiked connecting scaffold without using cement, is a significant scientific contribution of the Poznan bioengineering and clinical research team to the international biomedical engineering, in particular to biomechanical engineering and orthopaedic biomechanics.

Prof. Dr. Danuta Jasinska-Choromanska, PhD, Eng.
Faculty of Mechatronics
and School of Biomedical Engineering
Warsaw University of Technology, Warsaw, Poland

Preface

The aim of the monograph is to present the most significant results concerning the developed prototype of the biomimetic Multi-Spiked Connecting Scaffold (MSC-Scaffold) fixing in the periarticular bone of the components of a new generation of entirely non-cemented resurfacing arthroplasty (RA) endoprostheses, obtained by our bioengineering team (composed of researchers from the Poznan University of Technology, the Poznan University of Medical Sciences, and the Kazimierz Wielki University in Bydgoszcz) during the realization of two research projects of the Ministry of Science and Higher Education (Poland)/the National Science Centre Poland carried out by us in 2005–2015 at two faculties of the Poznan University of Technology (No. 4T07C05629 – at the Faculty of Machines and Transport, in the Chair of Machine Design Fundamentals, and No. NN518412638 – at the Faculty of Chemical Technology, in the Department of Process Engineering of the Institute of Chemical Technology and Engineering).

Completed research tasks of the above-mentioned research projects concerned: designing the prototype biomimetic MSC-Scaffold for a new generation of non-cemented resurfacing arthroplasty endoprostheses, manufacturing of preprototypes of the MSC-Scaffold in the Selective Laser Melting (SLM) technology of powders of titanium alloys, bioengineering laboratory and numerical experiments and pilot experiments in an animal model (hip and knee joints of swines of the Polish Large White breed) carried out with the permission of the Local Ethics Committee in Poznan in the surgical operating room of a veterinary clinic cooperating with the Laboratory of Microsurgery, Chair and Clinic Rehabilitation at the Wiktor Dega Orthopaedic and Rehabilitation Clinical Hospital of the Poznan University of Medical Sciences (Poland). The realization of bioengineering tasks was led by Professor Ryszard Uklejewski, PhD Eng., PhD MD (head of the above-mentioned research projects of the Ministry of Science and Higher Education/the National Science Centre Poland, the National Centre for Research and Development expert), and the realization of the pilot experimental studies in an animal model was led by Professor Piotr Rogala, PhD MD, an orthopaedic surgeon from the Wiktor Dega Orthopaedic and Rehabilitation Clinical Hospital of the Poznan University of Medical Sciences, author of a patented concept of a new generation of resurfacing arthroplasty endoprosthesis of the hip joint and other joints. Dr. P. Rogala in 1995 started scientific cooperation in the field of orthopaedic biomechanics with Assoc. Prof. Dr. R. Uklejewski who worked at the time in the Department of Mechanics and Acoustics of Porous Materials at the Acoustoelectronics Centre of the Institute of Fundamental Technological Research of the Polish Academy of Sciences (IPPT PAN), Poznan Branch.

Since 2003, following the invitation from the Poznan University of Technology, an interdisciplinary bioengineering and clinical research team was created under the supervision of Prof. Dr. R. Uklejewski, in the following years composed of scientists from three universities: (1) the Poznan University of Technology – from the Chair of Machine Design Fundamentals at the Faculty of Machines and Transport, from the Department of Process Engineering of the Institute of Chemical Technology and Engineering at the Faculty of Chemical Technology, and the Department of Technology Design of the Institute of Mechanical Technology at the Faculty of Machine Construction and Management (now Faculty of Mechanical Engineering), (2) the Poznan University of Medical Sciences – from the Clinic of Spine Surgery, Orthopaedics and Traumatology and the Chair and Clinic of Rehabilitation of the Wiktor Dega Orthopaedic and the Rehabilitation Clinical Hospital of the Poznan University of Medical Sciences, and (3) the Kazimierz Wielki University in Bydgoszcz – from the Department of Fundamentals of Medical Bioengineering, Institute of Technology at the Faculty of Mathematics, Physics and Technology.

The major published scientific papers that present the main results of the research projects of the Ministry of Science and Higher Education (Poland)/the National Science Centre Poland (No. 4T07C05629 and No. NN518412638) and their continuation, based on which this monograph was written, are papers: Ch.3 [46], Ch.4 [10–12], Ch.5 [2,3], Ch.6 [2,3,38], Ch.7 [19], Ch.8 [26]. The authors of these papers are members of two teams realizing the above-mentioned research projects; the monograph was developed and edited by the principal investigator of the above-mentioned research projects and the two key coinvestigators of these projects. As a result of extending the thematic scope of two research tasks included in the schedules of the above-mentioned research projects, the following two PhD theses have been completed: Ch.5 [1], Ch.6 [1].

Ryszard Uklejewski
Piotr Rogala
Mariusz Winiecki

Acknowledgements

The authors of this monographic study would like to thank the Deans and Vice-Deans of the Faculty of Chemical Technology and the Faculty of Mechanical Engineering (formerly the Faculty of Machine Construction and Management and the Faculty of Machines and Transport) as well as the Rector and Vice-Rectors of the Poznan University of Technology (Poland) for inviting us and kindly patronizing our scientific and didactic cooperation in the field of biomedical engineering within the structures of the Poznan University of Technology in the years 2005–2022 /cf. Appendix 2/. In particular, we would like to thank: Prof. Dr. Janusz Mielniczuk, the Vice-Dean for Science of the Faculty of Machines and Transport, Prof. Dr. Marian Dudziak, the Head of Chair of Machine Design Fundamentals; from the Faculty of Chemical Technology: Prof. Dr. Stefan Kowalski, Member of the Polish Academy of Sciences and the Head of the Department of Process Engineering, Prof. Dr. Krzysztof Alejski, the Dean of the Faculty, Prof. Dr. Adam Voelkel, the Head of the Institute of Chemical Technology and Engineering; from the Faculty of Mechanical Engineering and Management: Prof. Dr. Jan Żurek, the Vice-Rector of the Poznan University of Technology and the Dean of the Faculty, and Prof. Dr. Olaf Ciszak, the Vice-Dean (and the Dean) for inviting us to cooperate in organizing and conducting engineering studies in Biomedical Engineering at the Poznan University of Technology, and for cooperation in conducting a PhD student (Poznan University of Technology graduate) in Biomedical Engineering at the Warsaw University of Technology.

Ryszard Uklejewski
Piotr Rogala
Mariusz Winiecki

About the authors

Ryszard Uklejewski, PhD, Eng., PhD, MD is a Professor of Biomedical Engineering. He received an MSc from the Poznan University of Technology, Poland (1974), and a PhD at the Lodz University of Technology (in Electromechanics, 1979), and studied mathematics (1976–1980) at the University of Lodz, Poland. He is also a qualified medical doctor (1996, Poznan University of Medical Sciences, Poland), and received the PhD in Medicine (in Endocrinology) at the University of Medical Sciences in Poznan (2010). He worked (1974–1996) in the Department of Mechanics and Acoustics of Porous Materials at the Institute of Fundamental Technological Research, Polish Academy of Sciences. In 1995 he received the Habilitation in Biomedical Engineering from the Institute of Biocybernetics and Biomedical Engineering, Polish Academy of Sciences with a thesis on bioelectromechanics of porous bone filled with physiological viscous ionic fluid. He works (1997 till now) at the Kazimierz Wielki University in Bydgoszcz (Poland) as the Head of the Department of Medical Bioengineering Fundamentals in the Institute of Technology, currently in Chair of Constructional Materials and Biomaterials at the Faculty of Materials Engineering. His main research areas are structural-biomechanical bio-compatibility of bone-implant interface on the basis of the modern two-phase poroelastic biomechanical model of bone tissue and of the theory of poroelastic materials, bone tissue biomechatronics, and the endocrinology of growing human skeleton. He is the author of more than 180 research publications, the inventor of the patent on the non-invasive method of determination of density and poroelastic parameters of osteoporotic long bones, and the head of two research projects of the Polish Ministry of Science and the National Science Centre Poland on the development of prototypes of non-cemented resurfacing arthroplasty endoprostheses (invented by Professor P. Rogala), realized in the Poznan University of Technology. He is a member of the American Biographical Institute Research Association, the European Federation for Research in Rehabilitation, Polish Society for Biomaterials, a former member of AAAS and NYAS (for at least ten years) and is included in "2000 Outstanding Scientists of the 20th Century" by the International Biographical Centre, Cambridge, UK (ISBN: 0948875682).

Piotr Rogala, MD, PhD is an Associate Professor of Orthopaedic Surgery in the Department of Spine Surgery, Oncologic Orthopaedics and Traumatology of the Poznan University of Medical Sciences (Poland) and in the Institute of Health Sciences, State School of Higher Education in Gniezno (Poland) with more than 30 years of international clinical experience (France, Tunisia, Republic of South Africa), and the orthopaedic biomechanics consultant in the Department of Medical Bioengineering Fundamentals, Kazimierz Wielki University in Bydgoszcz (Poland). He is the inventor and patent owner of the new model of resurfacing arthroplasty endoprostheses and the author of the original concept of the multi-spiked connecting scaffold (MSC-Scaffold) for fixation of resurfacing arthroplasty components in surrounding bone with minimally invasive operating procedures. He is a member of several international scientific associations (European Federation of National Associations of Orthopaedics and Traumatology, European Orthopaedic Research Society, European Federation for Research in Rehabilitation, etc.). He is particularly interested in orthopaedic biomechanics, the etiopathology of adolescent idiopathic scoliosis, and clinical genetics of bone diseases. He is the author of more than 170 research publications, the head of two research projects of the Polish Ministry of Science in the field of clinical orthopaedics and genetics, and is included in Encyclopaedia Britannica, USA.

Mariusz Winiecki, PhD, Eng., is an Assistant Professor in the Chair of Constructional Materials and Biomaterials at the Faculty of Materials Engineering at the Kazimierz Wielki University in Bydgoszcz, Poland. In 2001 he received the MSc in Mechanical Engineering (specialization in Mechatronics) at the Poznan University of Technology, Poland, and in 2006 he received his PhD in Mechanical Engineering at the Poznan University of Technology, Poland, for the thesis on the investigation of the micro-geometric constructional properties of porous intraosseous implants and the influence of these properties on the strength of the bone-implant model fixation (PhD supervisor: Prof. R. Uklejewski). In 2007 he finished Postgraduate Studies in the field of Biomaterials Engineering at the AGH University of Science and Technology in Cracow, Poland, and since 2007 is a member of the Polish Society for Biomaterials. His main research areas in the field of biomaterials engineering are the engineering of bone-implant interfacing, design and implant surface functionalization towards improving the conditions for osseointegration. He has achievements in works of the interdisciplinary research group that has designed, prototyped, and manufactured in the selective laser melting technology, and developed through bioengineering research the essential innovation in fixation of components of a new generation of entirely cementless resurfacing hip arthroplasty endoprostheses in the subchondral trabecular bone by means of the biomimetic multi-spiked connecting scaffold – he was a key investigator in two research projects of the Polish Ministry of Science and the National Science Centre Poland, concerning the development of prototypes of non-cemented resurfacing arthroplasty endoprosthesis, realized at the Poznan University of Technology. He is the author of more than 90 scientific papers.

Introduction

The aim of the monograph is to present the most significant results concerning the developed prototype of the biomimetic Multi-Spiked Connecting Scaffold (MSC-Scaffold) fixing in the periarticular bone of the components of a new generation of entirely non-cemented resurfacing arthroplasty (RA) endoprostheses, obtained by our bioengineering team during the realization of two research projects of the Ministry of Science and Higher Education (Poland)/the National Science Centre Poland. Completed research tasks of these research projects concerned: designing the prototype biomimetic MSC-Scaffold for a new generation of non-cemented resurfacing arthroplasty endoprostheses, manufacturing of preprototypes of the MSC-Scaffold in the Selective Laser Melting (SLM) technology of powders of titanium alloys, bioengineering laboratory and numerical experiments and pilot experiments in an animal model.

Chapter 1 describes the currently used cement-based hip joint resurfacing arthroplasty endoprostheses in the background of previous designs of resurfacing endoprostheses. It also discusses the most common types of postoperative complications of this arthroplasty, caused by the method of fixation of the femoral component of modern resurfacing endoprostheses in the bone with the use of cement and a short stem.

Chapter 2 presents the concept of an entirely non-cemented and stemless method of fixation of the components of resurfacing endoprostheses of the hip joint in the bone using the biomimetic MSC-Scaffold and the consequences of this innovative fixation method for the transfer of biomechanical loads in the implant-bone system.

Chapter 3 presents the design, rapid prototyping, and manufacturing of the prototype biomimetic multi-spiked connecting scaffold (MSC-Scaffold) for a new generation of non-cemented resurfacing arthroplasty endoprostheses, including bioengineering CAD design and modelling, methods and effects of the electrical discharge machining of the MSC-Scaffold spikes, stereolithography prototyping of the MSC-Scaffold spikes, prototyping and manufacturing of titanium alloy powders of the MSC-Scaffold preprototypes, and a prototype of the total hip resurfacing endoprosthesis in the selective laser melting (SLM) technology, developed and carried out post-production treatment of the bone-contacting surface of the MSC-Scaffold preprototypes manufactured in the SLM technology, as well as reverse engineering the working prototype of partial resurfacing knee arthroplasty endoprosthesis manufactured in the SLM technology for experimental implantations in an animal model.

Chapter 4 presents the completed research task concerning the structural and osteoconductive functionalization of the interspike space of the prototype MSC-Scaffold. The theoretical basis for the evaluation of the pro-osteoconductive potential of the MSC-Scaffold is provided. Results of evaluating the possibility of forming the structural-osteoconductive properties of the MSC-Scaffold are presented, as well as the course and results of the preliminary biological evaluation in cell culture of the MSC-Scaffold preprototypes after the structural-osteoconductive functionalization of their interspike space, with the course and results of the pilot study of the preprototypes of the structurally functionalized MSC-Scaffold in an animal model.

Chapter 5 concerns the formation of the osteoinductive and osseointegrating properties of the bone-contacting surface of the MSC-Scaffold by electrochemical deposition (ECD) of calcium phosphates (CaPs). The chapter presents the results of preliminary attempts to modify the bone-contacting surface of the MSC-Scaffold preprototypes by ECD of CaPs carried out at constant current densities. It describes the process and the results of CaP potentiostatic ECD on the surface of spikes with the subsequent immersion of the MSC-Scaffold preprototypes in a simulated body fluid (SBF). The results of research in human osteoblasts culture on the calcium phosphate-coated prototype MSC-Scaffolds, as well as the results of the evaluation of their biointegration with bone as implanted under the articular surface of swine knee joints are presented.

Chapter 6 describes the biomechanical studies of the bone-implant system concerning the design of the structural and biomechanical properties of the considered multi-spiked connecting scaffold (MSC-Scaffold) carried out in the biomechanical tests on a universal testing machine and applying numerical simulation analysis. The chapter presents numerical studies of the influence of the geometric features of the MSC-Scaffold on the distribution of mechanical stresses in the periprosthetic bone, and the course and results of the experimental validation of the numerical model representing the initial intraoperative embedding in the periarticular bone of the prototype MSC-Scaffold providing entirely cementless fixation of the components of the resurfacing arthroplasty endoprostheses with the bone.

Chapter 7 presents the course and results of the pilot studies on the prototype MSC-Scaffold for entirely non-cemented resurfacing arthroplasty endoprostheses in an animal model. These studies included the experimental determination of an appropriate surgical approach to the hip and knee joints in a swine and the verification of ten experimental animals of a working prototype of partial resurfacing knee arthroplasty endoprosthesis implanted in the periarticular bone via the MSC-Scaffold.

Chapter 8 contains the results of a pilot study on human femoral heads obtained from postoperative material from patients with osteoarthritis who were surgically treated with Total Hip Arthroplasty (THA), conducted with the approval of the Bioethics Committee of the Poznan University of Medical Sciences concerning the quantitative microtomographic evaluation of the impact of embedding the prototype multi-spiked connecting scaffold (MSC-Scaffold) in the subchondral trabecular bone on the density of human femoral heads and their compressive strength.

Chapter 9 contains a summary of the monograph, conclusions, and final remarks. The developed prototype of the multi-spiked connecting scaffold (MSC-Scaffold) will allow us to move on to the next stage – surgical clinical trials conducted during the experimental treatment of patients with osteoarthritis by means of resurfacing arthroplasty with the use of a new generation of entirely non-cemented resurfacing endoprostheses, whose components will be fixed in the periarticular bone via the biomimetic MSC-Scaffold prototype developed by our bioengineering and clinical research team.

1 Characteristics of contemporary hip resurfacing arthroplasty endoprostheses and their possible postoperative complications

Hip resurfacing arthroplasty involves replacing the acetabular and femoral articular surfaces of the hip joint without damaging the medullary canal of the femur. Usually, this procedure is recommended for patients with, among others, osteoarthritis (OA), traumatic arthritis, juvenile idiopathic arthritis, rheumatoid arthritis, necrosis of the femoral head, tumours around the joint, and in patients under 65 years of age whose life expectancy exceeds the average life expectancy with long-stem total hip arthroplasty [1,2]. The main indication for joint replacement is a degenerative disease of joints involving mainly articular cartilage – osteoarthritis, which affects over 20% of people over 55 years of age [3,4]. Osteoarthritis has been ranked by the World Health Organization as the second leading cause of disability and is a major social issue in many countries. The treatment of choice is surgical replacement of the diseased joint with an endoprosthesis.

Due to the degenerative changes in the articular cartilage, in the case of traditional long-stem total hip arthroplasty, not only damaged articular cartilage but also often a large part of the healthy periarticular trabecular bone of the femoral head and femoral neck is removed. The removed cartilage and bone tissue are replaced with a metal structure. Due to the much higher (by 10–100 times) values of elastic parameters of metal alloys used for endoprostheses compared to the trabecular bone, during mechanical loads of the joint, the peri-implant bone in the periarticular area practically does not transfer mechanical loads – it is a non-physiological load transfer in the area of the peri-implant bone characterized by the formation of so-called *stress shielding* zones in the bone, causing resorption of bone tissue (osteolysis), and extensive destruction of the surrounding periprosthetic bone, loosening and migration of endoprosthesis components, and even bone fractures within the artificial joint [4–22].

Early design solutions for resurfacing arthroplasty endoprostheses included Smith (1917), Smith-Petersen (1923), Willey (1938), Albee and Pearson (1940–1944), Urist (1951), and Laing (1960) [23,24]. However, these solutions failed within a short time

DOI: 10.1201/9781003364498-1

1

due to surgical problems such as lack of permanent fixation or loosening of the endoprosthesis components, necrosis, rapid wear, and an intense reaction of tissues to wear particles. All of these endoprostheses were discontinued mainly due to the low biocompatibility of the biomaterials used at that time (Teflon®, celluloid, Bakelite, Pyrex® glass, polyethylene), the lack of good long-term fixation, high friction wear, and intensive tissue reaction to abrasive wear particles [25]. In the 1960s and early 1970s, attempts made to implant resurfacing endoprostheses designed by Charnley (1961), Müller (1968) (Figure 1.1), and Wagner and Freeman (1976) generally failed. These solutions had promising early postoperative results, but with longer follow-up, the failure rate reached 35% [26]. These failures were caused by loosening of the acetabular and femoral components, as well as fractures of the femoral neck resulting from the migration and penetration of implants (endoprostheses components) into the cancellous bone, and necrosis of the head and femoral neck vessels [26]. Bone cement was used to fix the components of these endoprostheses to the periarticular bone. Due to clinical results, this generation of hip resurfacing endoprostheses was abandoned in the mid-1980s.

Resurfacing arthroplasty has been experiencing a renaissance since the early 1990s. The first to present the results of arthroplasty with this generation of resurfacing arthroplasty endoprostheses was McMinn (1991), the precursor to both the Cormet Hip Resurfacing System and the Birmingham Hip Resurfacing System. At the same time, Amstutz began a series of innovations that culminated in the Conserve® Plus resurfacing hip system [27]. These endoprostheses differed from their predecessors in materials, fixation technique, component thickness, and component size options. The suggested advantages of these implants included more durable fixation, less wear, better bone tissue protection, and a lower risk of complications, especially fractures and sprains. Their clinical study has shown broader

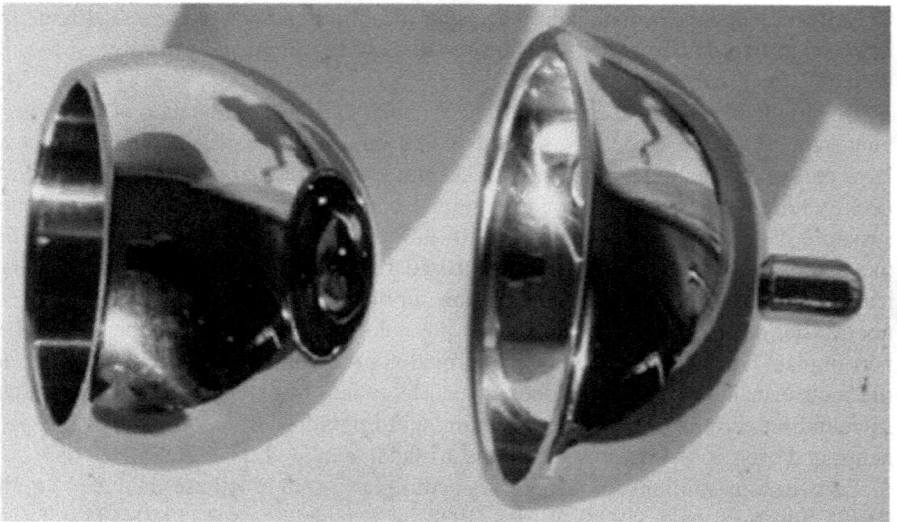

FIGURE 1.1　Müller's resurfacing endoprosthesis (1968).

and most interesting data on the observation and survival of surface implants [28,29]. Clinical observations of contemporary resurfacing arthroplasty endoprostheses (Figure 1.2) show several complications in the form of cracks and/or fractures of the femoral neck, as well as displacement and migration of the components of these endoprostheses (Figure 1.3), as well as fractures of the short stem of the femoral component (see Figure 20.111b in [30]).

In all currently used resurfacing endoprostheses designs (e.g., Birmingham Hip Resurfacing (BHR) prosthesis, Conserve® Plus hip resurfacing prosthesis, Cormet™ hip resurfacing prosthesis, Durom hip resurfacing prosthesis, ICON hip resurfacing prosthesis, BIOMET ReCap hip resurfacing prosthesis, DePuy Articular Surface Replacement (ASR™) hip resurfacing prosthesis, ESKA hip resurfacing prosthesis), the femoral component is fixed in the bone via bone cement and a short stem embedded in the area of the femoral neck [30]. Examples of contemporary resurfacing arthroplasty endoprostheses are shown in Figure 1.2.

Clinical studies show that cement has never guaranteed the correct and long-term fixation of these endoprostheses in the bone – the resorption of periarticular bone tissue, loosening in the bone-cement-implant interface, and the migration of endoprosthesis components and femoral fractures are the most common (approximately 75%) of the observed complications of the currently used cement resurfacing arthroplasty. This technique of fixation of the femoral component of hip resurfacing arthroplasty endoprostheses is the most common reason for postoperative complications. Also

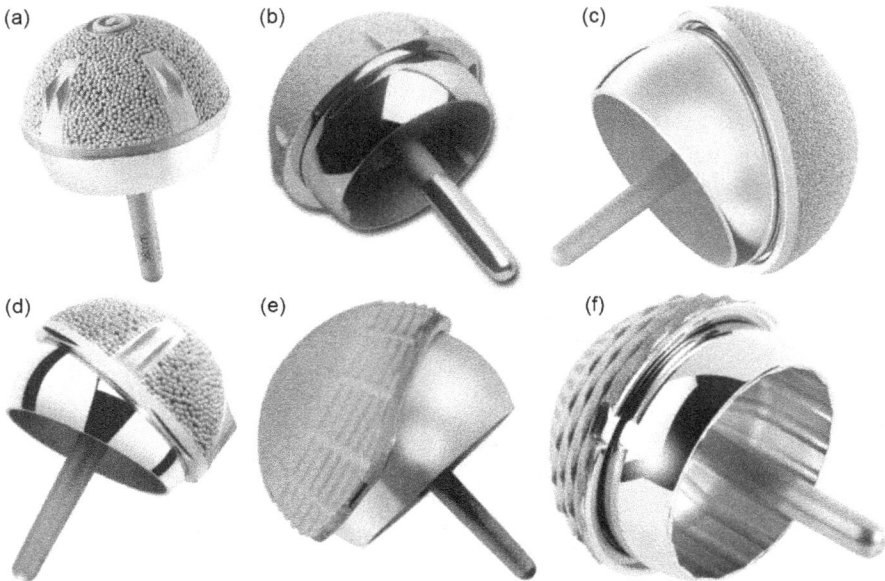

FIGURE 1.2 Examples of resurfacing arthroplasty endoprostheses used today: (a) Birmingham Hip Resurfacing System; (b) Cormet 2000™ Hip Resurfacing System; (c) DePuy ASR Hip Resurfacing System; (d) ICON Hip Resurfacing System; (e) ROMAX® Hip Resurfacing System; (f) Tornier DynaMoM Hip Resurfacing System.

due to the stress shielding zones in the vicinity of the short stem of the femoral component, loosening and migration occur (see Figure 28.42f in [30]).

In the case of cemented resurfacing hip arthroplasty, cement initially secures the femoral component of the endoprosthesis but penetrates deep into the cancellous bone of the femoral head – the zone of cement penetration (see Figure 1.4) occupies more than 30% of the total volume of the femoral head and causes local blood circulation insufficiency, which consequently leads to weakening of the internal microstructure of the cancellous bone of the femoral head and results in various complications [31]. Examples of radiographs showing the most common complications, such as loosening and migration of the femoral component and femoral neck fracture, are presented in Figure 1.3.

The design solutions of hip endoprostheses currently available on the market correspond to various survival rates with five-year follow-up, ranging from 97.1% (one of the best) to 80.9% (the worst) [1]. For this reason, there have been concerns about the safety of some of these resurfacing arthroplasty endoprostheses, leading, among others, to the withdrawal of DePuy Articular Surface Replacement (ASR™) (DePuy Orthopedics Inc., Warsaw, IN, USA) due to its high percentage of postoperative complications [32]. A femoral neck fracture is a common cause of early hip resurfacing arthroplasty failure, accounting for up to 35% of required revision surgeries [33,34], while aseptic loosening of the femoral or acetabular components is another common cause of hip resurfacing arthroplasty failure [35,36]. Aseptic bone necrosis (osteonecrosis) after hip resurfacing arthroplasty, described primarily in failures attributed to periprosthetic fractures or suggested as the cause of a periprosthetic fracture [37], is also interpreted as an effect associated with fixation of endoprosthesis components with the use of cement [38] or as a result of intraoperative damage to the vessels that supply the femoral head [39]. The thermal effect accompanying cement polymerization causes severe damage to the peri-implant tissue leading to the collapse of the femoral head [40,41]. Moreover, as already mentioned, during implantation of the femoral hip resurfacing arthroplasty endoprosthesis component, large amounts of

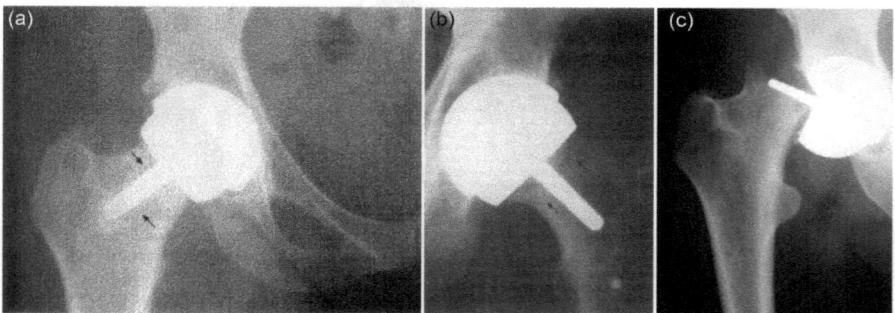

FIGURE 1.3 X-rays showing typical complications after cemented hip joint resurfacing arthroplasty using the Birmingham Hip Resurfacing (BHR) implant example: (a) loosening and migration of the femoral component; (b) stress fracture of the femoral neck; (c) hip fracture.

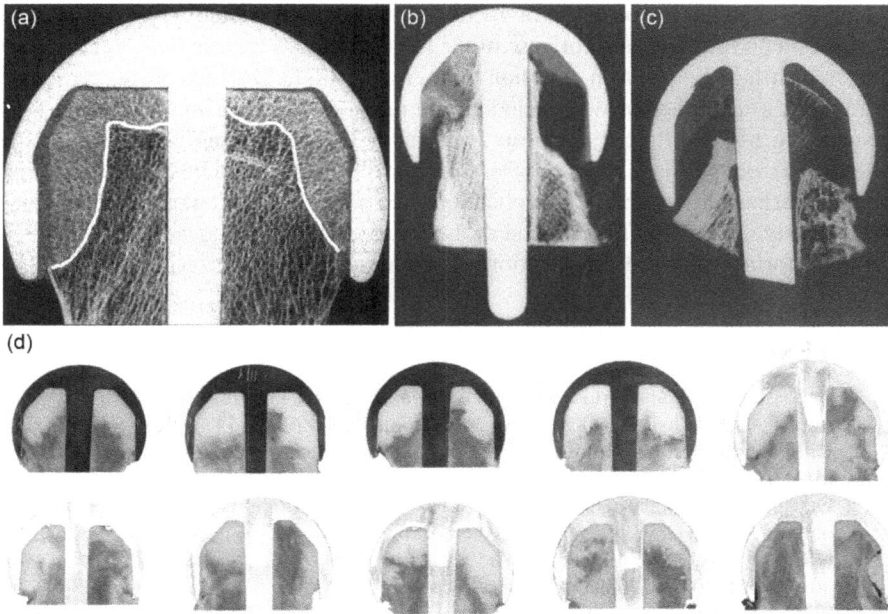

FIGURE 1.4 Radiographs of the femoral component attached with polymethacrylate cement: (a) status after implantation, cement penetrating into the pores of the periarticular cancellous bone takes up a significant volume (bright areas) of the femoral heads – the cement penetration zone in the femoral head covers more than one-third of the volume of this head; (b and c) exemplary long-term effects – extensive bone resorption in the femoral head area, resulting in the formation of large resorptive cavities [30]; (d) exemplary cross sections of the BHR endoprosthesis showing the diversity/unevenness of cement penetration and distribution.

cement are forced into the cancellous bone of the femoral head, forming a thick cement mantle there [42].

Aseptic bone necrosis has been reported to occur primarily in the early and mid-term periods of postoperative hip failure and may refer to the impaired blood supply to the femoral head or thermal injury during surgery [43]. According to Zustin et al. [43] who histologically analysed a series of 123 bone-implant samples (with five different endoprostheses systems of resurfacing like ASR by DePuy Orthopedics Inc., Birmingham Hip Resurfacing by Smith & Nephew, Cormet of Corin Group PLC, DUROM by Zimmer Inc., and ReCAP of Biomet Inc.) collected from patients with a preoperative diagnosis other than osteonecrosis, the osteonecrosis was found in 88% of cases and was associated with 60% of periprosthetic fractures. Eighty-five of the 123 examined revisions were for periprosthetic fractures, 8% due to acetabular loosening, and the remaining 23% for other reasons, such as groin pain from the femoral component; 60% of these periprosthetic fractures showed complete bone necrosis proximal to the fracture line and were defined as post-necrotic fractures. Most of the bone-implant samples collected showed histologically advanced aseptic necrosis, which was found to be the cause of 46% of all failures associated with post-necrotic periprosthetic fractures and collapse of the femoral head. Periprosthetic necrosis can be demonstrated by positron emission tomography (PET) [44]. According to Steiger et al. [45], after infection was excluded, the main causes of primary revision after resurfacing hip arthroplasty are hip fractures (43%), loosening/lysis (32%), metal allergic reactions (7%), and pain (6%). Consequently, due to the possible occurrence of these serious postoperative complications, the primary revision of hip resurfacing arthroplasty concerning the revision of the femoral component occurs in 62% of all cases performed in the above-mentioned procedures' primary revisions [45].

REFERENCES

1. Cadossi, M.; Tedesco, G.; Sambri, A.; Mazzotti, A.; Giannini, S. Hip resurfacing implants. *Orthopedics*. 2015; 38(8): 504–9. doi:10.3928/01477447-20150804-07.
2. Hing, C.; Back, D.; Shimmin, A. Hip resurfacing: indications, results, and conclusions. *Instr Course Lect*. 2007; 56: 171–8.
3. Dettmer, M.; Pourmoghaddam, A.; Kreuzer, S.W. Comparison of patient-reported outcome from neck-preserving, short-stem arthroplasty and resurfacing arthroplasty in younger osteoarthritis patients. *Adv Orthop*. 2015; 2015: 817689. doi:10.1155/2015/817689
4. Recommendations for the medical management of osteoarthritis of the hip and knee: 2000 update. American College of Rheumatology Subcommittee on Osteoarthritis Guidelines. *Arthritis Rheum*. 2000; 43(9): 1905–15. doi:10.1002/1529-0131(200009)43: 9<1905::AID-ANR1>3.0.CO;2-P
5. Amstutz, H.C.; Le Duff, M.J. Eleven years of experience with metal-on-metal hybrid hip resurfacing: a review of 1000 conserve plus. *J Arthroplasty*. 2008; 23(6 Suppl 1): 36–43. doi:10.1016/j.arth.2008.04.017
6. Amstutz, H.C.; Campbell, P.A.; Le Duff, M.J. Fracture of the neck of the femur after surface arthroplasty of the hip. *J Bone Joint Surg Am*. 2004; 86(9): 1874–7. doi:10.2106/00004623–200409000-00003
7. Asaad, A.; Hart, A.; Khoo, M.M.; Ilo, K.; Schaller, G.; Black, J.D.; Muirhead-Allwood, S. Frequent femoral neck osteolysis with Birmingham mid-head resection resurfacing arthroplasty in young patients. *Clin Orthop Relat Res*. 2015; 473(12): 3770–8. doi:10.1007/s11999-015-4348-0. Erratum in: *Clin Orthop Relat Res*. 2015; 473(12): 3985.
8. Aulakh, T.S.; Rao, C.; Kuiper J.-H.; Richardson, J.B. Hip resurfacing and osteonecrosis: results from an independent hip resurfacing register. *Arch Orthop Trauma Surg*. 2010; 130: 841–5. doi:10.1007/s00402-009-0963-0
9. Bose, V.C.; Baruah, B.D. Resurfacing arthroplasty of the hip for avascular necrosis of the femoral head: a minimum follow-up of four years. *J Bone Joint Surg Br*. 2010; 92(7): 922–8. doi:10.1302/0301-620X.92B7.23639
10. Falez, F.; Favetti, F.; Casella, F.; Panegrossi, G. Hip resurfacing: why does it fail? Early results and critical analysis of our first 60 cases. *Int Orthop*. 2008; 32(2): 209–16. doi:10.1007/s00264-006-0313-6
11. Huo, M.H.; Parvizi, J.; Gilbert, N.F. What's new in hip arthroplasty. *J Bone Joint Surg Am*. 2006; 88(9): 2100–13. doi:10.2106/JBJS.F.00595
12. Huo, M.H.; Stockton, K.G.; Mont, M.A.; Bucholz, R.W. What's new in total hip arthroplasty. *J Bone Joint Surg Am*. 2012; 94(18): 1721–7. doi:10.2106/JBJS.L.00620
13. Itayem, R.; Arndt, A.; Daniel, J.; McMinn, D.J.; Lundberg, A. A two-year radiostereometric follow-up of the first generation Birmingham mid head resection arthroplasty. *Hip Int*. 2014; 24(4): 355–62. doi:10.5301/hipint.5000136

14. Kim, P.R.; Beaulé, P.E.; Laflamme, G.Y.; Dunbar, M. Causes of early failure in a multicenter clinical trial of hip resurfacing. *J Arthroplasty.* 2008; 23(6 Suppl 1): 44–9. doi:10.1016/j.arth.2008.05.022

15. Marker, D.R.; Seyler, T.M.; Jinnah, R.H.; Delanois, R.E.; Ulrich, S.D.; Mont, M.A. Femoral neck fractures after metal-on-metal total hip resurfacing: a prospective cohort study. *J Arthroplasty.* 2007; 22(7 Suppl 3): 66–71. doi:10.1016/j.arth.2007.05.017

16. Morgan, D.; Myers, G.; O'Dwyer, K.; Thomas, A.M. Intertrochanteric fracture below Birmingham Hip Resurfacing: Successful non-operative management in two cases. *Injury Extra.* 2008; 39(9): 313–5. doi:10.1016/j.injury.2008.04.007

17. Munro, J.T.; Masri, B.A.; Duncan, C.P.; Garbuz, D.S. High complication rate after revision of large-head metal-on-metal total hip arthroplasty. *Clin Orthop Relat Res.* 2014; 472(2): 523–8. doi:10.1007/s11999-013-2979-6

18. Pailhé, R.; Sharma, A.; Reina, N.; Cavaignac, E.; Chiron, P.; Laffosse, J.M.; Hip resurfacing: a systematic review of literature. *Int Orthop.* 2012; 36(12): 2399–410. doi:10.1007/s00264-012-1686-3

19. Russell, R.D.; Estrera, K.A.; Pivec, R.; Mont, M.A.; Huo, M.H. What's new in total hip arthroplasty. *J Bone Joint Surg Am.* 2013; 95(18): 1719–25. doi:10.2106/JBJS.M.00764

20. Shimmin, A.J.; Back, D. Femoral neck fractures following Birmingham hip resurfacing: a national review of 50 cases. *J Bone Joint Surg Br.* 2005; 87(4): 463–4. doi:10.1302/0301–620X.87B4.15498

21. Shimmin, A.J.; Bare, J.; Back, D.L. Complications associated with hip resurfacing arthroplasty. *Orthop Clin North Am.* 2005; 36(2): 187–93, doi:10.1016/j.ocl.2005.01.002

22. Spencer, S.; Carter, R.; Murray, H.; Meek, R.M. Femoral neck narrowing after metal-on-metal hip resurfacing. *J Arthroplasty.* 2008; 23(8): 1105–9. doi:10.1016/j.arth.2007.10.014

23. Amstutz, H.C.; Le Duff, M.J. Hip resurfacing: a 40-year perspective. *HSS J.* 2012; 8(3): 275–82. doi:10.1007/s11420-012-9293-9

24. Amstutz, H.C.; Le Duff, M.J. Hip resurfacing: history, current status, and future. *Hip Int.* 2015; 25(4): 330–8. doi:10.5301/hipint.5000268

25. Menge, M. Seven years of experience in MoM resurfacing: results and open questions, in: Benazzo, F.; Falez, F.; Dietrich, M. (Eds.): *Bioceramics and Alternative Bearings in Joint Arthroplasty. Ceramics in Orthopaedics.* Steinkopff, 2006. doi:10.1007/978-3-7985-1635-9_5

26. Indelli, P.F.; Veins, N.; Dominguez, D.; Kitaoka, K.; Vail, T.P. In vitro biomechanical properties of a hip resurfacing system, in: Benazzo, F.; Falez, F.; Dietrich, M. (Eds.): *Bioceramics and Alternative Bearings in Joint Arthroplasty. Ceramics in Orthopaedics.* Steinkopff, 2006. doi:10.1007/978-3-7985-1635-9_9

27. Streicher, R.M. Hip Resurfacing – a superior articulation concept?, in: Benazzo, F.; Falez, F.; Dietrich, M. (Eds.): *Bioceramics and Alternative Bearings in Joint Arthroplasty. Ceramics in Orthopaedics.* Steinkopff, 2006. doi:10.1007/978-3-7985-1635-9_7

28. Amstutz, H.C.; Beaulé, P.; Dorey, F.J.; Le Duff, M.J.; Campbell, P.A.; Gruen, T.A. Metal-on-metal hybrid surface arthroplasty: two to six-year follow-up study. *J Bone Joint Surg Am.* 2004; 86(1): 28–39.

29. Daniel, J.; Pynsent, P.B.; McMinn, D.J. Metal-on-metal resurfacing of the hip in patients under the age of 55 years with osteoarthritis. *J Bone Joint Surg Br.* 2004; 86(2): 177–84. doi:10.1302/0301–620x.86b2.14600

30. De Smet, K.; Campbell, P.; Van Der Straeten, C. (Eds.): *The Hip Resurfacing Handbook. A Practical Guide to the Use and Management of Modern Hip Resurfacings.* Woodhead Publishing, Sawston, Cambridge, 2013.

31. Howald, R.; Kesteris, U.; Klabunde, R.; Krevolin, J. Factors affecting the cement penetration of a hip resurfacing implant: an in vitro study. *Hip Int.* 2006; 16(Suppl 4): 82–9. doi:10.5301/hip.2008.5209

32. Hug, K.T.; Watters, T.S.; Vail, T.P.; Bolognesi, M.P. The withdrawn ASR™ THA and hip resurfacing systems: how have our patients fared over 1 to 6 years?. *Clin Orthop Relat Res.* 2013; 471(2): 430–8. doi:10.1007/s11999-012-2547-5

33. Davis, E.T.; Olsen, M.; Zdero, R.; Smith, G.M.; Waddell, J.P.; Schemitsch, E.H. Predictors of femoral neck fracture following hip resurfacing: a cadaveric study. *J Arthroplasty.* 2013; 28(1): 110–6. doi:10.1016/j.arth.2012.05.015

34. Matharu, G.S.; McBryde, C.W.; Revell, M.P.; Pynsent, P.B. Femoral neck fracture after Birmingham Hip Resurfacing Arthroplasty: prevalence, time to fracture, and outcome after revision. *J Arthroplasty.* 2013; 28(1): 147–53. doi:10.1016/j.arth.2012.04.035

35. Haughom, B.D.; Erickson, B.J.; Hellman, M.D.; Jacobs, J.J. Do complication rates differ by gender after metal-on-metal hip resurfacing arthroplasty? A systematic review. *Clin Orthop Relat Res.* 2015; 473(8): 2521–9. doi:10.1007/s11999-015-4227-8

36. Amstutz, H.C.; Le Duff, M.J. Aseptic loosening of cobalt chromium monoblock sockets after hip resurfacing. *Hip Int.* 2015; 25(5): 466–70. doi:10.5301/hipint.5000251

37. Steffen, R.T.; Foguet, P.R.; Krikler, S.J.; Gundle, R.; Beard, D.J.; Murray, D.W. Femoral neck fractures after hip resurfacing. *J Arthroplasty.* 2009; 24: 614–9. doi:10.1016/j.arth.2008.04.008

38. Gill, H.S.; Campbell, P.A.; Murray, D.W.; De Smet, K.A. Reduction of the potential for thermal damage during hip resurfacing. *J Bone Joint Surg Br.* 2007; 89(1): 16–20. doi:10.1302/0301-620X.89B1.18369

39. Steffen, R.T.; Fern, D.; Norton, M.; Murray, D.W.; Gill, H.S. Femoral oxygenation during hip resurfacing through the trochanteric flip approach. *Clin Orthop Relat Res.* 2009; 467(4): 934–9. doi:10.1007/s11999-008-0390-5

40. Scheerlinck, T.; Delport, H.; Kiewitt, T. Influence of the cementing technique on the cement mantle in hip resurfacing: an in vitro computed tomography scan-based analysis. *J Bone Joint Surg Am.* 2010; 92(2): 375–87. doi:10.2106/JBJS.I.00322

41. Girard, J. Is it time for cementless hip resurfacing? *HSS J.* 2012; 8(3): 245–50. doi:10.1007/s11420-012-9295-7

42. Baker, R.; Whitehouse, M.; Kilshaw, M.; Pabbruwe, M.; Spencer, R.; Blom, A.; Bannister, G. Maximum temperatures of 89°C recorded during the mechanical preparation of 35 femoral heads for resurfacing. *Acta Orthop.* 2011; 82(6): 669–73. doi:10.31 09/17453674.2011.636681

43. Zustin, J.; Sauter, G.; Morlock, M.M.; Rüther, W.; Amling, M. Association of osteonecrosis and failure of hip resurfacing arthroplasty. *Clin Orthop Relat Res.* 2010; 468(3): 756–61. doi:10.1007/s11999-009-0979-3

44. Ullmark, G.; Sundgren, K.; Milbrink, J.; Nilsson, O.; Sörensen, J. Osteonecrosis following resurfacing arthroplasty. *Acta Orthop.* 2009; 80(6): 670–4. doi:10.3109/ 17453670903278258

45. de Steiger, R.N.; Miller, L.N.; Prosser, G.H.; Graves, S.E.; Davidson, D.C.; Stanford, T.E. Poor outcome of revised resurfacing hip arthroplasty. *Acta Orthop.* 2010; 81(1): 72–6. doi:10.3109/17453671003667176

2 Idea of entirely non-cemented implantation of the components of hip resurfacing arthroplasty endoprostheses with the multi-spiked connecting scaffold

Achieving a biomechanically stable and durable fixation between two different biomaterials, artificial and natural (i.e. biological tissue), is a challenge for the bioengineering design of artificial joints. If metal endoprostheses have been implanted in the periprosthetic bone, the physiological transfer of the load that occurs in the natural joints and the area of the periarticular tissue is disturbed to a greater or lesser extent. In particular, large differences in structural and mechanical properties between the constructional materials of the implant and the periprosthetic bone tissue result in a greater part of the mechanical load being borne by the implant. It results in underloading of the periprosthetic bone tissue and the so-called local osteoporosis resulting from underloading (disuse osteoporosis).

The hyaline cartilage of the articular cartilage of the diarthrodial joints is connected to the cancellous periarticular bone by the subchondral bone, which consists of the subchondral bone plate and the subchondral spongiosa [1–3]. A subchondral bone plate is a single unit formed by two mineralized layers: the calcified region of hyaline cartilage and the layer of lamellar bone. The calcified cartilage extends for a varying distance to the marrow cavity, where it is remodelled and replaced by woven or lamellar bone. This lamellar subchondral bone is similar to the supporting trabeculae, which are predominantly perpendicular to the joint surface and are crossed at right angles by finer trabeculae. The subchondral bone with its supporting trabeculae forms the system of interdigitations interlocking with the trabeculae of the periarticular cancellous bone, and in this way, it constitutes a specific transition zone that fixes *in vivo* the articular cartilage of the diarthrodial joints into the

DOI: 10.1201/9781003364498-2

periarticular cancellous bone. The system of subchondral bone interdigitations that interpenetrate the trabeculae of cancellous bone provides a gradual structural transition between the two dissimilar morphological structures of the joint – articular cartilage and periarticular trabecular bone tissue of the epiphysis. Figure 2.1 presents the author's diagram (based on the results [1–3]) of the hyaline articular cartilage and the subchondral bone with interdigitations that overlap with the trabeculae of the cancellous periarticular bone.

The biomimetic multi-spiked connecting scaffold (MSC-Scaffold) mimics the interdigitations of the subchondral bone that penetrate the intertrabecular marrow cavities of the periarticular cancellous bone. Filling the interspike spaces of the biomimetic MSC-Scaffold with ingrowing trabecular bone *in vivo* will allow recreating the shape and microstructure of cancellous bone tissue to a similar degree, which is not possible in the case of traditional long-stem hip arthroplasty and cemented resurfacing arthroplasty. As a consequence of this biomimetic fixation system of components of a new generation of non-cemented resurfacing arthroplasty endoprostheses within the periarticular bone, it can be assumed that the distribution of the mechanical load in the periarticular bone will be similar to that found in the periarticular bone of a natural hip joint.

The original concept of the MSC-Scaffold in the form of a spike-palisade system connecting the components of resurfacing arthroplasty endoprostheses with the intertrabecular space of the cancellous periarticular bone by Piotr Rogala [4–6] allows initial fixation of the components of these endoprostheses in the bone, inducing bone tissue ingrowth into the interspike pore space within the MSC-Scaffold,

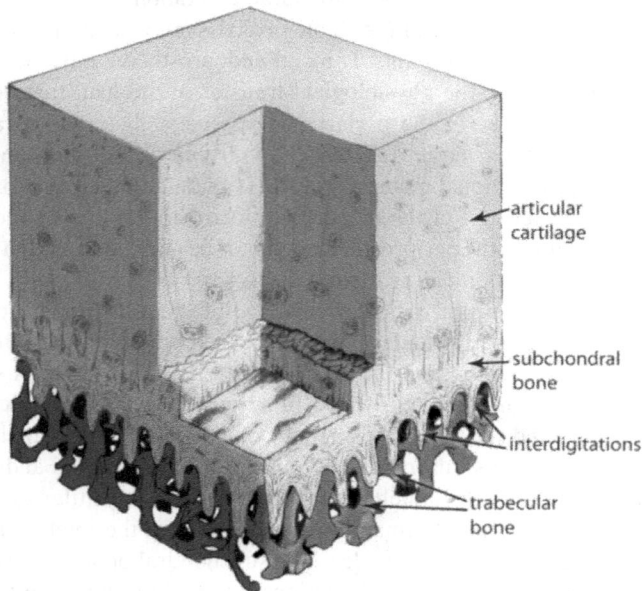

FIGURE 2.1 A diagram showing the hyaline cartilage and the subchondral bone with its interdigitations, anchoring among the trabeculae of the cancellous bone tissue.

resulting in the so-called osseointegration of the bone with the implant and ensuring long-term fixation of the components of resurfacing endoprostheses in the periarticular bone. The polygonal spikes of the MSC-Scaffold are inserted by the surgeon into the bone up to a certain depth (initial fixation), and the remaining space between the spikes will be filled in the postoperative period by the bone tissue that grows there (biological fixation). This is not possible in the case of currently used hip resurfacing arthroplasty endoprostheses.

The method of fixation of the components of resurfacing arthroplasty joint endoprostheses with the use of the MSC-Scaffold allows for a radical change in approach to the design solutions of endoprostheses used in hip arthroplasty, i.e. a departure from the currently used long-stem endoprostheses and even greater revision endoprostheses (implanted when the long-stem endoprosthesis fails) to a biomimetic, entirely non-cemented model, saving the periarticular bone tissue. Here, only the diseased cartilage tissue of the femoral head and acetabulum is replaced, saving the epiphyseal bone elements usually removed in the traditional long-stem arthroplasty of the hip joint. It also assumes the maximum elimination of micromotions between the implants and the bone, while simultaneously ensuring a stress field in the vicinity of the bone-implant fixation similar to the stress distribution occurring in physiological conditions (so that stress shielding – a practically deformation-free zone in the area surrounding the implant, with values of deformation well below physiological values, which causes bone loss around the implant and leads to its loosening – does not occur).

The MSC-Scaffold further ensures non-cemented fixation of the components of resurfacing arthroplasty endoprostheses of the hip joint in its most physiological form, thereby potentially eliminating several possible complications related to the use of bone cement.

During the implantation of the biomimetic MSC-Scaffold in the intertrabecular space of the cancellous bone, the spikes cause controlled destruction of its structure at the desired osteoinductive level, thus stimulating adaptive remodelling and bone tissue growth in the interspike space. The MSC-Scaffold spikes are supported in the trabecular bioconstruction of the cancellous bone, which results in more effective absorption of dynamic mechanical loads, and increases the biomechanical strength of the fixation of the components of the resurfacing arthroplasty endoprostheses in bone tissue, protecting them from spraining and loosening.

The prototype resurfacing arthroplasty endoprosthesis of the hip joint with the MSC-Scaffold, as demonstrated in Figure 2.2, consists of the acetabular component (1) and the femoral component (2).

The femoral component (2) has an annular supporting surface (9) located below the transverse axis of the acetabular component (2) on a plane perpendicular to its longitudinal axis and a spherical border surface (10) with polygonal spikes (11) and the central spike (12), whose axis coincides with the longitudinal axis of the femoral component of the endoprosthesis (2). Polygonal spikes (11) and central spike (12) are in the form of pyramids and have common base edges with adjacent spikes (11) and are of different lengths. The ratio of the radius of the circle circumscribed at the base of the spike – a regular pyramid – to the height of the pyramid is at least 1:5. Different lengths and arrangements of the polygonal spikes (4) and (11) contribute to an easy, even, and gradual embedding in the cancellous bone to the depth determined by the contact between the bone and the edge (6) and the bearing surface (9), respectively. The edge (6) and the bearing surface (9) are supported on the acetabulum and the cortical edge of the femur, respectively.

The acetabular component (1) has an outer spherical cap (3) equipped with polygonal spikes (4) and a cut whose circular surface (5) defined by an edge (6) is perpendicular to the symmetry of the axis of the acetabular component. The pyramid-shaped polygonal spikes (4) share base edges with adjacent spikes, but are of different lengths. The heights of the polygonal spikes do not extend beyond the edge (6),

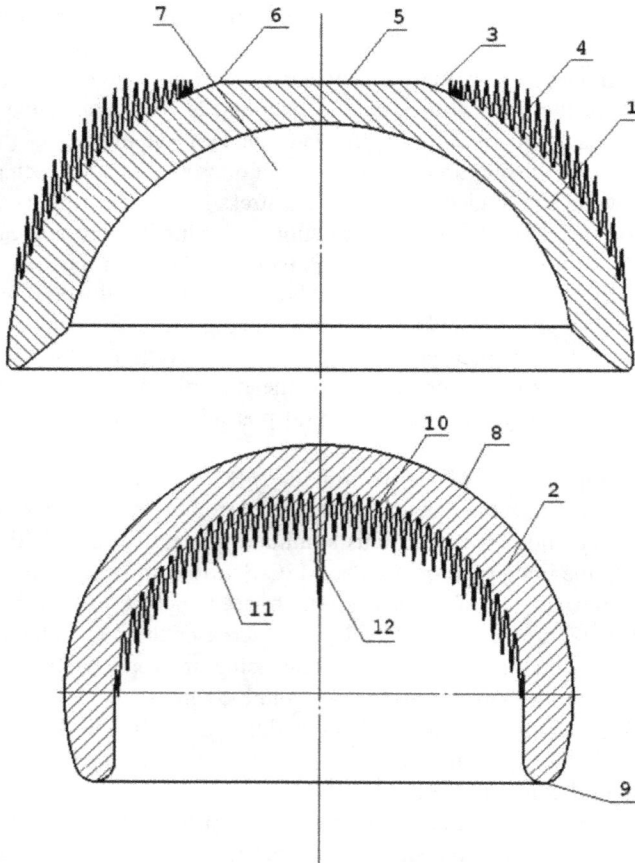

FIGURE 2.2 A sketch of the components of the hip joint resurfacing endoprosthesis with the MSC-Scaffold in the cross section: (1) acetabular component, (2) femoral component, (3) spherical boundary surface of the acetabular component, (4) polygonal spikes on the outer boundary surface of the acetabular component, (5) circular bearing surface, (6) edge lying in a plane perpendicular to the axis of the acetabular component, (7) cap, (8) the outer surface of the femoral component, (9) the annular bearing surface of the acetabular component, (10) spherical border of the femur, (11) polygonal spikes on the inner border of the femoral part, (12) central spike.

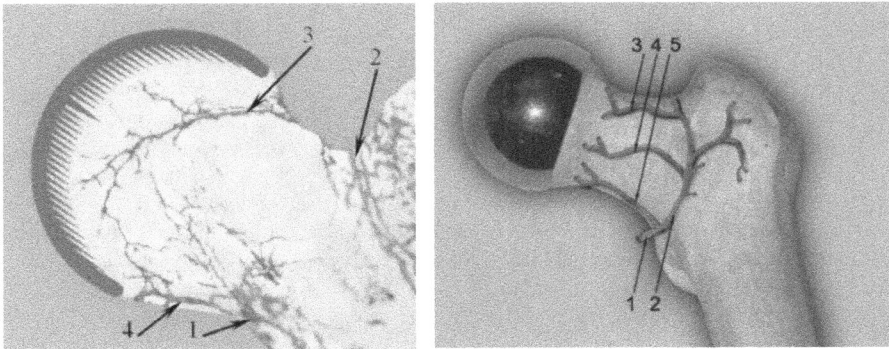

FIGURE 2.3 Author's diagram showing the femoral component of the hip joint resurfacing endoprosthesis *in situ* and intact arterial vascularization of the femoral head: (1) circumflexa femoris lateralis, (2) artery – ascending branch (1), (3) upper branch, (4) front branch, (5) lower branch.

and the ratio of the radius of the circle circumscribed at the base of the pyramid to the height is at least 1:5. The acetabular component is equipped with a cap (7), which houses the femoral part, being a segment of a sphere with an external surface (8).

Fixation of the implant with a biomimetic MSC-Scaffold is intended to ensure the load transfer in the implant-bone system similar to that occurring in a natural joint, so it can be expected that almost physiological biodynamics and bone tissue remodelling around the implant will be ensured and the desired osteoconduction can be reasonably expected, i.e. promotion of bone tissue ingrowth into the interspike space of the MSC-Scaffold. The macro-dimensions of the bearing part (see (9) in Figure 2.2) of the acetabular component of the endoprosthesis are to preserve the posterolateral and medial epiphyseal femoral arteries (subcapsular arteriae retinaculares: superior and inferior) of the femoral head (Figure 2.3), which is why the physiological blood supply and the proper potential for remodelling of the trabecular bone of the femoral head are preserved.

Our prototype of the biomimetic MSC-Scaffold ensuring fixation of the components of resurfacing arthroplasty endoprostheses with cancellous periarticular bone can be used in osteoarticular surgery procedures of all joints in humans and animals, in particular in resurfacing arthroplasty of the hip joint, knee joint, elbow joint, shoulder joint, ankle joints, hand and foot joints, as well as the implantation of artificial intervertebral discs [7].

REFERENCES

1. Madry, H.; van Dijk, C.N.; Mueller-Gerbl, M. The basic science of the subchondral bone. *Knee Surg Sports Traumatol Arthrosc.* 2010; 18(4): 419–33. doi:10.1007/s00167-010-1054-z
2. Villegas, D.F.; Hansen, T.A.; Liu, D.F.; Donahue, T.L. A quantitative study of the microstructure and biochemistry of the medial meniscal horn attachments. *Ann Biomed Eng.* 2008; 36(1): 123–31. doi:10.1007/s10439-007-9403-x

3. Milz, S.; Putz, R. Quantitative morphology of the subchondral plate of the tibial plateau. *J Anat.* 1994; 185: 103–10.
4. Rogala, P. Endoprosthesis. EU Patent No. EP072418 B1, 22 December 1999.
5. Rogala, P. Acetabulum Endoprosthesis and Head. U.S. Patent US5,911,759 A, 15 June 1999.
6. Rogala, P. Method and Endoprosthesis to Apply This Implantation. Canadian Patent No. 2,200,064, 1 April 2002.
7. Rogala, P.; Uklejewski, R.; Winiecki, M.; Mielniczuk, J.; Auguściński, A. The concept and geometrical model of modern endoprosthesis concerning minimal invasive total hip resurfacing arthroplasty (THRA). *Mach Dyn Probl.* 2006; 30(4): 89–96.

3 Design, rapid prototyping, and manufacturing of the biomimetic multi-spiked connecting scaffold prototype for non-cemented resurfacing endoprostheses

3.1 BIOENGINEERING CAD DESIGN AND MODELLING

As part of the research, geometric CAD models of the MSC-Scaffold preprototypes for non-cemented resurfacing arthroplasty endoprostheses have been designed to perform all tasks covered by the research project schedules (No. 4T07C05629 and No. NN518412638).

In the first stage, certain steps were taken to identify and compare the technological possibilities of manufacturing the MSC-Scaffold prototype described above with the use of Electrical Discharge Machining (EDM) methods and Selective Laser Melting (SLM) technology, as well as other available techniques for Direct Metal Fabrication, such as Selective Laser Sintering (SLS) and Electron Beam Melting (EBM).

This chapter presents the effects of prototyping the spikes of the MSC-Scaffold using 3D stereolithography. It also presents issues of post-production processing of the MSC-Scaffold for non-cemented resurfacing arthroplasty endoprostheses. The subsequent tasks within the schedules of both research projects (described in subsequent chapters of the monograph) required modelling and manufacturing of research samples (including working preprototypes) of specific shapes and sizes dictated by the conditions of the experiments, intended for:

- laboratory tests of embedding preprototypes of the MSC-Scaffold in the periarticular cancellous bone of swine femoral heads on a universal testing machine,

DOI: 10.1201/9781003364498-3

- analysis of the possibility of formation of the structural and osteoconductive potential of the interspike space of the prototype MSC-Scaffold,
- the research leading to the development of an effective post-production treatment of the bone-contacting surface of the prototype MSC-Scaffold with the use of abrasive blasting,
- an initial test of calcium phosphate modification of the bone-contacting surface of the MSC-Scaffold preprototypes using electrochemical cathodic deposition carried out at constant current density values,
- the study of the process of calcium phosphate modification of the MSC-Scaffold surface through electrochemical cathodic deposition carried out at constant values of the electric potential with the subsequent immersion of the MSC-Scaffold preprototypes in a simulated body fluid (SBF),
- pilot implantation of the MSC-Scaffold preprototypes into the articular subchondral layer in experimental animals (swine),
- a biological evaluation in human osteoblasts of preprototypes of the MSC-Scaffold with the calcium phosphate modified surfaces,
- evaluation of the biointegration of the calcium phosphate-coated MSC-Scaffold implanted in swine,
- experimental determination of appropriate surgical approaches to the hip and knee joints in swine,
- verification of a working prototype of partial resurfacing knee endoprosthesis implanted in bone through the MSC-Scaffold in ten experimental animals.

During all of these stages, the results of previous research conducted chronologically according to approved schedules were taken into account on an ongoing basis and in a consistent manner.

Two important aspects have played a key role in the bioengineering design of the MSC-Scaffold for non-cemented resurfacing endoprostheses. On the one hand, the bioengineering aspect is creating the appropriate conditions of the prototype MSC-Scaffold to promote the osteoconduction process of the periarticular bone to the interspike space of this MSC-Scaffold. On the other hand, the technological aspect is to meet the requirements of the manufacturing technology chosen to manufacture the MSC-Scaffold based on experimental comparative studies, as well as taking into account the limitations arising from the selected technology.

We have taken into account that the bone tissue that grows in the interspike space of the MSC-Scaffold will embed (anchor) the implant in the periarticular bone and simultaneously increase the total surface (lateral surface of the spikes) of contact with the bone tissue at the same time, which will adaptively optimize the load transfer in the implant-bone system and the distribution of stresses in the periarticular bone. To achieve biomechanical compatibility with bone, the MSC-Scaffold, which transfers the load to the peri-implant cancellous bone, should be designed so that, by increasing the contact surface between the implant and bone, it should ensure that the micro-movements between the implant and bone are as limited as possible during postoperative rehabilitation.

The total contact area between bone and implant, according to the patents [1–3], should be at least seven times larger than the articular surface of the head and the acetabulum of the endoprosthesis to allow loading of the artificial joint shortly after implantation. To this end, the geometric dimensions of the MSC-Scaffold spikes should be such that the ratio between the nominal height of the spike (H_n) and the radius (R) of the circle circumscribed at its base is 5 to 1 ($H_n/R = 5:1$) [1–3].

The size of the MSC-Scaffold spikes that mimic the so-called interdigitations of the subchondral bone should be modified to provide early postoperative mechanical stabilization of the components of the resurfacing endoprosthesis, allowing the patient to fully load the joint shortly after surgery. Ensuring the proper conditions within the MSC-Scaffold to promote the osteoconduction process, in particular, the optimal spacing between the edges of spike bases, should provide a volume of the interspike space that suffices for restoring vascularity between these spikes and consequently enable effective ingrowth and mineralization of the newly formed bone tissue.

In the first stage of the design of the spikes, the subject of the investigation was the selection of the most advantageous geometric shape of the spikes for the MSC-Scaffold taking into account the value of the implant-bone contact area increase factor [4]. The analysis of the value of this factor was carried out for a single spike, assuming its geometry in the form of a pyramid based on various regular polygons and a cone. Figure 3.1 presents a diagram of the implant-bone contact area increase factor for spikes that have the shape of a regular pyramid, whose base is, respectively, an equilateral triangle, square, hexagon, octagon, and decagon, and for cone-shaped spikes.

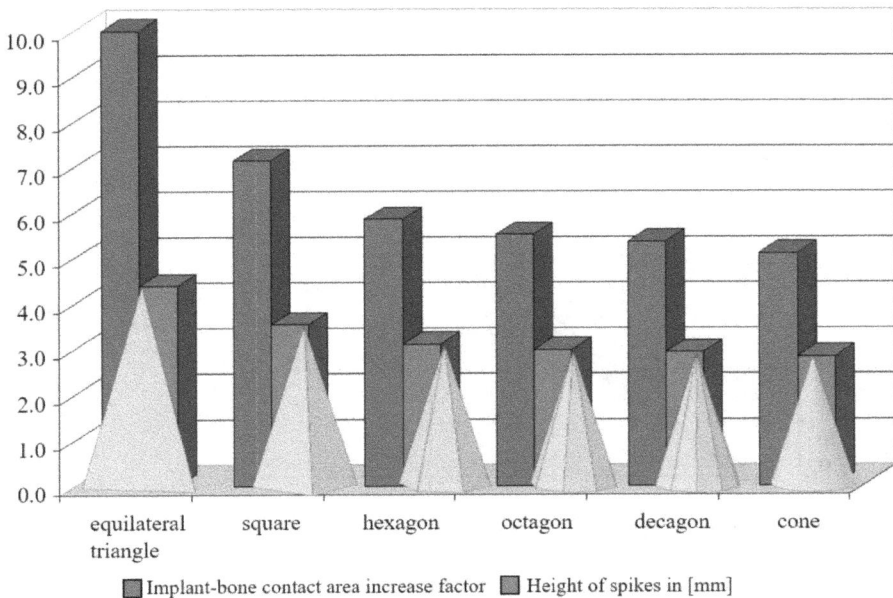

FIGURE 3.1 The values of the implant-bone contact area increase factor for the spikes of the MSC-Scaffold in the shape of a regular pyramid with an equilateral triangle, square, hexagon, octagon, and decagon at the bases, and cone-shaped spikes.

As can be seen from Figure 3.1, the most favourable value of the implant-bone contact area increase factor was obtained for pyramid-shaped spikes with an equilateral triangle and a square as a base. The same tendency is maintained for the value of the H_n/R ratio – increasing from 1 to 9, as indicated in Figure 3.2. On this basis, further analysis was carried out only for the pyramid-shaped spikes with an equilateral triangle, square, and hexagon at the base.

In the next step, an analysis was carried out for fragments of the MSC-Scaffold in the shape of a circle (ø16 mm, ø32 mm, and ø48 mm), whose surface was filled with spikes in the shape of the above-mentioned pyramids, i.e. with an equilateral triangle, square, and hexagon at the base, according to the four proposed arrangements as indicated in Figure 3.3a. The values of the implant-bone contact area increase factor for the proposed spike configuration systems are presented in the form of a diagram in Figure 3.3b.

The results presented in Figure 3.3 indicate the validity of choosing the configuration of the spikes of the MSC-Scaffold where the spikes are pyramid-shaped with the equilateral triangle at the base, and secondly where the spikes are pyramid-shaped with the square at the base and arranged in a rectangular configuration.

The structural compatibility analysis of the proposed MSC-Scaffold anchoring the implant with the periarticular trabecular bone of the animal femoral head was the next step to adjust the arrangement of the spikes, the geometric shape of the base of the spikes, the dimensions of the base edge, and the H_n/R ratio. Thus, based

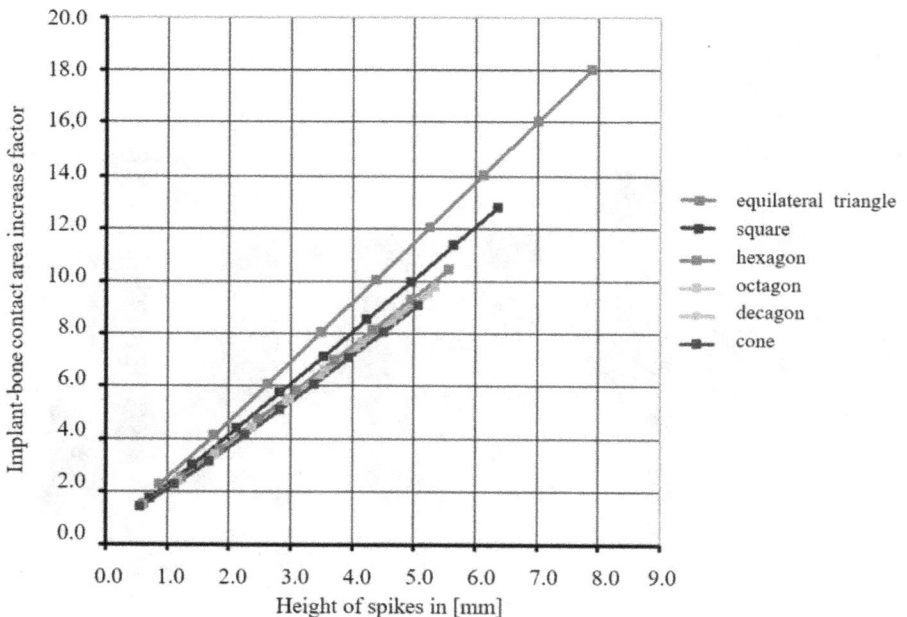

FIGURE 3.2 The values of the implant-bone contact area increase factor for the MSC-Scaffold spikes that have the form of regular pyramids and for cone-shaped spikes as a function of the height of these spikes.

(a)

(b)

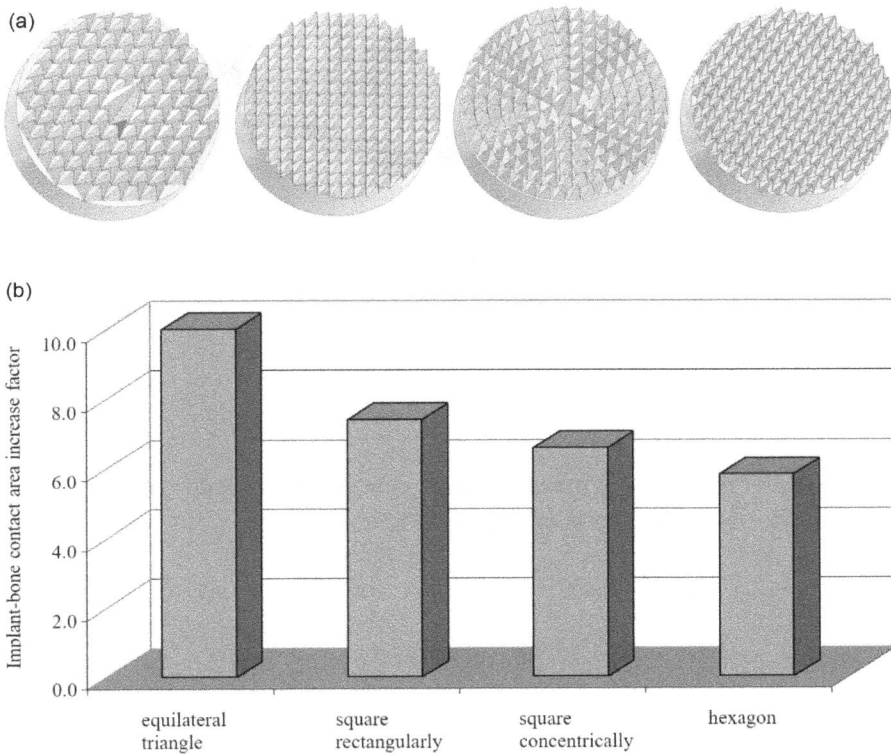

FIGURE 3.3 Proposals of different spike layouts for the MSC-Scaffold: (a) examples from left to right – pyramids with the following bases: an equilateral triangle at the base, a square (rectangular), a square (concentric), and hexagon; (b) values of the implant-bone contact area increase factor for the proposed spike arrangements.

on microscopic observation and measurements of the microstructure of the animal trabecular bone, we have carried out an analysis by adjusting the size and configuring the spikes to the intertrabecular porosity of the periarticular cancellous bone.

Four swine femurs have been obtained from a local slaughterhouse from four different animals of the same age and weight. Fresh bone samples were stored in a 0.9% NaCl bath at 4°C. The femoral head was then cut into 2-mm-thick sections with a low-speed diamond saw and digested in a 5% KOH solution for seven days to remove organic fragments from the pore space. In the following stages, the samples were dehydrated in a series of alcohols (70%, 95%, ≥99.8% ethanol) for 6 hours for every concentration, and then degreased in 99.8% acetone for 6 hours, after which the samples were dried at a temperature of 60°C overnight. The samples of dry bone, an exemplary cut, and an exemplary SEM image (Vega 5135, Tescan, Czech Republic) of a cancellous bone have been presented in Figure 3.4.

The measurements of the mean pore size, mean pore spacing, and pore surface area in the intertrabecular porosity compartment were performed with the AxioVision software (Zeiss, Germany); the results are shown in Table 3.1.

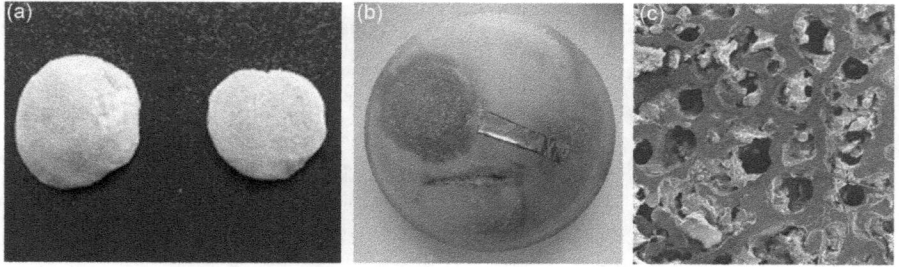

FIGURE 3.4 Dry bone samples (a), exemplary cut (b), and SEM microphotograph of the microstructure of the cancellous bone of the swine femoral head (c).

TABLE 3.1

The results of the porosity measurements concerning the intertrabecular space of the cancellous bone of the swine femoral head

Number of Microsections	Area (mm²)	Mean Size (mm)	Mean Distance (mm)
1	0.147	0.512	0.551
2	0.186	0.505	0.623
3	0.207	0.526	0.672
4	0.205	0.506	0.634
5	0.192	0.494	0.595
6	0.284	0.615	0.681
7	0.225	0.573	0.679
8	0.126	0.375	0.469
9	0.142	0.401	0.612
Mean ± SD	0.19 ± 0.05	0.50 ± 0.07	0.61 ± 0.07

The radius of the circle circumscribed at the base of a pyramid should be consistent with the mean pore size of the intertrabecular pore space in the animal cancellous bone. The results presented in Table 3.1 indicate that the value should be at least 0.50 ± 0.07 mm.

To match the size and arrangement of the MSC-Scaffold spikes with the irregular microstructure of the intertrabecular porosity in bone, optimization was performed with the use of the trabecular bone marrow lacunae and the spikes' coincidence index. This index was defined as the ratio of the number of spike tips that coincide with the pores of the intertrabecular porosity interval in the animal cancellous bone to the total number of spikes in the SEM micrograph of the cancellous bone taken from the animal femoral head (Figure 3.5).

Due to the rotational symmetry of the components of the hip endoprosthesis, only the concentric arrangements of spikes were analysed – in the shape of a pyramid with an equilateral triangle and a square at the base.

Figure 3.6 presents the relationship between the mean values of the trabecular bone marrow lacunae and spikes' coincidence index for spikes having a base where the radius of the circle circumscribed on the base (equilateral triangle and square) ranged from 0.4 to 0.7 mm.

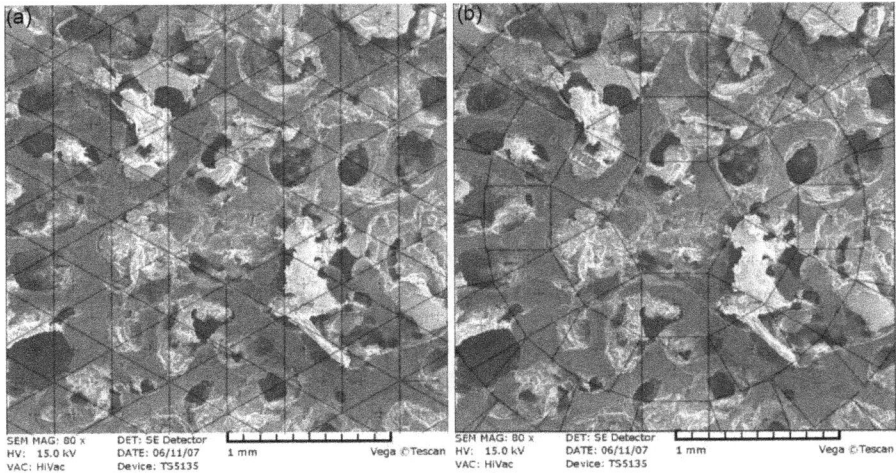

FIGURE 3.5 Contours of the spike bases of the analysed spike arrangements of the MSC-Scaffold plotted on the SEM image of the cancellous bone; a system of spikes made of (a) pyramids with an equilateral triangle at the base and (b) pyramids with a square at the base in a concentric arrangement.

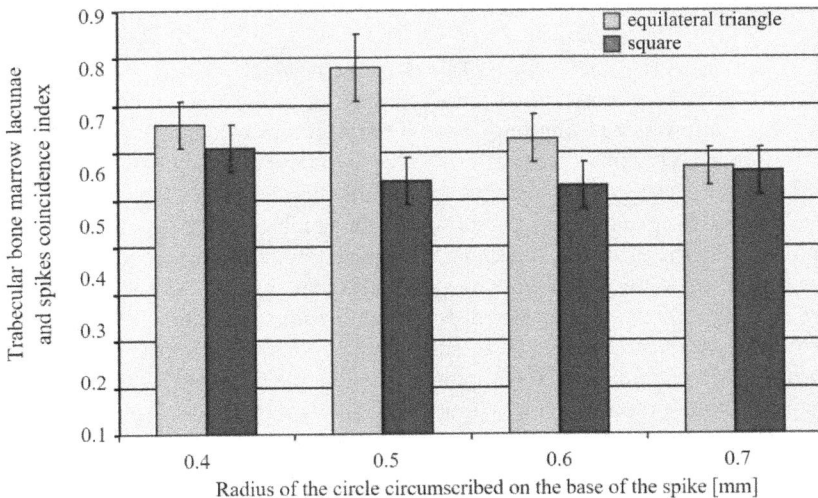

FIGURE 3.6 The coincidence index between the trabecular bone marrow lacunae and the spikes of the MSC-Scaffold for the system of polygonal spikes with the base in the form of an equilateral triangle and a square with the radius of the circle circumscribed on their base ranging from 0.4 to 0.7 mm.

For further research, the MSC-Scaffold preprototypes were modelled in the shape of fragments representing the central part of the femoral component of the hip joint resurfacing endoprosthesis located around the axis of this component.

Research on the prototype of the hip joint resurfacing endoprosthesis was planned to be carried out in an animal model – a swine of the Polish Large White breed. The diameter of the femoral head in a swine of this breed weighing 100–120 kg (according to own measurements) is 30.5 mm on average. This value was adopted as the nominal dimension for the diameter of the friction pair elements in the prototype endoprosthesis, and the remaining dimensions of the solid CAD models of both components were adjusted accordingly.

The parameterization method thus adopted will in the future allow: (1) design the components of the endoprosthesis in various dimensional variants, calculated according to the gradation of the size of the hip joint representative of the human population, and (2) adjusting the dimensions of the endoprosthesis components to the dimensions of the joint components and periarticular areas of the patient's hip joint as specified according to radiological scan.

Ultimately, the cap thickness for both the prototype of the acetabular component (component fixed in the pelvic bone) and the prototype of the femoral component (component implanted in the surgically prepared femoral head) was established as 3 mm. In the solid CAD model for both components of the prototype resurfacing endoprosthesis of the hip joint, the thickness was increased, taking into account the technological allowances for the shaping and finishing treatment of both components of the prototype endoprosthesis. Since, based on the analysis of the current state of knowledge in the field of manufacturing technologies, we have predicted that the selected method would be one of the additive methods consisting of melting metal powder grains, the allowances A were estimated according to the following formula:

$$A = A_{acc} + A_{th} + A_{gr} + A_{snd} + A_{tmp} \qquad (3.1)$$

where: A_{acc} – allowance taking into account the accuracy of the production method, A_{th} – allowance taking into account the average thickness of the melted powder grains and the resulting surface roughness of the details directly after the melting process, A_{gr} – allowance for grinding, A_{snd} – allowance for sandblasting, A_{tmp} – allowance taking into account the influence of temperature during the melting process.

For further finishing work, we have designed the technological handles shown in Figure 3.7. The acetabular component is provided with a gripping element (1) in the form of a cylinder with a height of at least 8 mm and a supporting surface of at least 1.5 mm wide (2); in the femoral component – below the diameter – there is an internal gripping seat in the form of a cylinder with a height of at least 5 mm (3).

The solid CAD models of the femoral and acetabular components of the prototype resurfacing endoprosthesis have been designed in Autodesk Inventor Professional 9.0 as revolving solids resulting from the rotation of a specific contour around an axis coplanar to that contour. As a result of the full rotation of the contours, both components of the surface of the hip joint endoprosthesis are spherical. For the femoral component, the MSC-Scaffold is on the inner surface of the base cap of the

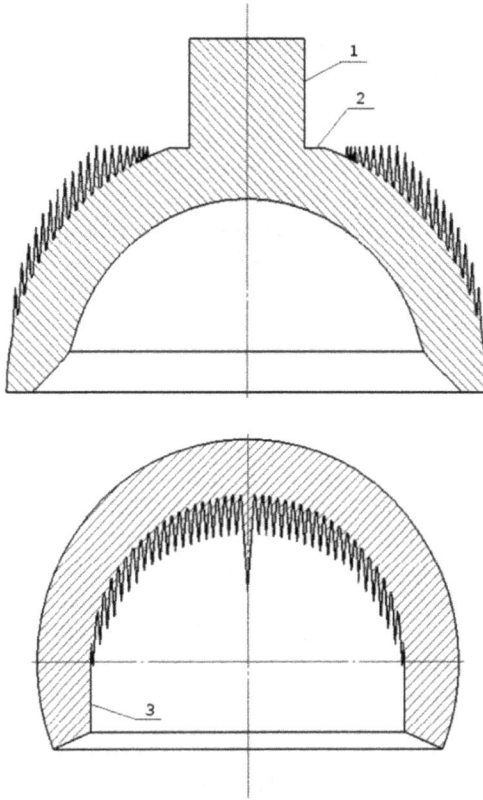

FIGURE 3.7 A cross section of the final form of CAD models of the components of the prototype hip joint resurfacing endoprosthesis (acetabular and femoral) with the designation of the technological handles: (1) grip pin, (2) abutment surface, (3) grip socket.

component, and for the acetabular component, the MSC-Scaffold is on the surface of the outer base cap of that component.

In CAD modelling of the MSC-Scaffold, we have used a circular pattern function, which allows duplicating a single solid element (spike) on a circle around the indicated axis of rotation and according to a given value of the spacing between the duplicated elements.

The spikes are arranged concentrically around the axis of rotation of the femoral component (on the inner surface of the component base cap) and the acetabular component (on the outer surface of the component base cap), respectively. In the rotation axis of the femoral component, there is a central spike, which is higher than the other spikes. According to the assumptions of the patents [1–3], the polygonal spikes on both components of the resurfacing endoprosthesis should be distributed as densely as possible (i.e. they should have common base edges with adjacent spikes). To obtain a practically maximally dense arrangement of spikes in the prototypes manufactured with the SLM method, in the CAD model, it was necessary to arrange the spikes at a distance of approximately 100 μm from each other. Therefore, the distance between the edges of the individual polygonal spikes at both the circumference and radius was established at 100 μm. This value was taken as at least three times the average thickness of the melted layer in the SLM process (~30 μm).

In the femoral component, we have designed a system of spikes that has the shape of a regular pyramid with the base of a square with a side length of 0.5 mm and a nominal height H_n such that the ratio H_n/R was from 5:1 (in spikes located close to the central spike) to 10:1 (in the spikes furthest from the central spike).

The number of spikes in a circular pattern ranges from 8 in the circle closest to the central spike to 120 in the concentric circle farthest from the central spike. In the acetabular component, we have designed a similar arrangement of spikes with a height ranging, according to the H_n/R ratio, from 5:1 (in the spikes closer to the axis of rotation) to 10:1 (in the spikes furthest from the axis of rotation), with the proviso that the tips of the spikes do not extend beyond the plane where edge (6) lies (see Figure 2.2, Chapter 2). Therefore, in the three circles closest to this edge, we have spikes designed with a shorter side of the base – 0.25 mm. The number of spikes ranged from 90 in the circle closest to the axis of rotation to 180 in the circle farther from the axis of rotation of the acetabular component.

The spikes of the prototype MSC-Scaffold have the shape of a regular pyramid with a square in the base. The nominal height H_n of the spike in the solid CAD model is the same as the height of the pyramid. The H_n/R ratio of the spike – the ratio of the nominal height to the radius of the circle circumscribed to the base of the pyramid – should be at least 5 according to the patents' assumptions [1–3]. The spikes are designed along the arc representing the meridian of the cap – with 20 spikes on the acetabular component and 17 on the femoral component along the parallel of the cap. All edges of the base of the pyramid lie below the surface of the spherical cap in such a way that the two distal vertices of its sides lie on the surface of the spherical cap. The curves formed at the intersection of the spherical cap surface with the sidewall of the pyramid constitute the actual edge of the base of a single spike of the MSC-Scaffold, while the edges of adjacent spikes are to be adjacent to each other both radially and circumferentially.

In the solid CAD model of the femoral component of the prototype endoprosthesis of the hip joint, three geometric variants of the MSC-Scaffold spikes were designed concentrically around its axis of rotation. The spikes designed in the first 12 parallels (counting from the central spike) have an H_n/R ratio of 8, the spikes designed in the next five parallels have an H_n/R ratio of 9, and the spikes designed in the last three parallels near the equator of the cap have H_n/R ratio of 10. The nominal heights H_n of the spikes of the prototype MSC-Scaffold are 2.828 mm, 3.182 mm, and 3.536 mm, for H_n/R ratios of 8, 9, and 10, respectively.

Figures 3.8a and 3.8b show solid CAD models of the acetabular component and the femoral component of the resurfacing endoprosthesis of the hip joint with the MSC-Scaffold (together with the projected additions and technological handles), while Figures 3.8c and 3.8d present a solid CAD model of the preprototype of the MSC-Scaffold, reflecting the central fragment of the femoral component of the resurfacing endoprosthesis of the hip joint (marked in Figure 3.8b with the arrow).

Figure 3.9 presents solid CAD models with the representation of the STL triangle mesh (a file format created for 3D printing by stereolithography, Standard Tessellation Language) of the components of the prototype hip joint resurfacing endoprosthesis.

Due to the required spatial arrangement of the MSC-Scaffold spikes on the inner surface of the cap (which is a part of the spherical base cap of the component), it was not possible to model the MSC-Scaffold using simple pattern operations, i.e. a linear pattern, a circular pattern, or a pattern based on a curve or a fill pattern. To this end, a mathematical model was developed to describe the position of the centre of the base of each of the spikes. Such a model allows for the variation of such structural and geometric parameters of the MSC-Scaffold as the width of the spike base, the distance between consecutive circles (lines) on which the spikes are placed, the distance between the adjacent spikes within a given circle and the number of planned circles, as well as the variation of the radius of the base cap, on which the MSC-Scaffold is placed.

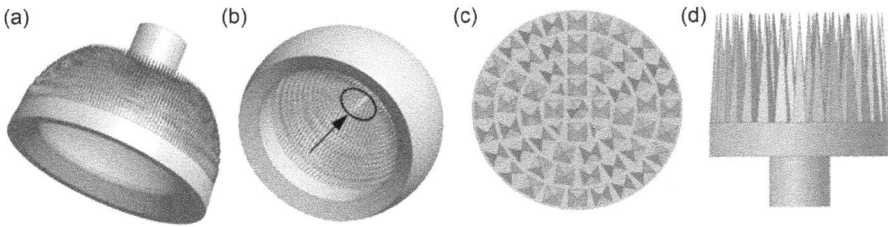

FIGURE 3.8   Three CAD models of two components of the prototype resurfacing endoprosthesis of the hip joint with the MSC-Scaffold with the designed allowances and technological grips: (a) acetabular component; (b) femoral component; and (c) top view and (d) side view of the MSC-Scaffold preprototype of the central fragment (marked with an arrow) of the femoral component.

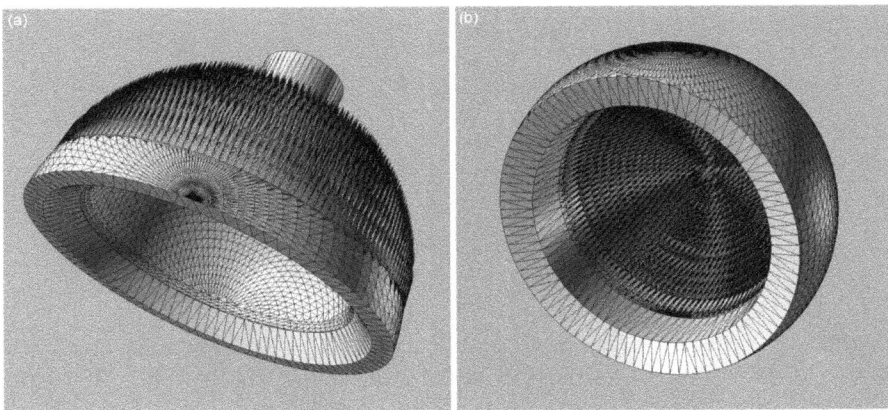

FIGURE 3.9   Representation of the STL triangle mesh of the components of the prototype endoprosthesis of the hip joint: (a) acetabular component, (b) femoral component.

For the planned experimental research carried out in the SolidWorks Premium 2013 x64 software, we have developed a solid CAD model in which the spikes of the prototype MSC-Scaffold were placed in a fragment of the spherical cap that is a section of the femoral component (Figure 3.10). Figure 3.11 presents the geometric relationships between the centres of the spike bases in the successive rows, and Figure 3.12 presents the geometric relationships between adjacent spikes within a given circle (row).

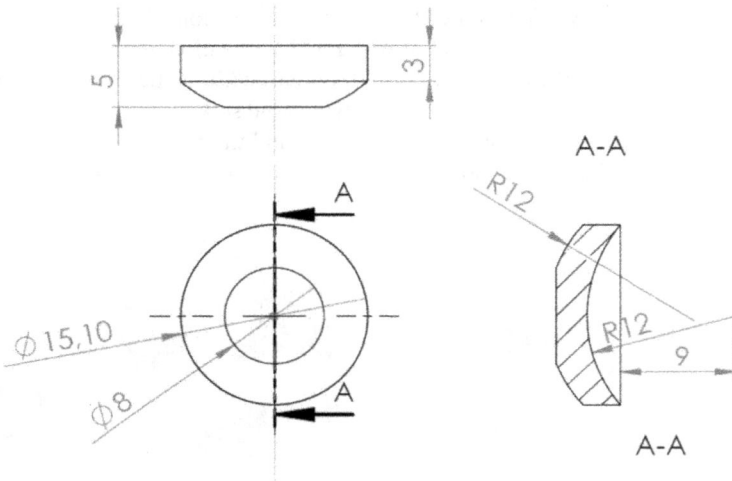

FIGURE 3.10 Technical drawing of a fragment of the base cap of the preprototype of the MSC-Scaffold.

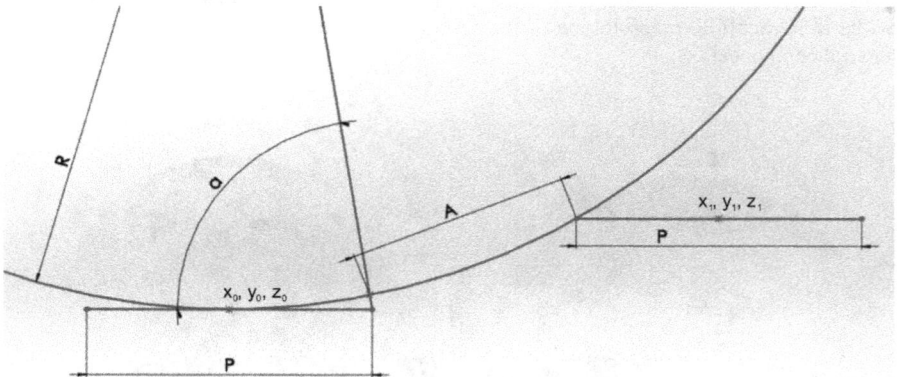

FIGURE 3.11 A diagram of geometric relationships between successive rows of the spike bases of the MSC-Scaffold; R – radius of the cap rounding on which the MSC-Scaffold was modelled, P – the width of the spike base, α – angle of inclination of the spike sidewall, A – the distance between consecutive circles (lines) on which the spikes are to be placed, (x_0, y_0, z_0) – the coordinates of a spike in the first circle (line), (x_1, y_1, z_1) – the coordinates of a spike in the next circle (line).

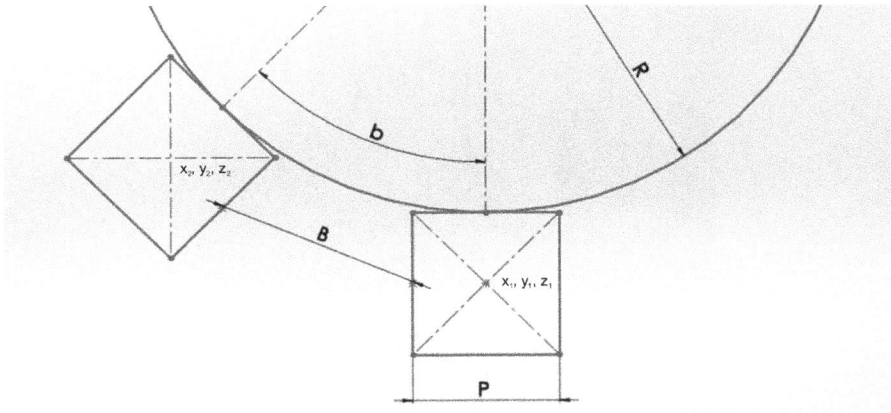

FIGURE 3.12 A diagram of the geometric relationships between the bases of adjacent spikes; R – the radius of the cap rounding on which the MSC-Scaffold was modelled, P – the width of the spike base, b – the angle between the centres of the spike bases, B – the distance between successive spikes in the circle (row), (x_1, y_1, z_1) – spike coordinates in the first circle (line), (x_2, y_2, z_2) – spike coordinates in the next circle (line).

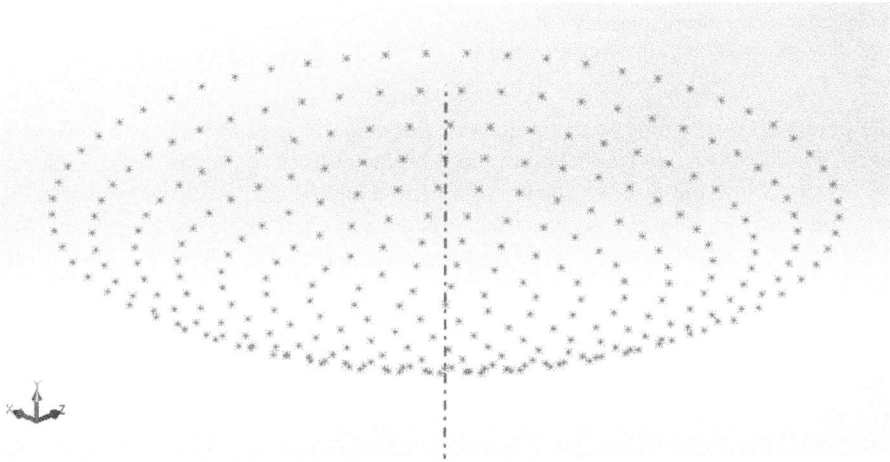

FIGURE 3.13 A 3D sketch of the distribution of the midpoints of the spike bases in the successive rows of the MSC-Scaffold, generated using a executive macro based on the coordinates calculated from the derived mathematical equation.

With the use of the basic trigonometric relationships, mathematical equations were determined to allow for the calculation of individual positions of the centres of the spike bases; we have designed a program generating the coordinates of characteristic points in the Wolfram Mathematica mathematical computing environment. After entering the quantities from Figure 3.11 and Figure 3.12, as well as the data such as the number of circles (rows) of spikes into the program syntax, the coordinates of

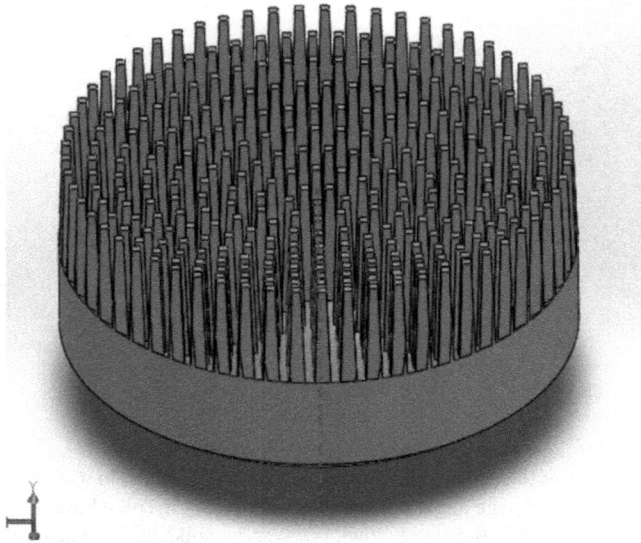

FIGURE 3.14 Solid CAD model of the prototype MSC-Scaffold, constructed using software generating the coordinates of the characteristic points (centres of the spike bases) and the executive macro allowing for the creation of a pattern of MSC-Scaffold based on a 3D sketch of the location of these centre points.

the points corresponding to the centres of the bases of individual spikes are calculated. These values can be written to the subsequent lines of the text file, which can be imported into the SolidWorks environment using the executive macro created in the same environment. In the resulting executive macro, we have implemented the loading of the coordinates of the spike base centres from the successive lines of the batch file and the creation of points distribution on the 3D sketch based on those lines. The result of this stage has been presented in Figure 3.13.

The combination of the CAD model of the spherical cap (Figure 3.10) and a 3D sketch of the midpoints allows for modelling the MSC-Scaffold by applying a pattern based on a sketch, as a result of which the first spike is modelled at a point located on the surface of the bottom of the cap and is duplicated at each of the generated points on the inner surface of the spherical cap representing the central part of the femoral component of the prototype resurfacing endoprosthesis of the hip joint. An exemplary solid CAD model of the MSC-Scaffold thus created is presented in Figure 3.14.

3.2 METHODS AND EFFECTS OF ELECTRO-EROSION MACHINING

The technological possibilities regarding traditional casting, machining, or subtractive manufacturing methods recognized and valid while realizing this task within the schedule of the research project indicated that with the current state of knowledge, it was not possible to produce the prototype of a resurfacing hip endoprosthesis with the MSC-Scaffold as a monolithic structure.

At first, it was necessary to make a prototype of a hip arthroplasty resurfacing endo-prosthesis for demonstration purposes. To that end, the die-sinking EDM was selected, and an attempt was made to manufacture a prototype made of chrome steel. However, it was possible to produce the MSC-Scaffold only with a much smaller number of spikes, comprising only 20% of what is proposed in patents [1–3]. Furthermore, the geometric structure of the prototype endoprosthesis produced in that manner did not reflect the patent requirements nor the shape and resolution reproduced in the solid CAD models (Figure 3.15).

We have undertaken further technological test trials for EDM and planned for two geometric structures. The first attempt consisted of the production of model spikes mounted on a plane, which were intended to be used in laboratory tests on a universal testing machine to embed the prototypes of the MSC-Scaffold in the periarticular cancellous bone of the swine femur. The second attempt involved the manufacturing of a prototype with a geometry that complies with the patents, that is, spikes located on a cylindrical surface. This test was conditional upon the positive results of the first attempt, for which we have made the following assumptions:

- wire-cut EDM was performed in steel,
- the spikes were designed in the form of pyramids with a square at the base,
- spikes were designed with three different heights of 5, 8, and 12 mm.

The manufacturing was carried out on a Robofil 290 EDM machine (Charmilles, Switzerland) (Figure 3.16). A brass-coated steel wire with a diameter of 0.25 mm was used. The parameters for electrical discharge machining are presented in Table 3.2.

Figure 3.17 presents a series of photos illustrating the working space of the wire-cut EDM machine, which shows the experimental geometric structure of the MSC-Scaffold fixed on a spindle of the indexing head during the machining process. Figure 3.18 shows three trial geometric structures of the MSC-Scaffold made by wire-cut EDM with spikes of various dimensions.

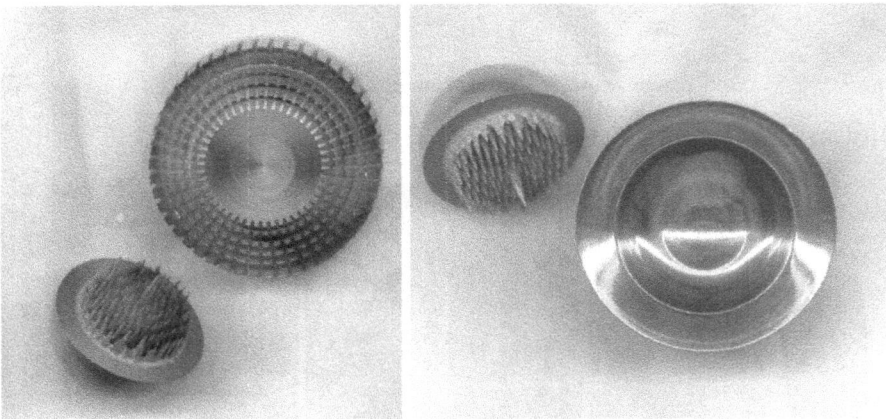

FIGURE 3.15 An early (unsuccessful) demonstration prototype of a hip joint resurfacing endoprosthesis, made for chrome steel using the die-sinking EDM.

TABLE 3.2

The parameters of wire-cut EDM

Parameter	Value
Time between 2 pulses	6 μs
Maximum linear feed	73.2 mm/min
Average operating voltage	48 V
Electrolyte pressure	11.5 bar
Machining mode	Isopulse roughing
Unloaded machining voltage	−80 V
Pulse duration	0.6 μs

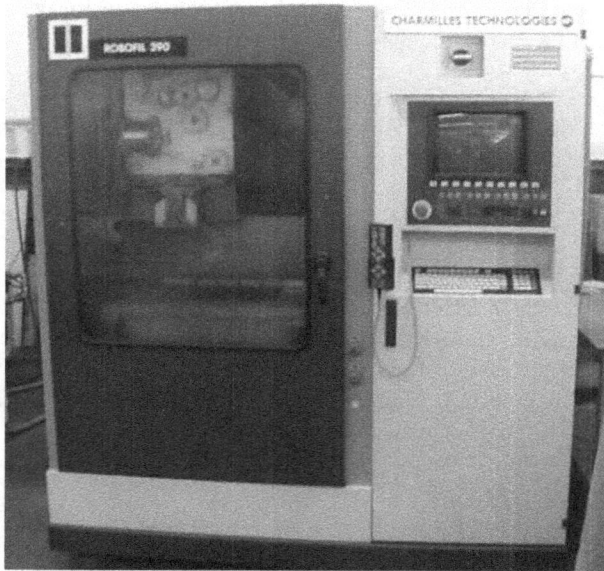

FIGURE 3.16   Robofil 290 EDM machine by the Swiss company Charmilles.

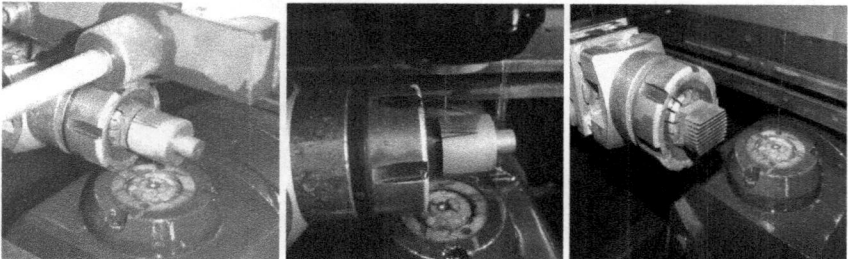

FIGURE 3.17   Wire-cut EDM of a trial geometric structure of the MSC-Scaffold; the illustrations present the cutting trajectory.

Tests have proven that it is possible to manufacture spikes with the required resolution and precision. Therefore, we have decided to try to create a fragment of the MSC-Scaffold on the cylindrical surface.

Technological trials of the manufacturing of the MSC-Scaffold for the hip joint resurfacing arthroplasty endoprosthesis on the inner surface of the semicylinder were carried out in two stages. The first stage is wire-cut EDM in the yz plane (Figure 3.19a), and the second stage is die-sinking EDM in the xy plane (Figure 3.19b). The tests were carried out using the EDA-25 EDM machine (Zakłady Mechaniczne Tarnów SA, Poland). To this end, a special precision copper electrode was made (Figure 3.19c). The treatment effects are presented in Figure 3.20.

It should be mentioned that the wire-cut EDM used in the first stage was only intended to speed up the process of spikes manufacturing, and the main goal was to observe the process and assess the effect of die-sinking EDM. During die-sinking EDM, quite intensive wear of the tool electrode was observed, which resulted in spike outline distortion at its base. In practice, therefore, it would be necessary to replace the tool electrode during the process or to recreate its shape by performing regeneration. There is a concern that after replacing the tool electrode, difficulties may arise in re-positioning it before continuing the manufacturing process, leading

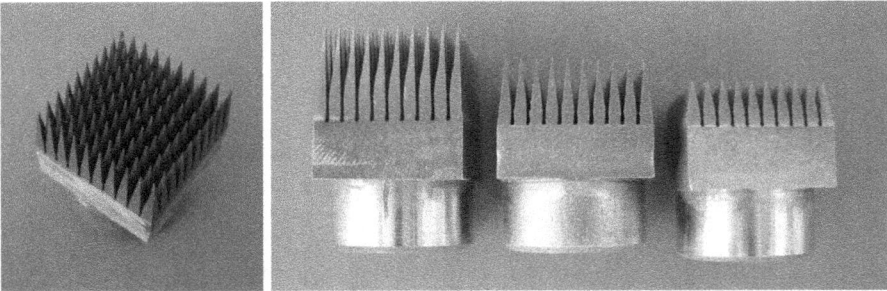

FIGURE 3.18 Trial geometric structures of the MSC-Scaffold of the prototype resurfacing endoprosthesis of the hip joint manufactured with the use of the wire-cut EDM method with three different heights of the spikes.

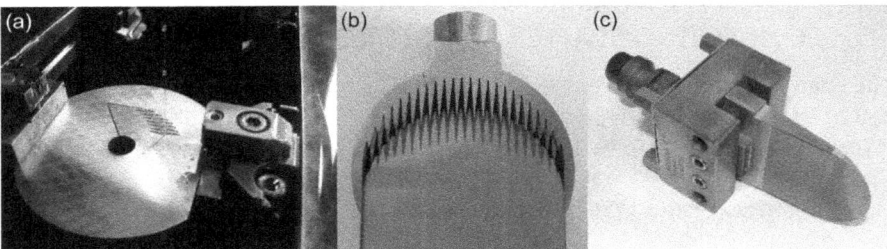

FIGURE 3.19 A two-stage process of manufacturing a prototype of a trial geometric structure of the MSC-Scaffold; (a) the step of cutting the cross-profile with a wire, (b) the step of die-sinking EDM, (c) the view of the tool electrode for die-sinking EDM.

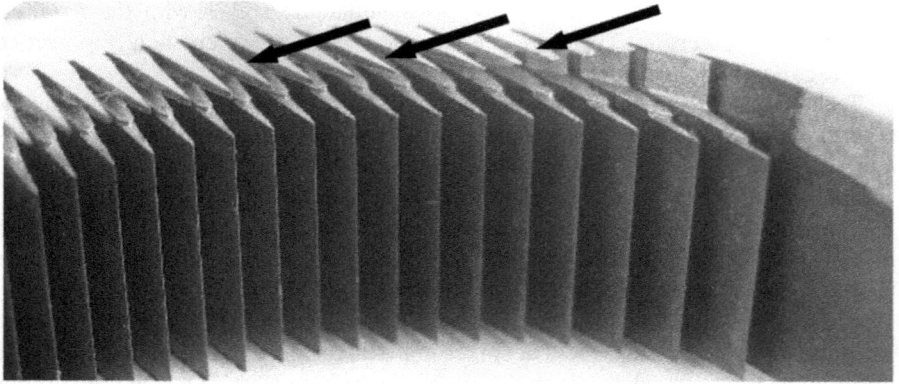

FIGURE 3.20 The geometric test structure of the MSC-Scaffold produced in the two-stage die-sinking EDM process.

to inaccuracies in the form of contour discontinuities. The disadvantage described above is a serious obstacle in accepting this method for possible serial production of spikes of the MSC-Scaffold in the prototype of the resurfacing endoprosthesis of the hip joint.

The technological trials of producing spikes with a stereometry compliant with the assumptions adopted for the concept of the MSC-Scaffold on the spherical surface of the femoral component of the resurfacing endoprosthesis by the die-sinking EDM have shown that it is possible to produce such structures; however, the process is time-consuming and costly. The wear of the tool electrode was found to be intense, the use of at least a few tools was required, and the machine was retooled several times. Therefore, this method can only be accepted for the production of single prototype copies; e.g. it is intended for experimental research but it is not suitable for mass production. Wire-cut EDM has proven its usefulness, but only for the production of spikes localized on a plane. Spikes on internal spherical surfaces, i.e. in the so-called femoral component of the resurfacing arthroplasty endoprosthesis of the hip joint, cannot be made using the EDM method.

3.3   PROTOTYPING SPIKES OF THE MULTI-SPIKED CONNECTING SCAFFOLD BY STEREOLITHOGRAPHY

The complete reproduction of the MSC-Scaffold geometry according to the concept described in the patents [1–3] was obtained by stereolithography (SLA). In Autodesk Inventor Professional 9.0, we have designed solid CAD models of:

- fragments of the MSC-Scaffold located on a flat surface (different spike arrangements),
- fragments of components of the hip joint resurfacing arthroplasty endoprosthesis with the MSC-Scaffold (located on the cylindrical surface),

• a prototype of a total hip resurfacing arthroplasty endoprosthesis with the MSC-Scaffold.

Based on these CAD models, 3D printouts of the above prototype structures were manufactured on a Viper Si2 SLA (3D Systems) printer with Accura SI 10 resin. The manufacturing was commissioned (in 2005) to the Department of Machine Technology and Production Automation at the Gdańsk University of Technology.

Fragments of the MSC-Scaffold in the form of 6 mm by 6 mm plates were characterized by two variants of structural and geometric spike arrangement. The first variant had 6 rows of 6 pyramids with a 1-mm square at the base and an H_n/R ratio of 5:1 to 10:1. In the case of the second variant of the manufactured prototype structures, the spikes were also planned in a rectangular configuration; spikes with the H_n/R ratio of 5:1 and 8:1 have been designed for separate plates. Regular pyramids had bases in the form of squares of the following lengths: 0.125, 0.25, 0.5, 1, and 2 mm. Examples of solid CAD models and the prototype structures of the MSC-Scaffold fragments printed based on such models are presented in Figure 3.21.

The manufactured semicircular spike structures represented the femoral and acetabular components of the prototype resurfacing endoprosthesis of the hip joint. Both components had six rows of regular pyramid-shaped spikes with a square at the base, a side length of 2 mm, and an H_n/R ratio of 8:1. Solid CAD models of the fragments of the components of the resurfacing endoprosthesis of the hip joint with the MSC-Scaffold (located on a cylindrical surface) and the 3D printouts manufactured based on these models are presented in Figure 3.22.

Figure 3.23 presents a solid CAD model and a demonstration prototype of a resurfacing arthroplasty endoprosthesis with the MSC-Scaffold produced based on this model with the use of the SLA method.

In the acetabular component of the endoprosthesis, the spikes have been designed in a system of 24 concentric circles on the outer surface of the spherical cap – from 88 spikes evenly spaced on the outermost inner circle to 225 spikes evenly spaced on the outermost circle. On the femoral component of the endoprosthesis, the spikes on the inner surface of the spherical base cap have been designed in a system of 29 concentric circles around the central cone-shaped spike – from 12 spikes evenly spaced on the outermost inner circle to 200 spikes evenly spaced on the outermost circle.

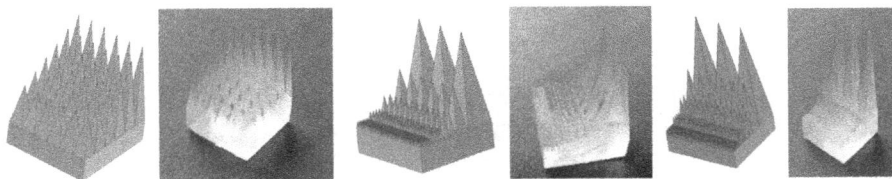

FIGURE 3.21 Examples of 3D CAD models and prototype structures of MSC-Scaffold fragments printed based on such CAD models for resurfacing endoprostheses.

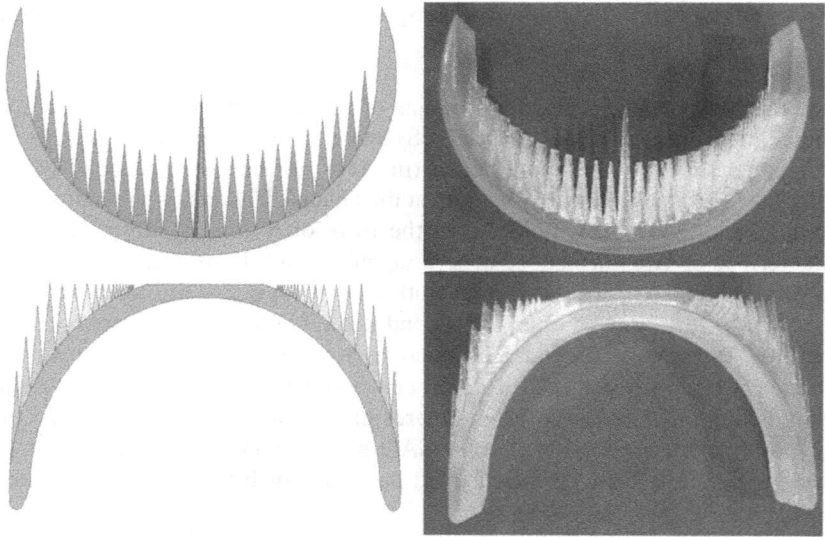

FIGURE 3.22 3D CAD models and 3D printouts of fragments of components of a prototype hip joint resurfacing endoprosthesis with the MSC-Scaffold (located on the cylindrical surface), generated on their basis using the SLA method.

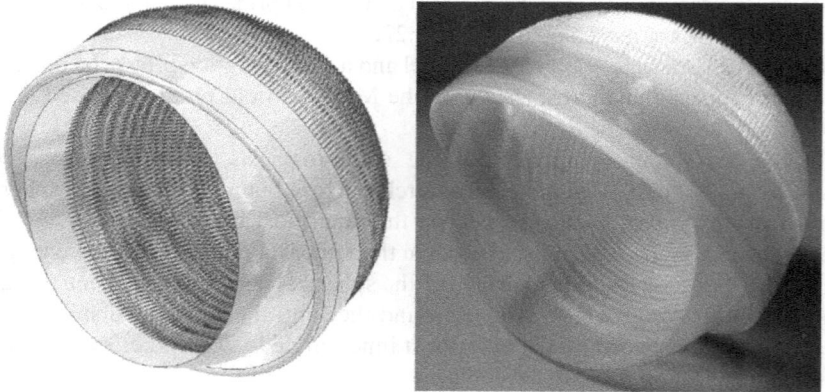

FIGURE 3.23 The solid CAD model and the resulting demonstration prototype of a resurfacing arthroplasty endoprosthesis with the MSC-Scaffold.

3.4 PROTOTYPING AND MANUFACTURING OF THE MULTI-SPIKED CONNECTING SCAFFOLD AND THE TOTAL HIP RESURFACING ENDOPROSTHESIS BY SELECTIVE LASER MELTING

The prototype of the resurfacing endoprosthesis with the MSC-Scaffold is a spectacular example of an orthopaedic implant whose manufacturing, as indicated in previous attempts, would not be possible without an additive manufacturing technologies.

The dynamic development of additive manufacturing processes allows for the formation of complex three-dimensional objects from powders of biocompatible metals or alloys, which provides new perspectives for advanced manufacturing and also for biomedical applications, e.g. orthopaedic intraosseous implants. Currently, to improve the viability of orthopaedic implants *in vivo* by increasing their structural and biomechanical biocompatibility with peri-implant bone tissue, and largely with the use of the above manufacturing technologies, it is possible to materialize and prototype structural elements that mimic the microstructure of natural biostructures.

Serially produced orthopaedic intraosseous implants (e.g. hip or knee endoprostheses) are, in general, manufactured by traditional methods of forging, casting, computer-aided subtractive manufacturing methods with the use of numerically controlled machine tools or powder metallurgy, including hot isostatic pressing (HIP), and in the technology of metal injection moulding (MIM) or powder injection moulding (PIM), ensuring high dimensional and shape accuracy of the manufactured elements [5–7]. These technologies, however, often fail if the implant component to be manufactured has a complex shape, containing thin-walled sections for which cutting/machining operations take a long time due to the need to remove a significant amount of material. In knee endoprostheses, up to 80% of the bar material used during the manufacturing process is converted into chips [8]. In several individual cases, when the need to manufacture patient-fit endoprosthesis components or when new design solutions are developed, the low efficiency and relatively high cost of conventional (subtractive) processing are highly disadvantageous.

In recent years, the production of freely formed solids (Solid Free-form Fabrication, SFF), also known as Rapid Prototyping (RP) or Layered Manufacturing (LM), Additive Manufacturing (AM) or Rapid Manufacturing (RM), or Direct Digital Manufacturing (DDM), is a new dynamic stage in the development of the production process [8]. Manufacturing free-form solids is a family of one-step processes involving layered shaping and material consolidation in powder or wire form, eliminating all machine tooling, and thus, reducing the time and costs of production [9]. Due to the additive character of these methods, they can be used to produce parts with a high complexity of shape directly according to the CAD model. These technologies allow for the manufacturing of custom-made components/implants, tailored to the needs of a specific patient, with the shape of such components formed by sintering or melting powder layers with a laser beam or with an electron beam. With these technologies, it is possible to build components from biocompatible metal powders or alloys, such as titanium and its alloys and cobalt-chrome alloys. Monodisperse metal or alloy powders with uniform microstructure for rapid solidification, desired in these technologies, became generally available only at the beginning of the 21st century [8].

In the case of SLM technology, the high energy density allows for the full melting of powders; therefore, the parts produced in this technology are characterized by a very high, close to theoretical, density [9,10]. Vandenbroucke and Kruth described the possibility of forming objects from biocompatible metal powders and alloys for biomedical applications in this technology [10]. For comparison purposes, the characteristics and research on another technology, EBM, that allows the shaping of components by full melting (according to the classification given by Kruth et al. [9]) were given by Murr et al. [9,11]. Support for this opinion can be found, for example, in the article by Leordean et al. [12], in which it was demonstrated that SLM process is promising in the production of personalized titanium implants. According to Gong et al. [13], although elements produced with the use of SLM technology (of Ti-6Al-4V powder), using optimal process parameters, have comparable properties (such as ductility, fatigue strength, or hardness) to elements produced with the use of EBM technology, some properties, such as the yield point and tensile strength, are higher than in the case of other DMM technologies [14,15].

It should be noted that the DMM technologies were little known at the turn of the 20th and 21st centuries and were not widely available – especially those that allow for the production of biocompatible metals and alloys: "(…) the range of commercially available metal powders suitable for use in SLM technology is still limited" [9].

Currently, DMM technologies such as SLM, SLS, and EBM offer the technological potential for the production of biomimetic porous structures or bone scaffolds [15–20]. This creates new possibilities for the bioengineering design of orthopaedic implants, e.g. spine implants [21], cranioplasty implants [22,23], oral and maxillofacial implants, finger joint implants [24,25], bone filling implants [26], nonstandard hip and knee implants [16,27] as well as dental implants [8,10].

Additive technologies allow the production of highly porous metal structures (porosity >80%) with precisely controlled microstructure, offering many new possibilities for the design of orthopaedic implants and implant coatings [28–40]. It is also possible to produce porous scaffolds with desired mechanical properties similar to the mechanical properties of a natural bone [41,42] and with the desired microstructure of interconnected pores with well-defined dimensions of the pores and the joints between them [22,43].

As part of the research, activities were carried out to identify and compare the technological possibilities of producing a prototype MSC-Scaffold with the use of SLM technology and other similar manufacturing methods available on the market – i.e. EBM and SLS.

The EBM technology, due to the microfolding of the lateral surface of the spikes and the large number of nonmelted metallic powder particles accumulated in the area between the spikes, has been assessed as practically unsuitable for use in the production of resurfacing endoprosthesis components with the MSC-Scaffold. The prototypes manufactured with the use of SLS technology had numerous material discontinuities on the lateral surface of the prototype MSC-Scaffold, as well as microcracks and micropores in the cross section, which prevents the recommendation of this technology for the production of prototypes of an entirely non-cemented resurfacing endoprosthesis with the MSC-Scaffold. Similar defects have not been found in the preprototypes of MSC-Scaffold made in SLM technology and subjected to metallographic tests. Figures 3.24 and 3.25 show, respectively, the negatively evaluated preprototypes of the MSC-Scaffold manufactured with the use of EBM and SLS technology.

The requirements for the production of full-density components having mechanical properties comparable to those made of homogeneous materials have directed our attention to the SLM technology. Based on our comparative experimental study [44] and data available in the literature, we concluded that this DMM technique can be considered suitable for the production of personalized biomimetic resurfacing endoprostheses with the MSC-Scaffold.

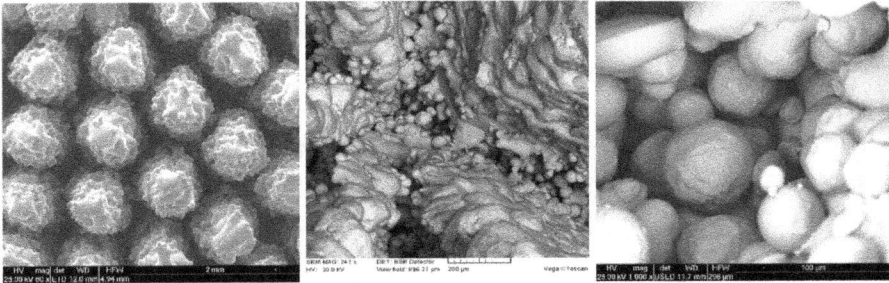

FIGURE 3.24 Negatively evaluated (due to the microfolding of the lateral surface of the spikes and a large number of nonmelted metallic powder particles accumulated in the area between the spikes) the preprototype of MSC-Scaffold produced in the EBM technology.

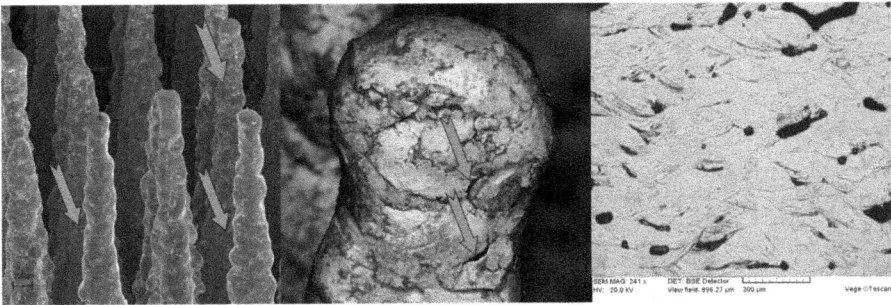

FIGURE 3.25 Negatively evaluated (due to numerous material surface discontinuities, as well as microcracks and micropores) preprototype of the MSC-Scaffold produced using the SLS method.

To assess the possibility of SLM technology for the manufacturing of MSC-Scaffold, we have designed several 3D CAD models with different dimensional and geometric variants. These preprototypes had an arrangement of spikes reproduced as in the central region of the femoral component, i.e. around the central polygonal spike. In the research stage, two types of regular pyramids (spikes) were selected for further prototyping of the components of the resurfacing endoprosthesis: (1) with equilateral triangles at the base and (2) with squares at the base (concentric system). The spikes were placed on round discs (⌀16 mm). Each of the pyramid systems had four variants of the length of the polygon side at the base: 0.5, 1.0, 1.5 and 2.0 mm, and H_n/R ratio values were 5:1, 7:1, and 9:1.

The SLM Tech Center (Paderborn, Germany) was subcontracted to manufacture 24 different preprototypes of the MSC-Scaffold in SLM technology of Ti-6Al-7Nb alloy on the ReaLizer SLM 100 machine. The set of preprototypes of the MSC-Scaffold produced using the SLM technology is presented in Figure 3.26. Examples of preprototypes for each geometric arrangement of spikes are presented in Figure 3.27.

SLM is a technique of layered material bonding that makes it possible to generate complex parts by selectively melting successive layers of metal powder on top of each

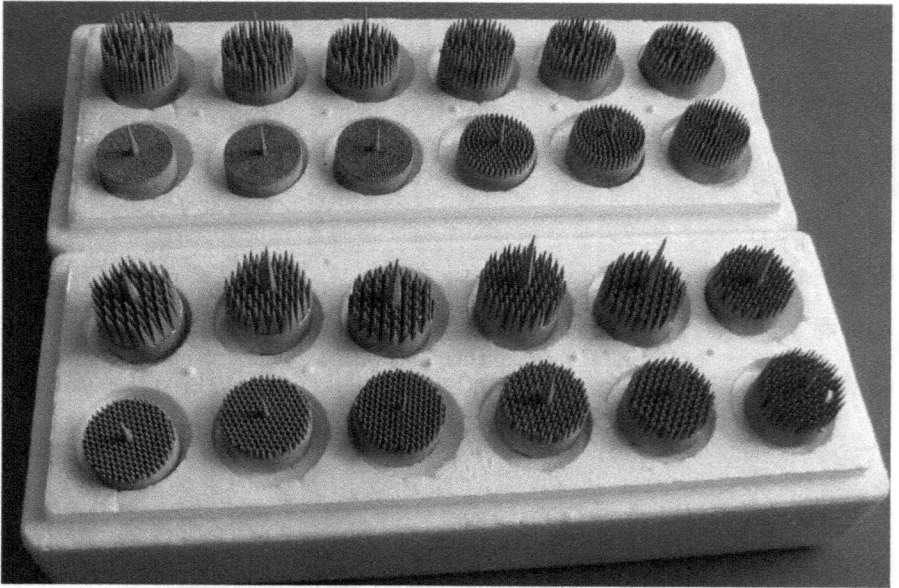

FIGURE 3.26   A set of 24 preprototypes of the MSC-Scaffold produced by SLM technology.

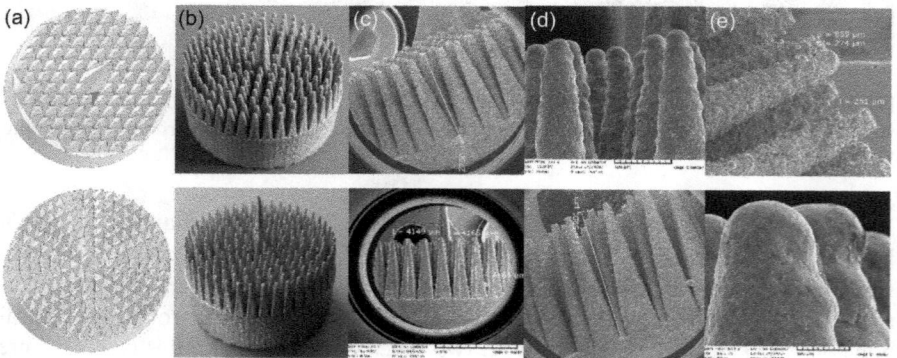

FIGURE 3.27   CAD models (a), SLM preprototypes of MSC-Scaffold (b), and SEM images of their spikes (c)–(e).

other with the use of thermal energy provided by a focused and computer-controlled laser beam. In each layer, the laser beam generates the outline of the part that is built up by melting the powder particles before the build plate is lowered and covered with a new powder layer. SLM is one of the commercially available technologies for producing metallic parts, typically having a large variety of geometric patterns and using various types of materials, including biocompatible titanium alloys and chromium-cobalt alloys. In SLM, the powder particles are fully melted. This process occurs in a powder bed. It begins by applying a thin powder layer to the substrate held in place by an adjustable platform. The laser then scans the surface of the powder, and the heat generated by the laser causes the powder particles to melt and form a drop (pool) of molten metal [8]. As the laser beam moves away from the pool, the molten material solidifies to form an element of the object geometry. After the layer is fully scanned and melted, the adjustable platform lowers and the next powder layer is spread over the previous layer and re-melted by the laser. A schematic diagram showing the principle of this process is presented in Figure 3.28.

The prototypes of the MSC-Scaffold for resurfacing endoprostheses of the hip joint were fabricated of Ti-6Al-7Nb alloy powder on a ReaLizer SLM 100 machine (MTT Technologies Group, Germany) equipped with the Nd:YAG laser. The grain size distribution of the powder was 5 to 50 µm; the average grain size of the Ti-6Al-7Nb alloy powder was 35 µm. The SEM image of the Ti-6Al-7Nb powder particles and the histogram of the size distribution (diameter) of the powder particles developed based on the series of SEM images are presented in Figure 3.29. During the SLM process of manufacturing a prototype of a hip joint resurfacing endoprosthesis with the MSC-Scaffold, the following parameters were used: layer thickness – 50 µm, scanning speed – 125 mm/s, construction speed – 4 cm³/h.

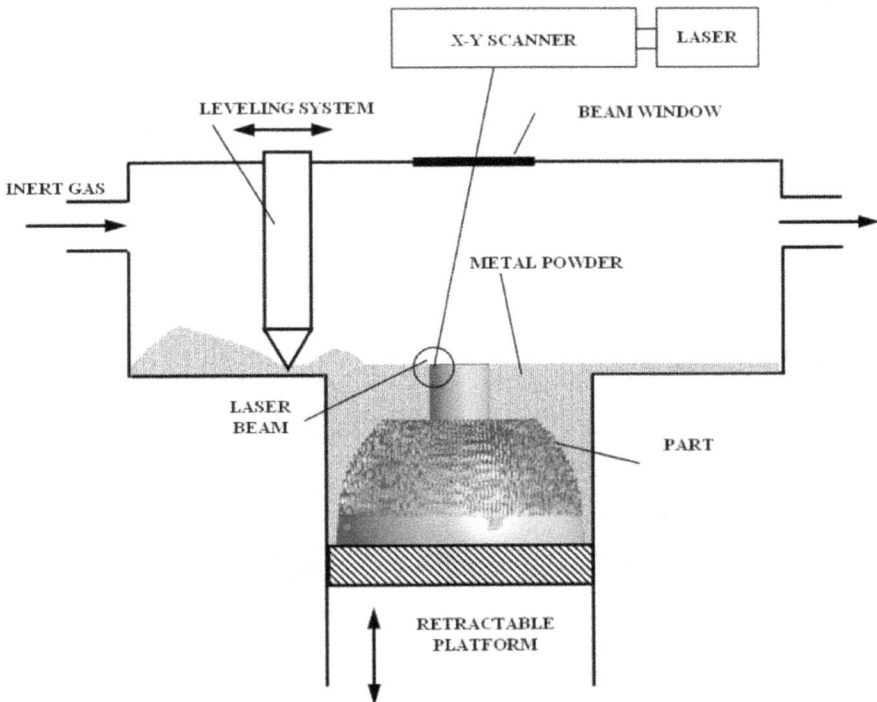

FIGURE 3.28   A schematic diagram showing the principle of selective laser melting (SLM) (Note: the actual proportions of the size of the generated component in relation to the SLM machine chamber differ from those presented in the diagram).

Due to titanium's high reactivity with environmental elements such as oxygen, nitrogen, carbon, and hydrogen, the SLM process occurs in a closed chamber, constantly flushed with argon gas to lower the oxygen level below 0.1%.

Figure 3.30 presents a prototype of a surface hip endoprosthesis with the MSC-Scaffold directly after removal from the SLM machine. The prototypes produced required finishing surface treatment, that is, turning, grinding, polishing, and lapping the articulating surfaces of the hip joint endoprostheses. We have designed

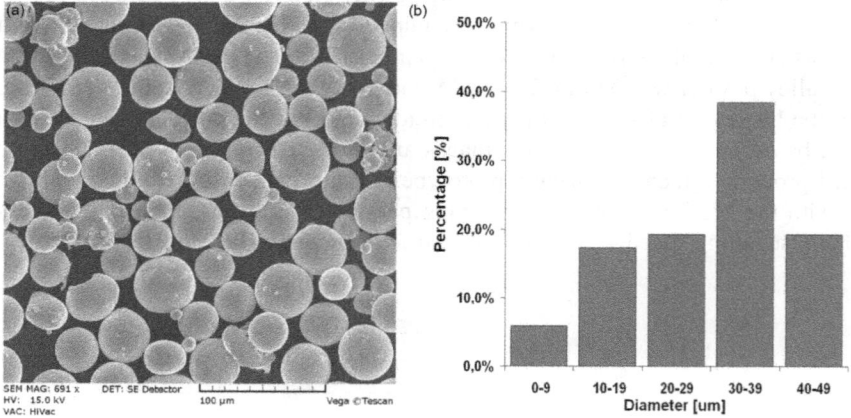

FIGURE 3.29 SEM images of Ti-6Al-7Nb powder particles used to produce SLM prototypes of a resurfacing endoprosthesis with the MSC-Scaffold (a) and a histogram of the size distribution (diameter) of powder particles based on a series of SEM images (b).

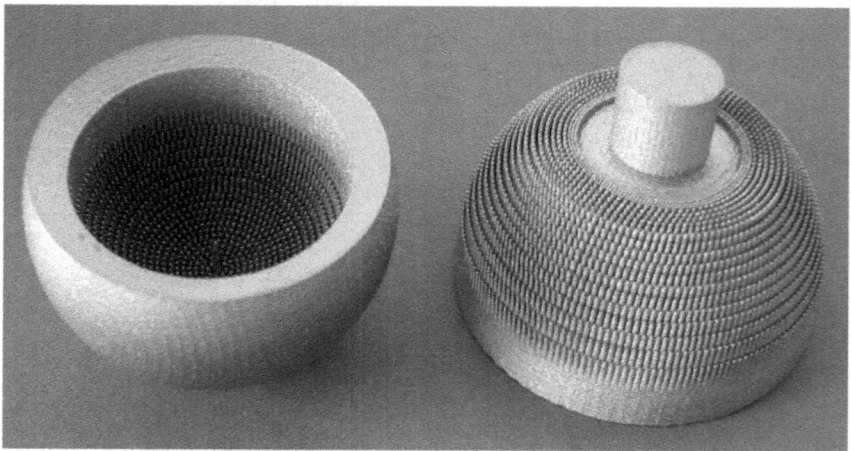

FIGURE 3.30 Prototypes produced in SLM technology required further precise processing (turning, grinding, polishing, lapping of the cooperating articulate surface of hip joint endoprostheses); visible technological handles allow precise surface finishing.

technological grips for surface finishing, which were then partially removed as part of the ongoing processing by wire-cut EDM.

Figure 3.31 presents the prototype of an endoprosthesis for hip joint resurfacing with the MSC-Scaffold after grinding and polishing the articulating surfaces. Figure 3.32a shows the spikes from the area marked with a square frame in Figure 3.31a, and Figure 3.32b shows a single spike in a close-up. To remove the nonmelted powder aggregates adhering to the surface of the spikes, we have used the method of micro glass beads blasting treatment.

To examine the density in the cross section, we prepared material samples of the manufactured prototype. As demonstrated in Figure 3.33, there are micropores in the cross section inside which loose or nonmelted powder particles can be found. These types of pores within the implant structure may be the source of the initiation and propagation of microcracks when this implant is subject to periodic loading [27] .

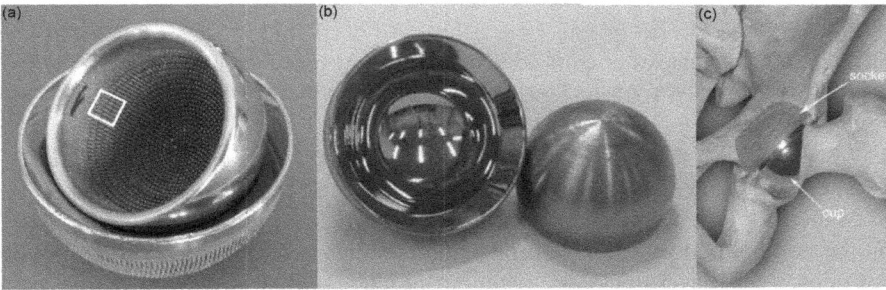

FIGURE 3.31   A prototype of a resurfacing endoprosthesis of the hip joint with the MSC-Scaffold: (a) and (b) after grinding and polishing the articulate surface, (c) illustratively in the hip joint.

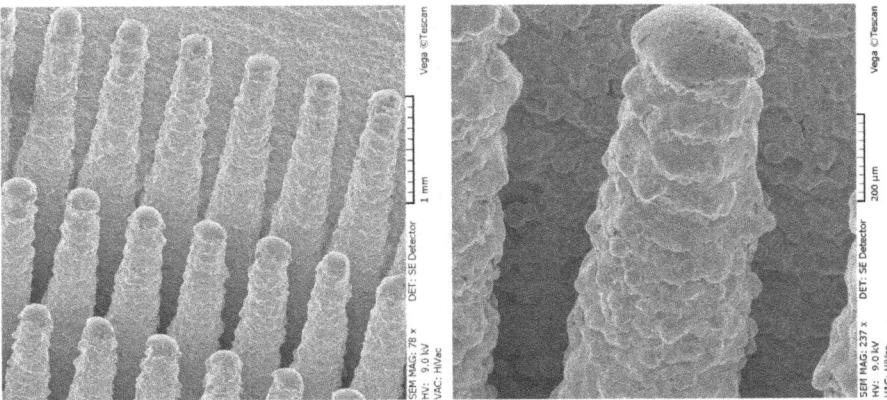

FIGURE 3.32   A fragment of the MSC-Scaffold (from the area marked with a square frame in Figure 3.31a) after blasting with glass microspheres; close-up of a single spike.

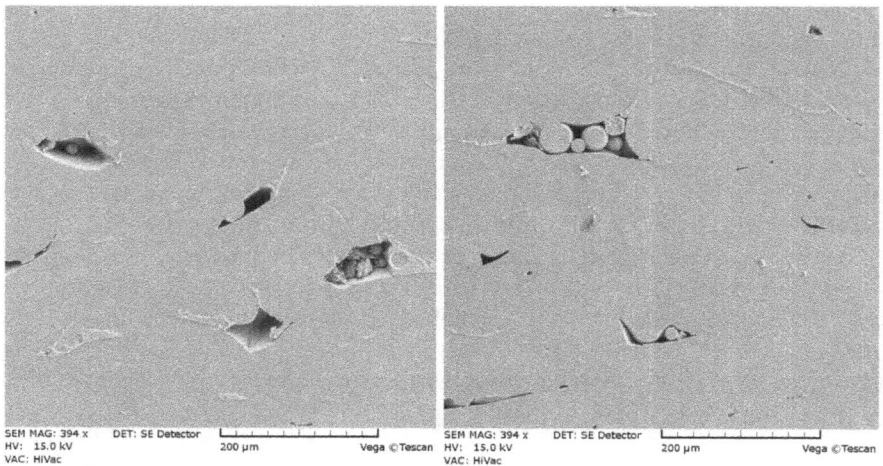

FIGURE 3.33 Examples of cross sections of the SLM prototype of a hip joint resurfacing endoprosthesis reveal zones of nonmelted material (pores, cavities), including nonmelted powder particles.

The occurrence of such pores within the surface of the details produced by the SLM method, including the nonmelted powder particles contained therein, is caused by the non-optimal selection of production parameters (such as laser beam power, scanning speed, layer thickness, scanning strategy, particle size, distribution, etc.). These are typical technological defects in structures produced using the SLM method [45]. The presence of such defects on the polished articulate surface of the endoprosthesis may disqualify the components of the endoprosthesis produced with this method from use due to the risk of accelerated wear causing the migration of wear particles to the surrounding living tissues. It follows that some optimization should be made in the selection of the parameters of the SLM process. This will allow the occurrence of pores in the cross section to be avoided and a homogeneous, coherent, and crack-free microstructure will be obtained. According to Sercombe et al. [27], to control the microstructure of the components produced with the use of the SLM method, we should consider the heat treatment of implant prototypes.

3.5 POST-PRODUCTION TREATMENT OF THE BONE-CONTACTING SURFACE OF THE MULTI-SPIKED CONNECTING SCAFFOLD

The SLM additive manufacturing process leaves numerous micro-residues on the bone-contacting surface of the tested MSC-Scaffold, in the form of not fully melted alloy powder particles and variously shaped splatted forms: spherical-like (adhering to almost the entire surface) and elongated, twisted, wire-like (occasional, mainly at the tips of the spikes and spaces between them). The presence of such undesirable technological micro-residues in medical devices intended for implantation poses a high risk of complications in the form of inflammation, which impede the proper healing of the implant. The necessity to guarantee the proper quality of the surface in the case of such unusual design solutions often requires the development of nonstandard technological tasks that are involved in post-production processing.

In the study of MSC-Scaffold, we have used various variants of preprototypes, designed as central fragments of the femoral component of the hip resurfacing endo-prosthesis and made of Ti-6Al-4V alloy with the use of SLM technology. Their man-ufacturing was subcontracted to the Center for New Materials and Technologies of the West Pomeranian University of Technology in Szczecin. Figure 3.34 presents an overview of the preparation of a file with CAD models of MSC-Scaffold preproto-types for additive formation – adding the necessary technological supports, through which the models will be printed on the plate mounted in the SLM working chamber. This step was performed in Magics 13.0 (Materialize HQ, Belgium).

Figure 3.35 depicts the main steps of the process of additive pre-prototyping of the MSC-Scaffold on an SLM machine (ReaLizer SLM 250, MTT Technologies).

An example preprototype of the MSC-Scaffold directly after manufacturing using SLM technology is presented in Figure 3.36. The SEM documentation presented in Figure 3.36 reveals numerous micro-residues in the form of not completely melted alloy powder particles and spherical-like spattering forms present on its entire bone-contacting surface. This is a normal phenomenon. These types of micro-residues are usually removed by abrasive blasting treatment.

SEM examination of the surface condition of MSC-Scaffold preprototypes man-ufactured in the SLM technology, whose example results have been presented in Figure 3.37, also revealed a few technological residues in the form of elongated,

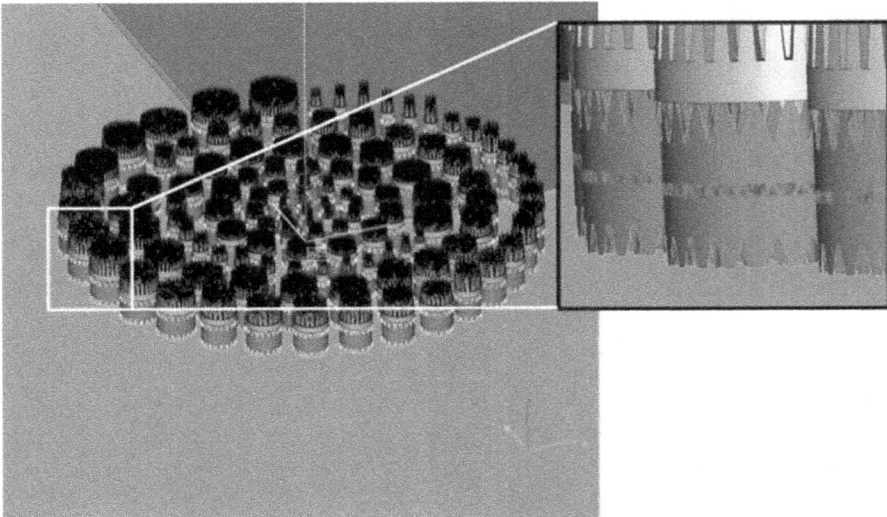

FIGURE 3.34 The stage of preparing a file with assemblage of CAD models of the MSC-Scaffold preprototypes for additive manufacturing on the SLM machine.

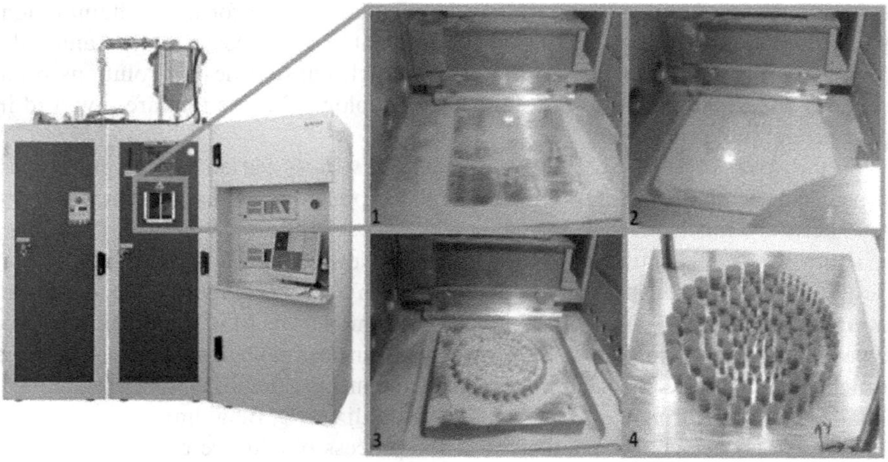

FIGURE 3.35 The main steps of the additive manufacturing process of the preprototypes of the MSC-Scaffold with the SLM machine (ReaLizer SLM 250, MTT Technologies): (1) selective laser melting of one of the first powder layers, (2) selective laser melting of one of the last powder layers, (3) cleaning of the produced nonmelted powder preprototypes, (4) as-manufactured preprototypes printed on board.

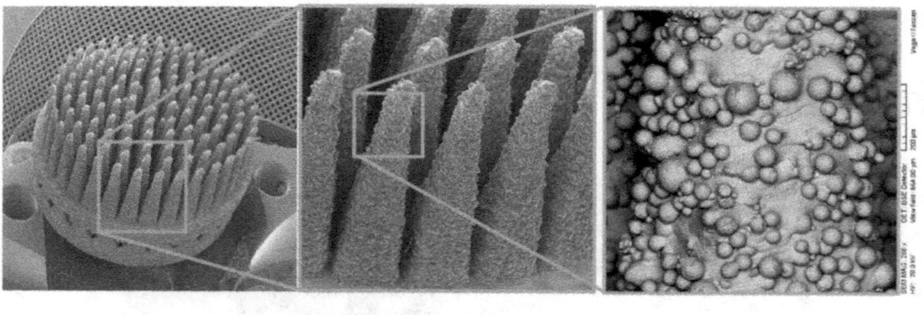

FIGURE 3.36 An example of the MSC-Scaffold preprototype directly after its production in the SLM technology.

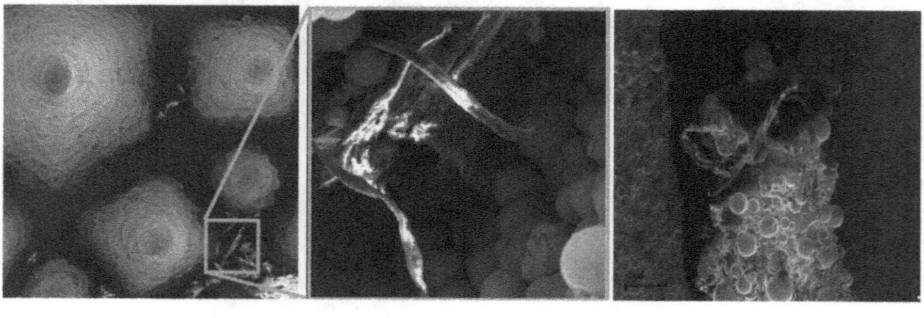

FIGURE 3.37 SEM documentation of micro-residues revealed in preprototypes directly after their production in SLM technology.

twisted, wire-like forms occurring sporadically at the tops of the spikes and in the space between the spikes.

Post-production processing of the original series of the preprototypes subject to testing, with the configuration of spikes that adopts a value of 100 μm for spacing between the bases of the spikes measured radially and circumferentially, carried out with abrasive blasting technology and with the use of glass beads (diameter ~40–70 μm), allowed for the removal of most of the micro-residues adhered to the surface; however, it was not possible to remove the micro-residues from the spaces directly at the base of the spikes. This is seen in Figure 3.38a. Arrows indicate numerous micro-residues remaining in the interspike areas of the MSC-Scaffold. SEM documentation (Figure 3.38b) presents a thoroughly cleaned lateral surface of the MSC-Scaffold spikes and spherical-like remains on the surface at the base of the spikes (Figures 3.38c and 3.38d).

The negative biological effect resulting from such a condition of the bone-contacting surface of the prototype MSC-Scaffold has been proven following pilot implantation of the MSC-Scaffold preprototypes into the articular subchondral layer of the knee joint in experimental animals (Polish Large White breed swine) [46]. Histopathological evaluation of the peri-implant bone obtained nine weeks after implantation revealed the presence of numerous metallic particles that cause inflammation in the peri-implant bone tissue. Figure 3.38d presents a cross section of a specimen of the peri-implant bone with an implant, where, due to the large number of metallic micro-residues, the desired biointegration of the peri-implant bone with the implant was not achieved. An analysis of the histopathological documentation and the preliminary evaluation of the preprototypes in human osteoblasts culture discussed in [46] both indicate that it is necessary to develop a more effective post-production surface treatment of the prototype MSC-Scaffold.

To increase the efficiency of post-production blasting treatment of the surface of the prototype MSC-Scaffold, tests were carried out with the use of abrasives such as White Fused Alumina and glass beads. Due to persistent difficulties in removing micro-residues from the space near to the spikes bases, it was decided to modify the MSC-Scaffold design variant, i.e. the spacing between the spike bases was increased to 200 μm (radially and circumferentially). The effects of experimental abrasive blasting of these preprototype design variants are presented in Figures 3.39a, 3.39b and 3.39d, 3.39e.

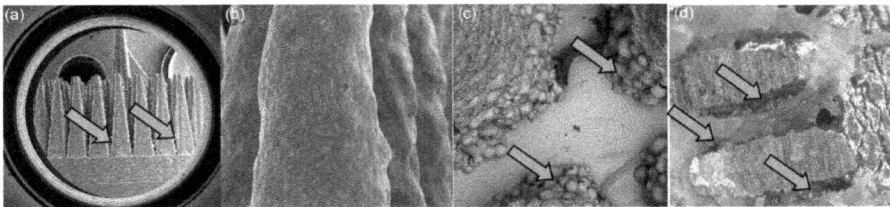

FIGURE 3.38 An example of the MSC-Scaffold preprototype manufactured in SLM technology as encountered after abrasive treatment with the use of micro glass beads with diameters of ~40–70 μm: (a); the lateral surface of MSC-Scaffold spikes (b); around the bases of the spikes (c); no visible biointegration of the bone with the implant due to the presence of metallic particles between the peri-implant bone and the implant (d).

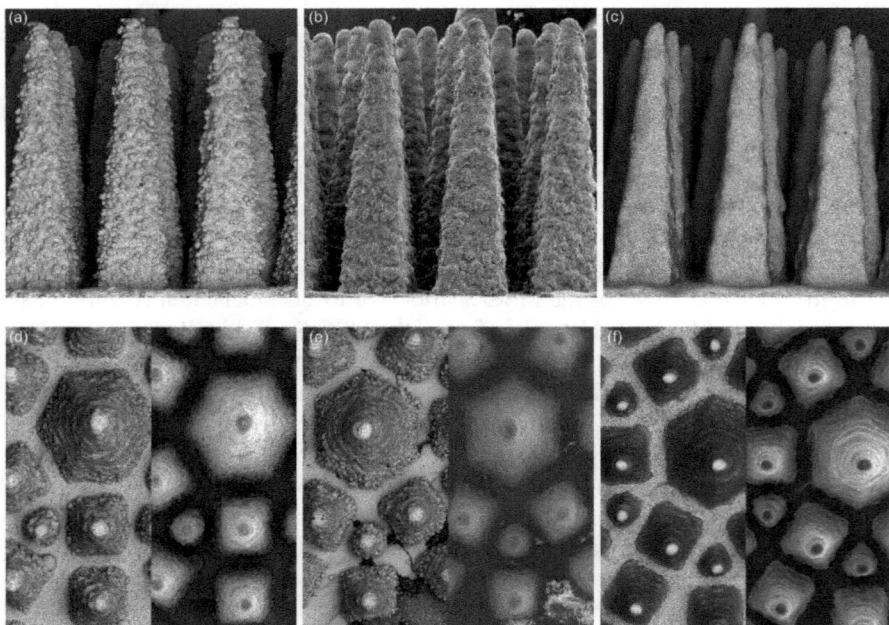

FIGURE 3.39 SEM documentation of the bone-contacting surface of the MSC-Scaffold preprototypes manufactured in SLM technology – side view, located on the cylindrical surface, and top view, respectively, after the experimental post-production treatment performed with the abrasive blasting technique using: (a) and (d) White Fused Alumina F220; (b) and (e) micro glass beads with a grain size of ~30–50 µm; (c) and (f) developed abrasive mixture.

The use of White Fused Alumina F220 allowed a slight smoothing of the MSC-Scaffold surface, but a significant amount of micro-residues remained on the entire lateral surface of the spikes (Figures 3.39a and 3.39d). The use of microspheres resulted in a smoother surface (Figures 3.39b and 3.39e) than with the use of electrocorundum; however, it was still not possible to completely remove the microdebris from the bottom of the MSC-Scaffold and the spikes' surface at the base of the spikes. After micro-beading, the lateral surface of the MSC-Scaffold spikes was still noticeably wavy.

During further research, and on the basis of the experience gained, we have developed an abrasive mixture composed of equal proportions of:

- White Fused Alumina F220 (~55–75 µm grain size),
- White Fused Alumina F320 (~30 µm ± 1.5% grain size),
- glass microbeads (~ 30 µm ± 10% grain size).

The addition of a smaller granulation abrasive agent to the mixture and sifting microbeads with a larger diameter were primarily intended to ensure better access of the abrasive agent to the tight spaces of the MSC-Scaffold at the base of the spikes.

The effects of post-production processing using this abrasive mixture are presented in Figures 3.39c and 3.39f. The SEM documentation shows that not only the

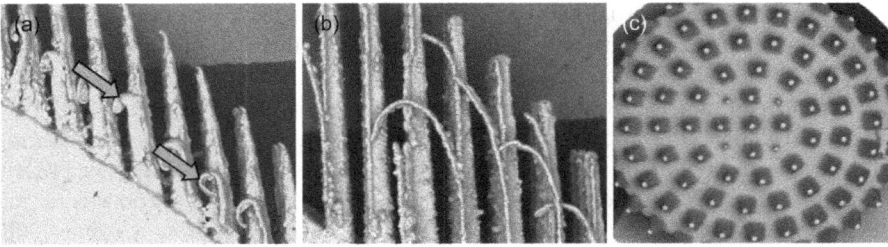

FIGURE 3.40 SEM documentation shows the unfavourable effects of too intensive post-processing: (a) and (b) curling of the spikes and (c) excessive abrasion.

lateral surfaces of the spikes of the prototype MSC-Scaffold were thoroughly cleaned of any residues, but so were the surfaces at the base of the spikes.

An important aspect of post-production abrasive blasting is the need to ensure constant process parameters. Nozzles made of high-quality cemented carbide, which for a long time retain the original diameter and profile of the outlet opening, allowed to maintain a repeatable and stable intensity of the abrasive stream.

The possibilities of influencing the effectiveness of post-production abrasive blasting include adjusting the distance of the abrasive jet outlet from the treated surface and the exposure time (process duration). Due to the ongoing visual inspection, adverse effects in the form of curling of the spikes have been observed if the adopted distance of the abrasive stream outlet from the surface of the processed preprototype was too short ($\approx$ 2–3 cm). Abrasive blasting carried out in this way guaranteed a short process duration (approximately 8–10 min per series), but it caused great destruction, also in the form of excessive abrasion of the spikes. The discussed unfavourable effects of experimental post-production processing are presented in Figure 3.40.

The occurrence of unfavourable effects was minimized by further tests, where the pressure value was reduced from 10 to 7 bar and the distance from the abrasive stream outlet from the surface of the processed preprototype was increased to 20 cm. The time of manual post-process abrasive blasting for a series of ten preprototypes with the use of the developed abrasive mixture was approximately 30 min, which allowed for obtaining a bone-contacting surface with the condition presented in Figures 3.39c and 3.39f, without the adverse effects visible in Figure 3.40.

As a result of the conducted experimental tests, an effective and repeatable method of cleaning the bone-contacting surface of the prototype MSC-Scaffold was developed with the use of an abrasive mixture with the composition proposed above and with individually selected parameters for post-production processing.

3.6 REVERSE DESIGN OF THE WORKING PROTOTYPE OF PARTIAL RESURFACING KNEE ARTHROPLASTY ENDOPROSTHESIS

In the case of traditional resurfacing arthroplasty of the knee joint, its components are implanted in the bone with bone cement and stabilized with pins designed in the femoral component, which are implanted in the holes drilled in the femoral condyles (e.g. Arthrex® iBalance Unicompartmental Knee Arthroplasty, MAKOplasty® Partial Knee

Resurfacing, Oxford® Partial Knee Resurfacing, etc.). Extensive penetration of cement into periarticular cancellous bone causes resorption of this periarticular bone tissue [47]. Between the implant and the bone, osseointegration is altered, resulting in micromovements and radiolucent lines (RLLs) appearing in radiological imaging [48]. Pain associated with the appearance of radiolucent lines is believed to be due to the loosening of the endoprosthesis component and usually leads to revision surgery over time [49,50]. Fixation of the non-cemented components of joint endoprostheses in the bone is associated with a lower incidence of micromovement complications and fewer revisions [50].

Figure 3.41, taking the knee joint as an example, schematically presents the hyaline cartilage tissue, the subchondral bone with interdigitations anchoring the cartilage tissue in the periarticular cancellous bone, and the biomimetic design solution constituting an innovative, entirely non-cemented, method of fixation in the periarticular bone of components of resurfacing joint endoprostheses (e.g. hip joint, knee joint) using the MSC-Scaffold.

The femur bone of the swine of the Polish Large White breed, harvested from a 9-month-old male weighing 87 kg, was used to build a three-dimensional CAD

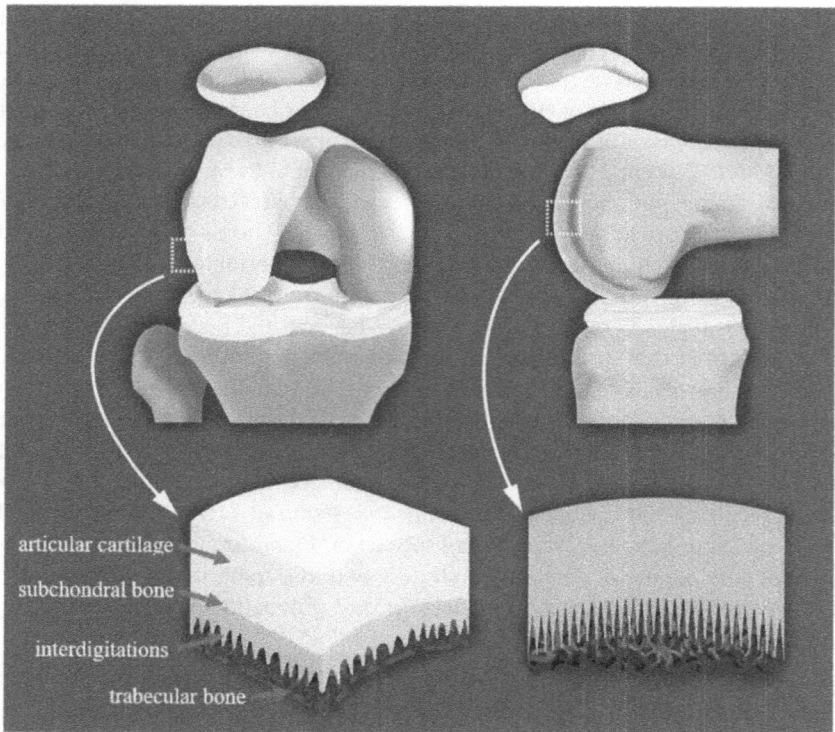

FIGURE 3.41 A diagram showing the hyaline cartilage, subchondral bone with interdigitations anchoring the cartilage in the periarticular cancellous bone, and the biomimetic method of fixation of the components of resurfacing joint endoprostheses with the use of the MSC-Scaffold.

model of a working prototype of partial resurfacing knee arthroplasty endoprosthesis with the MSC-Scaffold. Bone was obtained from a local slaughterhouse, then soft tissues were mechanically cleaned and preserved in a 6% formalin solution (formaldehyde in phosphate buffer) for one week.

Bone scanning was performed using an Atos Core high-precision 3D industrial scanner (GOM GmbH, Germany). Before scanning, the device was calibrated, the bone surface was degreased, dirt was removed, and the reference points were marked on its surface with markers (Figure 3.42).

To reflect the geometry of the entire bone, 15 measurements were taken at different locations. Individual exposures were automatically adjusted to each other using the scanner software. Finally, a point cloud saved in STL format was obtained. The processing of the scans consisting of the removal of noise caused by the scanning of environmental components, e.g. the table, filling in the defects in the scanned surfaces, and removal of artefacts was carried out in the GOM Inspect Professional software (GOM GmbH, Germany). In Figure 3.43 surface defects are visible in the so-called raw model. Missing fragments of the surface and other defects were repaired and checked using the so-called leak-tightness inspection.

The 3D digital model of bone was reconstructed with special emphasis on the precision of the dimensions within the surface of the lateral femoral condyle (Figure 3.44). The surface of the articular condyle, reconstructed as a cloud of points, was processed to remove noise and numerical errors. The isolated 3D model of the lateral femoral condyle is presented in Figure 3.45.

Subsequently, the lateral surface of the femoral condyle was extracted and imported into SolidWorks Premium 2013 x64 software in the form of an STL point cloud using the ScanTo3D plugin. Subsequently, the shell was constructed as the basis for the further design of a working prototype of partial resurfacing knee arthroplasty endoprosthesis with the MSC-Scaffold. During the import, the following corrections were made: the surfaces were smoothed by eliminating local pits, the edges were smoothed to obtain a more complete outline, and the number of components

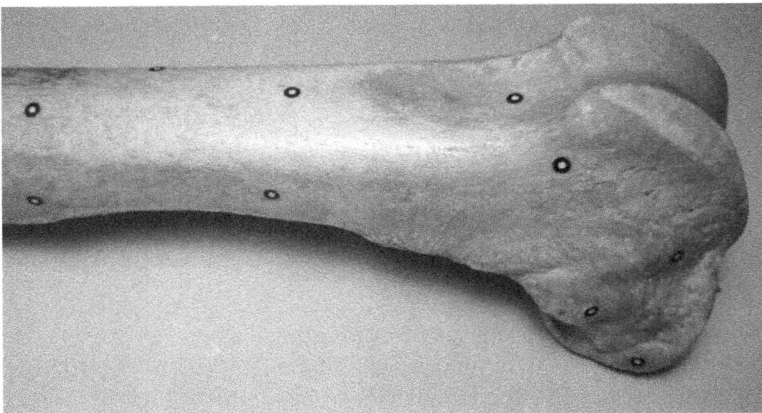

FIGURE 3.42 Swine femur prepared for optical scanning.

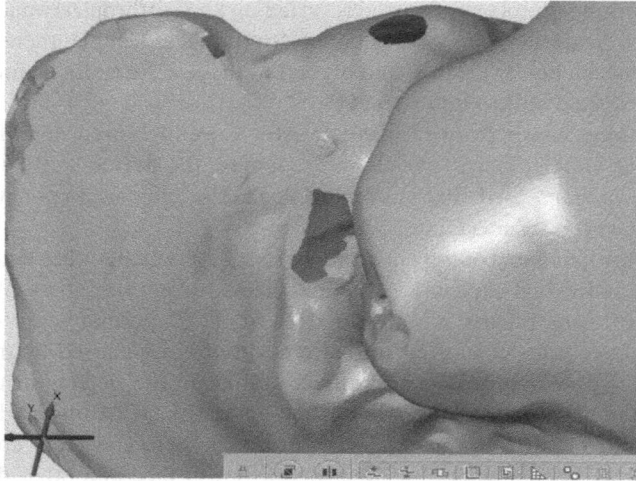

FIGURE 3.43   Screenshot with visible defects on the scan surface.

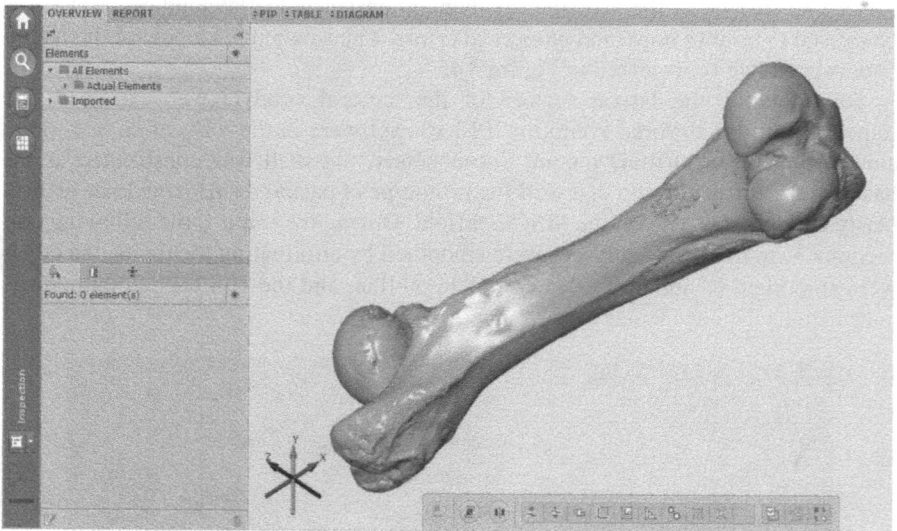

FIGURE 3.44   View of a screenshot of GOM Inspekt Professional software showing a three-dimensional digital model of a swine femur.

representing the surfaces was reduced by a uniform reduction, i.e. while maintaining a constant number of points on the surface. Figure 3.46 shows the triangle mesh representation of the swine lateral condyle surface imported into the SolidWorks Premium 2013 x64 software. In the next step, under the previous assumptions, the continuous surface was thickened by 2 mm in the direction normal to its surface inward (Figure 3.47), whereupon a cylindrical surface was generated to form a base on the inside for CAD modelling the MSC-Scaffold spikes.

CAD modelling of the MSC-Scaffold spikes commenced with determining the geometric centre on the cylindrical surface and modelling the first spike at this point. The geometric centre was determined at the intersection of the diagonals of the quadrilateral formed in the xy plane by joining the parallel projection of the extreme points of the endoprosthesis contour onto this plane, the xy plane being tangent to the cylindrical

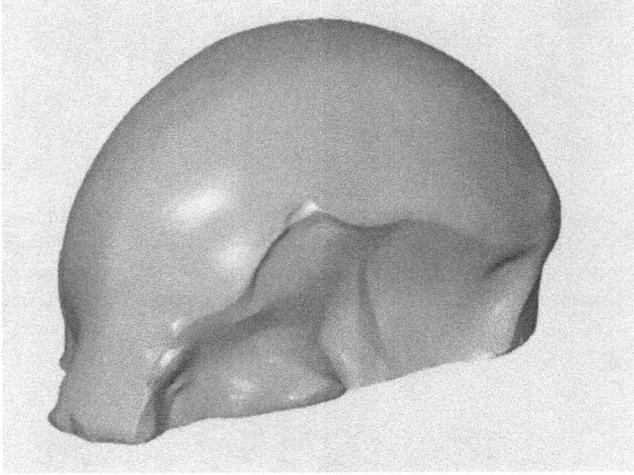

FIGURE 3.45 A fragment representing the lateral condyle extracted from a 3D digital model of a swine femur.

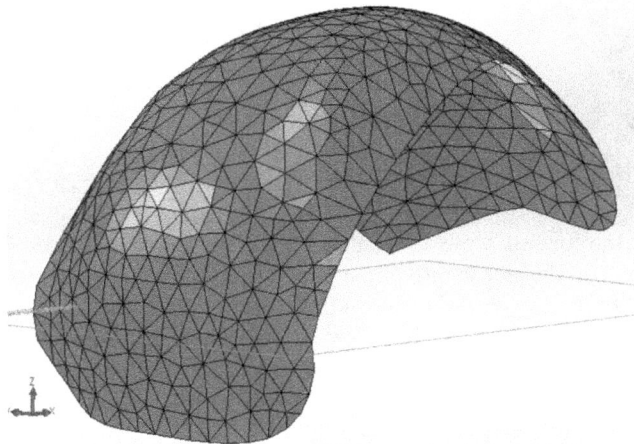

FIGURE 3.46 Representation of the triangle mesh of the lateral femoral condyle surface imported into SolidWorks Premium 2013 x64 software.

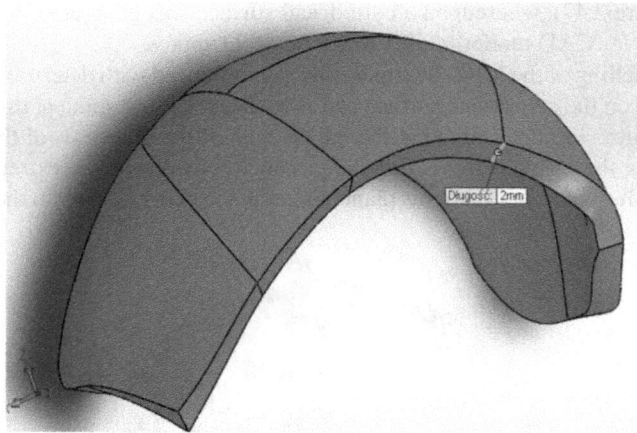

FIGURE 3.47   View of the base cap of the femoral component of the knee endoprosthesis after being added to the modelled surface of the lateral femoral condyle with a thickness of 2 mm normal to this surface. The thickness, measured for illustrative purposes with the use of a SolidWorks measurement tool, has been presented as the length of the indicated segment.

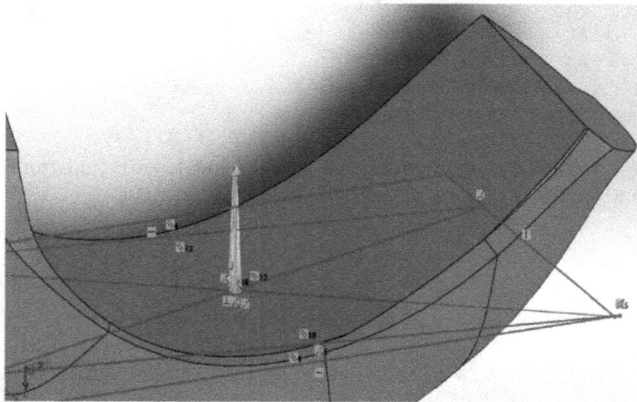

FIGURE 3.48   Modelling the first MSC-Scaffold spike.

surface inside the contour at the designated point of the geometric centre (Figure 3.48). In the CAD model, the side length of the base of the square-shaped spikes is 0.5 mm, and the centre of the base is positioned at the point in the previous step.

The spikes were designed in the shape of a truncated pyramid with the base of a square with a side length of 0.5 mm and the length of the side of the square at the top of the spike of 0.25 mm. The overall height of the spike in the CAD model was 4.5 mm. In the next step, the spikes were duplicated using the pattern creation tools – curve pattern and linear pattern. The distance between the base of the spikes was 350 μm in both directions. Figure 3.49 shows the stage of creating a curve pattern. The CAD model of the working prototype of partial resurfacing knee arthroplasty endoprosthesis with the MSC-Scaffold is presented in Figure 3.50. By scaling the original CAD model by ±10%, a series of prototype sizes of this working prototype was generated.

For further processing of the endoprosthesis component produced using SLM technology (grinding, polishing), a technological holder was designed to allow for the fixation of the component during processing. The CAD model also provides a 0.5 mm allowance for finishing, which includes the allowances for individual component treatments: removal of the support – 0.2 mm, grinding – 0.2 mm, and polishing – 0.1 mm.

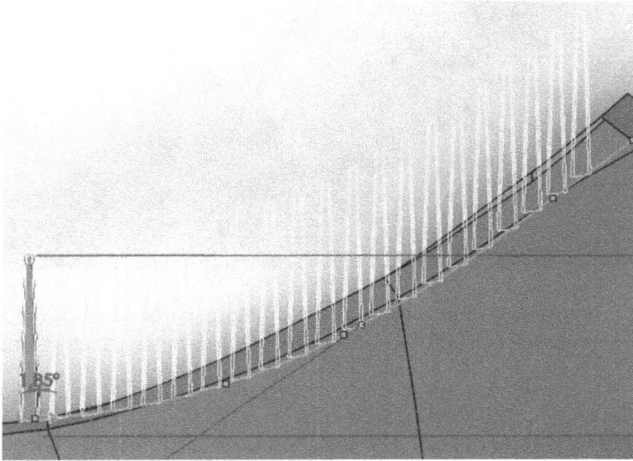

FIGURE 3.49   Spikes duplicated with the curve pattern tool.

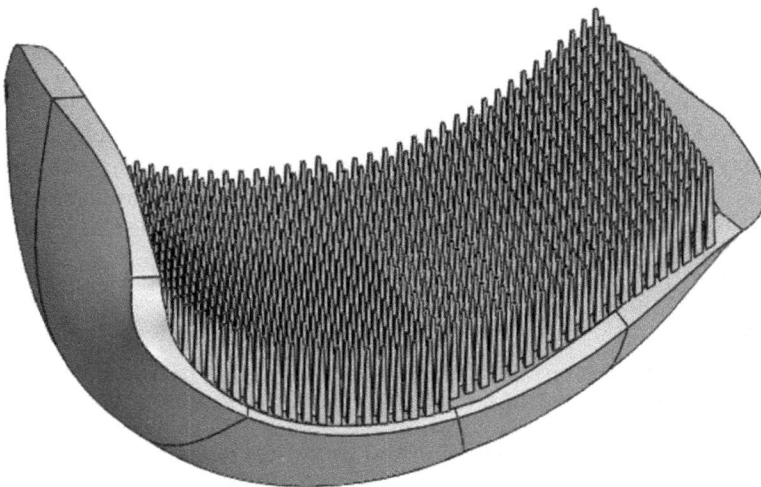

FIGURE 3.50   CAD model of a working prototype of partial resurfacing knee arthroplasty endoprosthesis with the MSC-Scaffold.

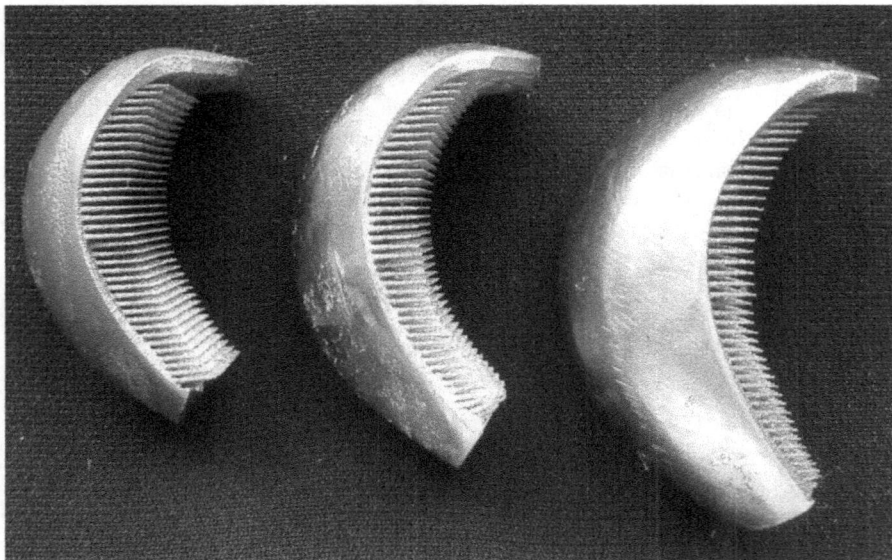

FIGURE 3.51 A range of sizes designed (CAD) and manufactured in the SLM technology of working prototype of partial resurfacing knee arthroplasty endoprostheses with the MSC-Scaffold.

The working prototype of partial resurfacing knee arthroplasty endoprosthesis with the MSC-Scaffold was produced using SLM technology on the ReaLizer SLM 250 machine (MTT Technologies Group, Germany) of Ti-6Al-4V powder. Their manufacturing was subcontracted to the Center for New Materials and Technologies of the West Pomeranian University of Technology in Szczecin. The following SLM process parameters were used: laser power – 100 W, fused layer thickness – 30 μm, laser spot size – 0.2 mm, scanning speed – 0.4 m/s, and energy density – 70 J/mm³. Post-production processing was carried out according to the developed methodology presented in Section 3.5.

Figure 3.51 presents the size series of the designed and SLM-manufactured working prototype of partial resurfacing knee arthroplasty endoprosthesis with the MSC-Scaffold. The articular surfaces of the manufactured prototype knee endoprosthesis were ground and polished, after which the technological handles were cut off by wire-cut EDM.

REFERENCES

1. Rogala, P. Endoprosthesis. EU Patent No. EP072418 B1, 22 December 1999.
2. Rogala, P. Acetabulum Endoprosthesis and Head. U.S. Patent US5,911,759 A, 15 June 1999.
3. Rogala, P. Method and Endoprosthesis to Apply This Implantation. Canadian Patent No. 2,200,064, 1 April 2002.
4. Mielniczuk, J.; Rogala, P.; Uklejewski, R.; Winiecki, M.; Jokś, G.; Auguściński, A.; Berdychowski, M. Modelling of the needle-palisade fixation system for the total hip resurfacing arthroplasty endoprosthesis. *Trans VŠB-TU Ostrava*, Metallurgical Series. 2008; 51(1): 160–6.

5. Long, M.; Rack, H.J. Titanium alloys in total joint replacement—a materials science perspective. *Biomaterials.* 1998; 19(18): 1621–39. doi:10.1016/s0142-9612(97)00146-4

6. Gibson, I. (Ed.): *Advanced Manufacturing Technology for Medical Applications.* Wiley, London, 2005.

7. Murr, L.E.; Quinones, S.A.; Gaytan, S.M.; Lopez, M.I.; Rodela, A.; Martinez, E.Y.; Hernandez, D.H.; Martinez, E.; Medina, F.; Wicker, R.B. Microstructure and mechanical behavior of Ti-6Al-4V produced by rapid-layer manufacturing, for biomedical applications. *J Mech Behav Biomed Mater.* 2009; 2(1): 20–32. doi:10.1016/j.jmbbm.2008.05.004

8. Santos, E.C.; Shiomi, M.; Osakada, K.; Laoui, T. Rapid prototyping of metal components by laser forming. *Int J Mach Tools Manuf.* 2006; 46(12–13): 1459–68. doi:10.1016/j.ijmachtools.2005.09.005

9. Kruth, J.-P.; Mercelis, P.; Van Vaerenbergh, J.; Froyen, L.; Rombouts, M. Binding mechanisms in selective laser sintering and selective laser melting. *Rapid Prototyping J.* 2005; 11(1): 26–36. doi:10.1108/13552540510573365

10. Vandenbroucke, B.; Kruth, J.-P. Selective laser melting of biocompatible metals for rapid manufacturing of medical parts. *Rapid Prototyping J.* 2007; 13(4): 196–203. doi:10.1108/13552540710776142

11. Murr, L.E.; Esquivel, E.V.; Quinones, S.A.; Gaytan, S.M.; Lopez, M.I.; Martinez, E.Y.; Medina, F.; Hernandez, D.H.; Martinez, E.; Martinez, J.L.; Stafford, S.W.; Brown, D.K.; Hoppe, T.; Meyers, W.; Lindhe, U.; Wicker, R.B. Microstructures and mechanical properties of electron beam rapid manufactured Ti-6Al-4V biomedical prototypes compared to wrought Ti-6Al-4V. *Mater Charact.* 2009; 60(2): 96–105. doi:10.1016/j.matchar.2008.07.006

12. Leordean, D.; Dudescu, C.; Marcu, T.; Berce, P.; Balc, N. Customized implants with specific properties, made by selective laser melting. *Rapid Prototyping J.* 2015; 21(1): 98–104. doi:10.1108/RPJ-11-2012-0107

13. Gong, H.; Rafi, K.; Gu, H.; Ram, G.; Starr, T.; Stucker, B. Influence of defects on mechanical properties of Ti-6Al-4V components produced by selective laser melting and electron beam melting. *Mater Des.* 2015; 86: 545–54. doi:10.1016/j.matdes.2015.07.147

14. Xu, W.; Brandt, M.; Sun, S.; Elambasseril, J.; Liu, Q.; Latham, K.; Xia, K.; Qian, M. Additive manufacturing of strong and ductile Ti-6Al-4V by selective laser melting via in situ martensite decomposition. *Acta Mater.* 2015; 85: 74–84. doi:10.1016/j.actamat.2014.11.028

15. Campanelli, S.L.; Contuzzi, N.; Ludovico, A.D.; Caiazzo, F.; Cardaropoli, F.; Sergi, V. Manufacturing and characterization of Ti6Al4V lattice components manufactured by selective laser melting. *Materials.* 2014; 7(6): 4803–22. doi:10.3390/ma7064803

16. Hrabe, N.W.; Heinl, P.; Flinn, B.; Körner, C.; Bordia, R.K. Compression-compression fatigue of selective electron beam melted cellular titanium (Ti-6Al-4V). *J Biomed Mater Res B Appl Biomater.* 2011; 99(2): 313–20. doi:10.1002/jbm.b.31901

17. Liu, F.; Ruey-Tsung, L.; Lin, W.; Liao, Y. Selective laser sintering of bio-metal scaffold. *Procedia CIRP.* 2013; 5: 83–7. doi:10.1016/j.procir.2013.01.017

18. Song, B.; Zhao, X.; Li, S.; Han, C.; Wei, Q.; Wen, S.; Liu, J.; Shi, Y. Differences in microstructure and properties between selective laser melting and traditional manufacturing for fabrication of metal parts: a review. *Front Mech Eng.* 2015; 10: 111–25 doi:10.1007/s11465-015-0341-2

19. Quan, Y.; Drescher, D.; Zhang, F.; Burkel, E.; Seitz, H. Cellular Ti6Al4V with carbon nanotube-like structures fabricated by selective electron beam melting. *Rapid Prototyping J.* 2014; 20(6): 541–50. doi:10.1108/RPJ-05-2013-0050

20. Van Bael, S.; Chai, Y.C.; Truscello, S.; Moesen, M.; Kerckhofs, G.; Van Oosterwyck, H.; Kruth, J.-P.; Schrooten, J. The effect of pore geometry on the in vitro biological behavior of human periosteum-derived cells seeded on selective laser-melted Ti6Al4V bone scaffolds. *Acta Biomater.* 2012; 8(7): 2824–34. doi:10.1016/j.actbio.2012.04.001

21. Hollander, D.A.; Wirtz, T.; Walter, M. von; Linker, R.; Schultheis, A.; Paar, O. Development of individual three-dimensional bone substitutes using "Selective Laser Melting". *Eur J Trauma.* 2003; 29: 228–34. doi:10.1007/s00068-003-1332-2

22. Hieu, L.C.; Bohez, E.; Vander Sloten, J.; Phien, H.N.; Vatcharaporn, E.; Binh, P.H.; An, P.V.; Oris, P. Design for medical rapid prototyping of cranioplasty implants. Rapid Prototyping J. 2003; 9(3): 175–86. doi:10.1108/13552540310477481

23. Hieu, L.C.; Zlatov, N.; Vander Sloten, J.; Bohez, E.; Khanh, L.; Binh, P.H.; Oris, P.; Toshev, Y. Medical rapid prototyping applications and methods. *Assem Autom.* 2005; 25(4): 284–92. doi:10.1108/01445150510626415

24. Gibson, I.; Cheung, L.K.; Chow, S.P.; Cheung, W.L.; Beh, S.L.; Savalani, M.; Lee, S.H. The use of rapid prototyping to assist medical applications. *Rapid Prototyping J.* 2006; 12(1): 53–8. doi:10.1108/13552540610637273

25. Singare, S.; Yaxiong, L.; Dichen, L.; Bingheng, L.; Sanhu, H.; Gang, L. Fabrication of customised maxillo-facial prosthesis using computer-aided design and rapid prototyping techniques. *Rapid Prototyping J.* 2006; 12(4): 206–13. doi:10.1108/13552540610682714

26. Hoeges, S.; Lindner, M.; Fischer, H.; Meiners, W.; Wissenbach, K. Manufacturing of bone substitute implants using selective laser melting, in: Vander Sloten, J.; Verdonck, P.; Nyssen, M.; Haueisen, J. (Eds.): *4th European Conference of the International Federation for Medical and Biological Engineering. IFMBE Proceedings*, vol. 22. Springer, Berlin, Heidelberg, 2009, 2230–4. doi:10.1007/978-3-540-89208-3_534

27. Sercombe, T.; Jones, N.; Day, R.; Kop, A. Heat treatment of Ti-6Al-7Nb components produced by selective laser melting. *Rapid Prototyping J.* 2008; 14(5): 300–4. doi:10.1108/13552540810907974

28. Facchini, L.; Magalini, E.; Robotti, P.; Molinari, A. Microstructure and mechanical properties of Ti-6Al-4V produced by electron beam melting of pre-alloyed powders. *Rapid Prototyping J.* 2009; 15(3): 171–8. doi:10.1108/13552540910960262

29. Ahmadi, S.M.; Yavari, S.A.; Wauthle, R.; Pouran, B.; Schrooten, J.; Weinans, H.; Zadpoor, A.A. Additively manufactured open-cell porous biomaterials made from six different space-filling unit cells: the mechanical and morphological properties. *Materials.* 2015; 8(4): 1871–96. doi:10.3390/ma8041871

30. Attar, H.; Calin, M.; Zhang, L.C.; Scudino, S.; Eckert, J. Manufacture by selective laser melting and mechanical behavior of commercially pure titanium. *Mater Sci Eng A.* 2014; 593: 170–7. doi:10.1016/j.msea.2013.11.038

31. Heinl, P.; Körner, C.; Singer, R. Selective electron beam melting of cellular titanium: mechanical properties. *Adv Eng Mater.* 2008; 10: 882–8. doi:10.1002/adem.200800137

32. Heinl, P.; Müller, L.; Körner, C.; Singer, R.F.; Müller, F.A. Cellular Ti-6Al-4V structures with interconnected macro porosity for bone implants fabricated by selective electron beam melting. *Acta Biomater.* 2008; 4(5): 1536–44. doi:10.1016/j.actbio.2008.03.013

33. Jonitz-Heincke, A.; Wieding, J.; Schulze, C.; Hansmann, D.; Bader, R. Comparative analysis of the oxygen supply and viability of human osteoblasts in three-dimensional titanium scaffolds produced by laser-beam or electron-beam melting. *Materials.* 2013; 6(11): 5398–409. doi:10.3390/ma6115398

34. Laptev, A.; Bram, M.; Buchkremer, H.; Stöver, D. Study of production route for titanium parts combining very high porosity and complex shape. *Powder Metall.* 2004; 47(1): 85–92. doi:10.1179/003258904225015536

35. Li, X.; Wang, C.; Zhang, W.; Li, Y. Fabrication and characterization of porous Ti6Al4V parts for biomedical applications using electron beam melting process. *Mater Lett.* 2009; 63(3–4): 403–5. doi:10.1016/j.matlet.2008.10.065

36. Mullen, L.; Stamp, R.C.; Brooks, W.K.; Jones, E.; Sutcliffe, C.J. Selective laser melting: a regular unit cell approach for the manufacture of porous, titanium, bone ingrowth constructs, suitable for orthopedic applications. *J Biomed Mater Res B Appl Biomater.* 2009; 89(2): 325–34. doi:10.1002/jbm.b.31219

37. Mullen, L.; Stamp, R.C.; Fox, P.; Jones, E.; Ngo, C.; Sutcliffe, C.J. Selective laser melting: a unit cell approach for the manufacture of porous, titanium, bone ingrowth constructs, suitable for orthopedic applications. II. Randomized structures. *J Biomed Mater Res B Appl Biomater.* 2010; 92(1): 178–88. doi:10.1002/jbm.b.31504

38. Murr, L.E.; Gaytan, S.M.; Medina, F.; Lopez, H.; Martinez, E.; Machado, B.I.; Hernandez, D.H.; Martinez, L.; Lopez, M.I.; Wicker, R.B.; Bracke, J. Next-generation biomedical implants using additive manufacturing of complex, cellular and functional mesh arrays. *Philos Trans A Math Phys Eng Sci.* 2010; 368(1917): 1999–2032. doi:10.1098/rsta.2010.0010

39. Parthasarathy, J.; Starly, B.; Raman, S.; Christensen, A. Mechanical evaluation of porous titanium (Ti6Al4V) structures with electron beam melting (EBM). *J Mech Behav Biomed Mater.* 2010; 3(3): 249–59. doi:10.1016/j.jmbbm.2009.10.006

40. Ponader, S.; von Wilmowsky, C.; Widenmayer, M.; Lutz, R.; Heinl, P.; Körner, C.; Singer, R.F.; Nkenke, E.; Neukam, F.W.; Schlegel, K.A. In vivo performance of selective electron beam-melted Ti-6Al-4V structures. *J Biomed Mater Res A.* 2010; 92(1): 56–62. doi:10.1002/jbm.a.32337

41. Campoli, G.; Borleffs, M.S.; Amin Yavari, S.; Wauthle, R.; Weinans, H.; Zadpoor, A.A. Mechanical properties of open-cell metallic biomaterials manufactured using additive manufacturing. *Mater Des.* 2013; 49: 957–65. doi:10.1016/j.matdes.2013.01.071

42. Imwinkelried, T. Mechanical properties of open-pore titanium foam. *J Biomed Mater Res A.* 2007; 81(4): 964–70. doi:10.1002/jbm.a.31118

43. Yavari, S.A.; Wauthlé, R.; Stok, J.V.; Riemslag, A.; Janssen, M.; Mulier, M.; Kruth, J.-P.; Schrooten, J.; Weinans, H.; Zadpoor, A.A. Fatigue behavior of porous biomaterials manufactured using selective laser melting. *Mater Sci Eng C.* 2013; 33(8): 4849–58. doi:10.1016/j.msec.2013.08.006

44. Uklejewski, R.; Winiecki, M.; Rogala, P. Technological issues of additive manufacturing of preprototypes of the multispiked connecting scaffold for non-cemented resurfacing arthroplasty endoprostheses. *Eng Biomater.* 2014; 17(128–9): 81–2.

45. Vilaro, T.; Abed, S.; Knapp, W. Direct manufacturing of technical parts using selective laser melting: example of automotive application, in: *Proc. of 12th European Forum on Rapid Prototyping*, 2008, France.

46. Uklejewski, R.; Rogala, P.; Winiecki, M.; Kędzia, A.; Ruszkowski, P. Preliminary results of implantation in animal model and osteoblast culture evaluation of prototypes of biomimetic multispiked connecting scaffold for noncemented stemless resurfacing hip arthroplasty endoprostheses. *Biomed Res Int.* 2013; 2013: 689089. doi:10.1155/2013/689089

47. Srinivasan, P.; Miller, M.A.; Verdonschot, N.; Mann, K.A.; Janssen, D. A modelling approach demonstrating micromechanical changes in the tibial cemented interface due to in vivo service. *J Biomech.* 2017; 56: 19–25. doi:10.1016/j.jbiomech.2017.02.017

48. Ritter, M.A.; Herbst, S.A.; Keating, E.M.; Faris, P.M. Radiolucency at the bone-cement interface in total knee replacement. The effects of bone-surface preparation and cement technique. *J Bone Joint Surg Am.* 1994; 76(1): 60–5. doi:10.2106/00004623-199401000-00008

49. Gulati, A.; Chau, R.; Pandit, H.G.; Gray, H.; Price, A.J.; Dodd, C.A.; Murray, D.W. The incidence of physiological radiolucency following Oxford unicompartmental knee replacement and its relationship to outcome. *J Bone Joint Surg Br.* 2009; 91(7): 896–902. doi:10.1302/0301-620X.91B7.21914

50. Pandit, H.; Liddle, A.D.; Kendrick, B.J.; Jenkins, C.; Price, A.J.; Gill, H.S.; Dodd, C.A.; Murray, D.W. Improved fixation in cementless unicompartmental knee replacement: five-year results of a randomized controlled trial. *J Bone Joint Surg Am.* 2013; 95(15): 1365–72. doi:10.2106/JBJS.L.01005

4 Structural and osteoconductive functionalization of the interspike space of the prototype multi-spiked connecting scaffold

4.1 ASSESSMENT OF THE PRO-OSTEOCONDUCTIVE POTENTIAL – THEORETICAL BASIS

Evaluation of the structural-osteoconductive functionality of the porous implant coatings and intraosseous scaffolds is conditioned by the formation of the microgeometric features of their pores [1–3]. These functional features of the microstructure of the porous coatings of implants and intraosseous scaffolds implanted in the periarticular bone without the use of cement are referred to as the so-called pro-osteoconductive potential and are conditioned by the microstructure. It is determined by the microstructural conditions of the interconnected pores, allowing for the effective growth of new bone tissue into the pore space, enabling the reconstruction or formation of basic units of the bone tissue biostructure, such as osteons or bone trabeculae, in cortical and cancellous bone tissue, respectively. Effective filling of the pores with the ingrown bone tissue and its mineralization induces the formation of functional bone-implant fixation, capable of permanently fulfilling the intended reconstructive and biomechanical function (i.e. load transfer) of the components of the artificial joint. In other words, the pro-osteoconductive potential of the implant pore microstructure is the potential for the effective promotion of bone tissue ingrowth and subsequent biointegration with the implant, ensuring the formation of a bone-implant fixation characterized by the long-term biomechanical stability and the ability to transfer loads of the artificial joint components to the bone.

In the case of porous-coated long-stem joint endoprostheses, the pro-osteoconductive functionality of their outer layer can be characterized by a set of parameters proposed for such an evaluation describing the microgeometry of porous coatings of orthopaedic implants in terms of their accessibility for bone tissue ingrowth [2,4,5] and by using the methodology for determining these parameters in research microtopography by surface profilometry [2,5].

DOI: 10.1201/9781003364498-4

To determine the pro-osteoconductive potential of the prototype MSC-Scaffold for the non-cemented fixation of components of resurfacing arthroplasty endoprostheses, an analogous structural analysis of its interspike space should be performed in terms of evaluating the structural-pro-osteoconductive functionality that ensures the expected osseointegration with periarticular trabecular bone tissue. To this end, the interspike space of the prototype MSC-Scaffold should have the proper conditions for penetration through the ingrown bone tissue, allowing the formation of vascularized and mineralized bone tissue.

The set of poroaccessibility parameters proposed for the evaluation of the structural and osteoconductive functionality of the outer layer of porous coatings [2,4] allows for the evaluation of the requirements regarding the ability to accept the ingrown bone tissue into the pores of such a coating (the so-called accessibility). These parameters describe the spatial, volumetric, and functional properties of porous coatings, which can be interpreted in terms of the properties mentioned above [2,4]. Table 4.1 presents a set of stereometric parameters for characterization of the poroaccessibility of the outer layers of porous coatings along with a proposal of equivalent parameters recommended for the analogous evaluation of the structural and osteoconductive properties of the MSC-Scaffold. Analogous to the concept of porosity, the structural accessibility of the prototype MSC-Scaffold for bone ingrowth is characterized by its pro-osteoconductive functionality, conditioned by the geometric features of its interspike space.

The effective height H_{ef} of the spikes of the MSC-Scaffold is the height of the spike protruding above the spherical base cap of the component (femoral or acetabular) on

---

TABLE 4.1

The set of stereometric parameters for characterization of the poroaccessibility of intraosseous implant porous coating outer layers and the equivalent parameters proposed for determination of the interspike structural and pro-osteoconductive potential in the MSC-Scaffold prototype

Poroaccessibility of the Intraosseous Implant Porous Coating Outer Layer Can Be Evaluated by the Following Parameter Set	The MSC-Scaffold Prototype Structural Accessibility for Ingrowing Bone Tissue Can Be Assessed by the Proposed Parameters Set
The effective pore depth p_{def}	The effective height H_{ef}
The representative pore size p_{Srep}	The representative interspike distance $D_{is\text{-}rep}$
The effective volumetric porosity ϕ_{Vef}	The relative volume fraction of the interspike space $\phi_{Vis\text{-}ef} = f(H_{ef}, D_{is\text{-}rep})$
The representative surface porosity ϕ_{Srep}	The relative surface fraction of the interspike compartment cross section $\phi_{Sis\text{-}rep} = f(D_{is\text{-}rep})$
The index of the porous coating outer layer space capacity V_{PM}	The index of the capacity of the interspike space $V_{is} = f(H_{ef}, D_{is\text{-}rep})$ (mm³/cm²)
The representative angle of the poroaccessibility Ω_{rep}	The representative angle of the interspike space osteoaccessibility $\Omega_{rep\text{-}is}$
The bone-implant interface adhesive surface enlargement index ψ	The bone-implant contact area increase index ψ_{is}

which it is located. It should be measured as the length of the segment coinciding with the spike axis, from its apex to the point intersecting the inner or outer arc that represents the meridian of the spherical base cap of the femoral component and the acetabular component of the resurfacing arthroplasty hip endoprosthesis, respectively.

The representative distance between the spikes $D_{is\text{-}rep}$ is the arithmetic mean of the distance between the spikes of the MSC-Scaffold measured at the predetermined height levels. In the case of the components of a hip joint resurfacing endoprosthesis, the spikes are arranged in a concentric pattern on circles representing the parallels of the spherical base cap at a fixed distance, both circumferentially and radially.

The relative area share of the interspike space in the cross section $\phi_{Sis\text{-}rep}$ is dependent upon the representative distance between the spikes of the MSC-Scaffold $D_{is\text{-}rep}$:

$$\phi_{Sis-rep} = f(D_{is-rep}) \tag{4.1}$$

and can be estimated as the ratio of the area of the interspike space in a given cross section to the total area over which the spikes are arranged. This parameter should be estimated as the arithmetic mean of the individual area fractions measured at the determined levels of the spike heights.

The three-dimensional parameters characterizing the volume features of the interspike space geometry of the MSC-Scaffold, both absolute and related to the unit area, can generally be estimated as the product of the base area of the spike and its height. Since the MSC-Scaffold spikes are designed as a parametrically ordered arrangement, the volume of the interspike space available for ingrowth of the cancellous bone tissue can be roughly estimated from the constant assumed value of the distance between the spike bases, projecting a representative distance between the spikes $D_{is\text{-}rep}$ and the measured effective height H_{ef} value of the spikes. Therefore, the relative volume fraction of the interspike space $\phi_{Vis\text{-}ef}$ in the MSC-Scaffold can be estimated as the ratio of the volume of the interspike space of the scaffold fragment subject to testing to the total volume of that scaffold, while the index of the interspike space capacity V_{is} determines the potential volume of the interspike space of the MSC-Scaffold available for the ingrowth of cancellous bone tissue related to the unit area of the fragment of the scaffold subject to testing. It can be defined by the following function:

$$V_{is} = f\left(H_{ef}, D_{is-rep}\right) \left[\text{mm}^3/\text{cm}^2\right]. \tag{4.2}$$

The representative angle of the osteoaccessibility of the interspike space $\Omega_{rep\text{-}is}$ is the angle of inclination of the sidewalls of the spike surfaces, which is equal to half of the vertical angle of a single spike Ω_i. It can be estimated using the following formula:

$$\Omega_{rep-is} = 90° - \Omega_i / 2. \tag{4.3}$$

In the case of a prototype MSC-Scaffold designed for both components of a hip joint resurfacing endoprosthesis, the value of this angle may be the same for all spikes or spikes designed for specific areas occupied by these spikes. Due to the high value of the H_n/R ratio of individual spikes of the MSC-Scaffold, the values of their vertical angles are relatively small; therefore, the influence of a representative angle of the osteoaccessibility of the interspike space $\Omega_{rep\text{-}is}$ has a practically negligible effect on the volume parameters determining the osteoconductive accessibility of the MSC-Scaffold.

The bone-implant contact area increase index ψ_{is} is the ratio of the lateral surface area of the spikes of the MSC-Scaffold, including the surface at the base of the spikes, to the total surface on which the spikes are located. Increasing the effective height H_{ef} of the MSC-Scaffold spikes manufactured using SLM technology significantly contributes to an increase in the value of this index. Regarding the conclusions presented in the work [5] and to the patents' assumptions for the resurfacing arthroplasty endoprosthesis [6–8], the parameter describing the increase of the implant-bone contact surface is one of the key structural parameters conditioning the promotion of bone tissue ingrowth. Its linear dependence on the effective height H_{ef} of the scaffold spikes was demonstrated in [9]; therefore, we can conclude that:

$$\psi_{is} = f(H_{ef}, \Omega_{rep-is}). \qquad (4.4)$$

Considering the above issues, as well as the mutual relation between the porosity parameters proven experimentally in [9], characterizing the pro-osteoconductive potential of the outer layers of porous coatings of intraosseous implants, it can be assumed that in the case of the MSC-Scaffold, combining the parameters proposed as equivalent to its analogous evaluation (V_{is} and H_{ef}) can be used interchangeably. Therefore, the structural osteoaccessibility of the prototype MSC-Scaffold, i.e. its pro-osteoconductive potential, will be dependent on the effective height H_{ef} of its spikes and the representative distance between the spikes $D_{is\text{-}rep}$.

Since patent specifications [6–8] regarding the method of fixation of components of resurfacing arthroplasty endoprostheses in the periarticular bone with the use of the MSC-Scaffold prototype do not assume a change in the representative distance between the spikes ($D_{is\text{-}rep}$), the analysis of the possibility of formation of the pro-osteoconductive potential of the interspike space of the prototype MSC-Scaffold manufactured using SLM technology will focus on the change of the effective height H_{ef} of the spikes of the prototype MSC-Scaffold.

4.2 FORMATION OF THE STRUCTURAL AND OSTEOCONDUCTIVE PROPERTIES OF THE MULTI-SPIKED CONNECTING SCAFFOLD

Analysing the possibility of formation of the pro-osteoconductive potential of the prototype MSC-Scaffold, the assumed increase in the interspike space volume achieved by increasing the nominal height H_n of the spikes was evaluated as for corresponding specimens manufactured using the SLM technology.

The prototype hip joint resurfacing endoprosthesis [10–12] manufactured in the SLM technology was evaluated for the structural and osteoconductive properties of the MSC-Scaffold using the confocal profilometry. The basic study has been carried out on a series of specific SLM preprototypes designed specifically for this purpose, representing fragments of the prototype MSC-Scaffold for both components (femoral and acetabular) of the resurfacing endoprosthesis of the hip joint, through a digital measurement of the effective height H_{ef} of its spikes.

To compare the prototype MSC-Scaffold with its theoretical CAD model, 3D confocal scanning and profile measurements have been performed with the Olympus Lext OLS 4000 microscope equipped with the MPLFLN·5 lenses (Olympus, Tokyo, Japan). Scanning was performed on adjacent areas of the MSC-Scaffold measuring 2,560 µm by 2,560 µm located along the radius of both components of the resurfacing endoprosthesis. Figures 4.1a and 4.1b show the components of the prototype hip joint resurfacing endoprosthesis manufactured using the SLM technology, where the measurement areas have been marked with square frames. Digital 2D and 3D representations of each scanned area have been subject to measurements with the use of software related to the confocal microscope. The profile lines have been drawn radially through the tops of the spikes, and on that basis, the effective height H_{ef} of the spikes and the radius of the base of the spikes R_x have been measured. The average values of the (H_{ef}/R_x) ratios were calculated and related to the values of the H_n/R ratios assumed in the CAD models. Figure 4.1c presents a fragment of the CAD model corresponding to the selected measurement area of the acetabular component of the resurfacing arthroplasty endoprosthesis along with the tip points of the prototype MSC-Scaffold. Since the MSC-Scaffold spikes are located on concentric parallels of the spherical base cap, Figure 4.1d presents the sequence of measurements for representative spikes lying on five consecutive parallels counted from the spherical axis of the base cap.

To create three-dimensional solids similar to the spherical sector of the base cap, the CAD models of the preprototypes representing fragments of the prototype MSC-Scaffold, the contours of the hip joint resurfacing endoprosthesis components were assigned with the feature of thickness. The prototype MSC-Scaffold spikes have been designed in a row along the arcs representing the meridians of the spherical sector of the cap. In each of the two designed series of preprototypes representing fragments of the MSC-Scaffold, changes have been introduced to improve the pro-osteoconductive functionality of the MSC-Scaffold fabricated using SLM technology by modifying the geometric design features of its spikes. In the first series, this functionality was theoretically improved in CAD models by changing the nominal height H_n of the spikes, while in the second series, the nominal height H_n of the spikes has not been changed, but the geometric shape of the spikes was changed by cutting the top of the pyramid and variation of the vertical angle of the spikes.

The first preprototype in the series is taken as the base for the entire series and has been labelled as FCS_I for the series representing the MSC-Scaffold of the femoral component and ACS_I for the series representing the MSC-Scaffold of the acetabular component. These preprototypes have been reconstructed based on CAD models of the hip joint resurfacing endoprosthesis prototype mentioned in [10–12].

In the CAD models of the first series of nine MSC-Scaffold preprototypes representing the femoral component of the hip joint resurfacing endoprosthesis (denoted as FCS_I-FCS_IX), we have assumed that the H_n/R ratio for the spikes would increase from 8, 9, and 10 to 16, 17, and 18 for three geometric variants of spikes for

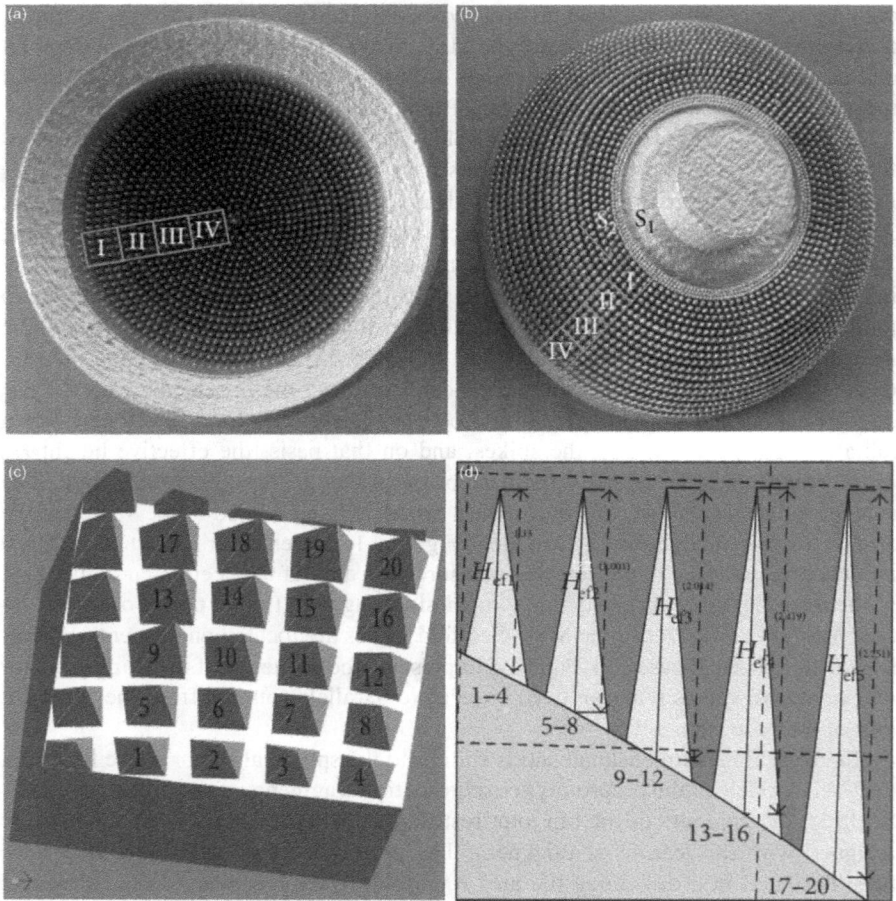

FIGURE 4.1 Femoral component (a) and acetabular component (b) of the SLM prototype of an entirely non-cemented resurfacing endoprosthesis of the hip joint – square frames represent areas of the MSC-Scaffold scanned and measured by confocal profilometry; fragment of the CAD model of the acetabular component of the resurfacing arthroplasty endoprosthesis corresponding to one of the MSC-Scaffold areas (c) and the spikes of the prototype MSC-Scaffold shown on the CAD model (d) in the view from the direction marked with an arrow and the letter S_2.

different areas of the cap. Similarly, for the preprototypes representing the acetabular component of the resurfacing endoprosthesis of the hip joint (designated as ACS_I-ACS_IX), we assumed that the H_n/R ratio for the spikes would increase from 10 to 18 for all spikes. The second series of nine MSC-Scaffold preprototype variants for both components of the resurfacing arthroplasty endoprosthesis has been designed based on the selected preprototypes from the first series: FCS_I, FCS_V, and FCS_VIII, and ACS_I, ACS_V, and ACS_VIII. In CAD models of this series, the spikes were designed in the shape of a truncated pyramid, where the side length of the square resulting from the truncation was 0.1, 0.2, and 0.3 mm, respectively, for each variant selected as the initial one.

The effect of improving the structural pro-osteoconductive functionality of the MSC-Scaffold, established in individual CAD models of the preprototypes, has been verified on the preprototypes manufactured based on these CAD models using SLM technology. At the same time, four sets of preprototypes have been produced of Ti-6Al-4V powder on a Renishaw AM250 machine (Renishaw plc, Great Britain). The process parameters used for production are: laser power – 150–200 W, layer thickness – 30 μm, laser spot size – 0.07 mm, scanning speed – 0.35–5.00 m/s, and laser energy density – 80–160 J/mm^3.

Figure 4.2a presents a collective CAD model of a set of preprototypes representing fragments of the femoral and acetabular components of the hip joint resurfacing endoprostheses with different geometric variants of the MSC-Scaffold, while the set of preprototypes produced based on this CAD model in SLM technology is presented in Figure 4.2b. The preprototypes were separated and sorted. Each copy was photographed in high resolution with a DSC-H1 digital camera (Sony, Japan). CAD models of the preprototypes from the first series are presented in Figures 4.3a and 4.4a, while the corresponding preprototypes manufactured in the SLM technology are presented in Figures 4.3b and 4.4b. CAD models of preprototypes from the second series are presented in Figures 4.5a and 4.6a, while the corresponding preprototypes manufactured in the SLM technology are presented in Figures 4.5b and 4.6b.

The effective height H_{ef} of the spikes of the MSC-Scaffold preprototypes manufactured using SLM technology was measured using ImageJ (National Institutes of Health, Bethesda, MD, USA). Before measurement, the software was calibrated using a scale photographed with the preprototypes. In CAD models, the effective height H_{ef} of the spikes was measured using a measurement tool available in Autodesk Inventor Professional 9.0.

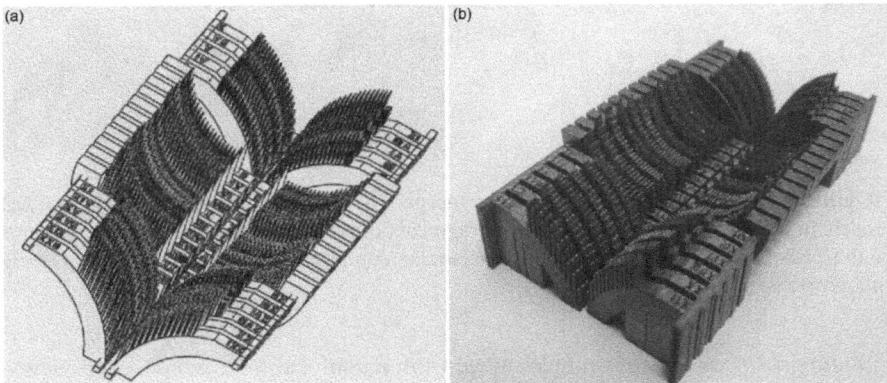

FIGURE 4.2 A collective CAD model (a) and a set of preprototypes (b) manufactured based on these CAD models in SLM technology, representing fragments of the femoral and acetabular components of the hip joint resurfacing arthroplasty endoprosthesis with different geometric variants of the prototype MSC-Scaffold.

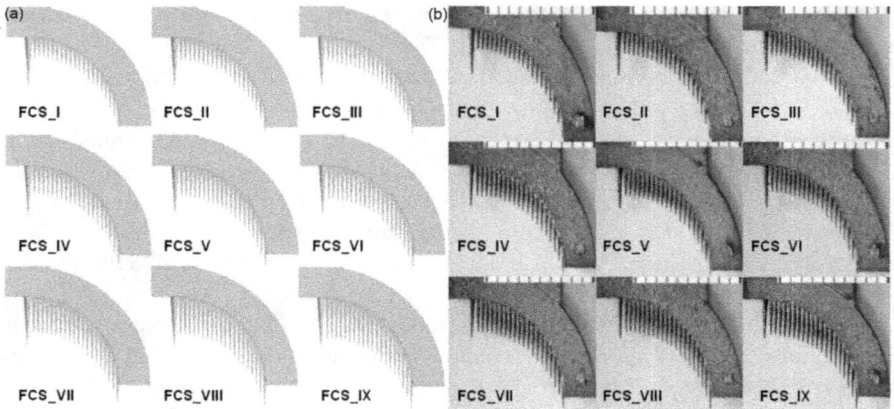

FIGURE 4.3 CAD models (a) and preprototypes (b) manufactured based on these CAD models in SLM technology, representing fragments of the first series of geometric variants of the prototype MSC-Scaffold of the femoral component of the hip joint resurfacing endoprosthesis.

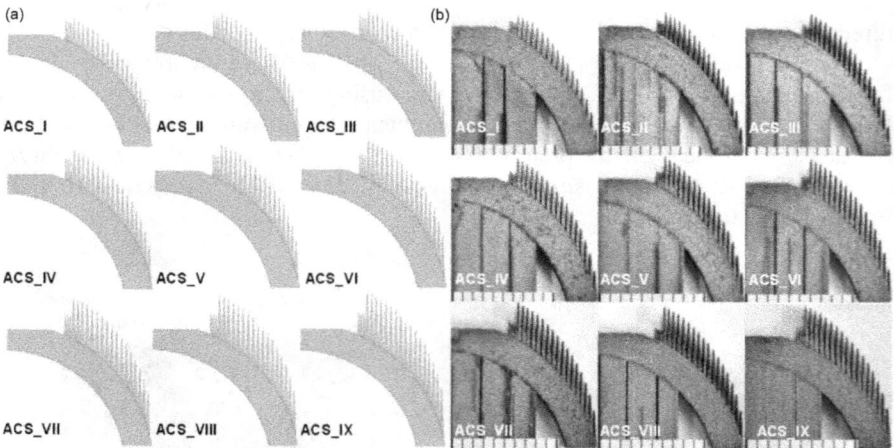

FIGURE 4.4 CAD models (a) and preprototypes (b) manufactured based on these CAD models in SLM technology, representing fragments of the first series of geometric variants of the prototype MSC-Scaffold of the acetabular component of the hip joint resurfacing endoprosthesis.

Figure 4.7 presents an example image from a confocal microscope – top view – of the tested area of the prototype MSC-Scaffold manufactured using SLM technology on the acetabular component of the prototype hip joint resurfacing arthroplasty endoprosthesis, its three-dimensional reconstruction, and a presentation of the method of measuring the effective height H_{ef} of the spikes on the profile passing through their vertices.

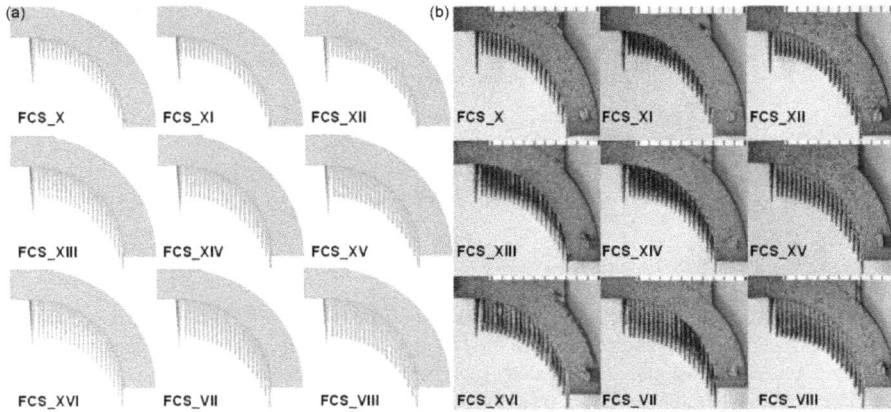

FIGURE 4.5 CAD models (a) and preprototypes (b) manufactured based on these CAD models in SLM technology represent fragments of the second series of geometric variants of the MSC-Scaffold prototype of the femoral component of the hip joint resurfacing endoprosthesis.

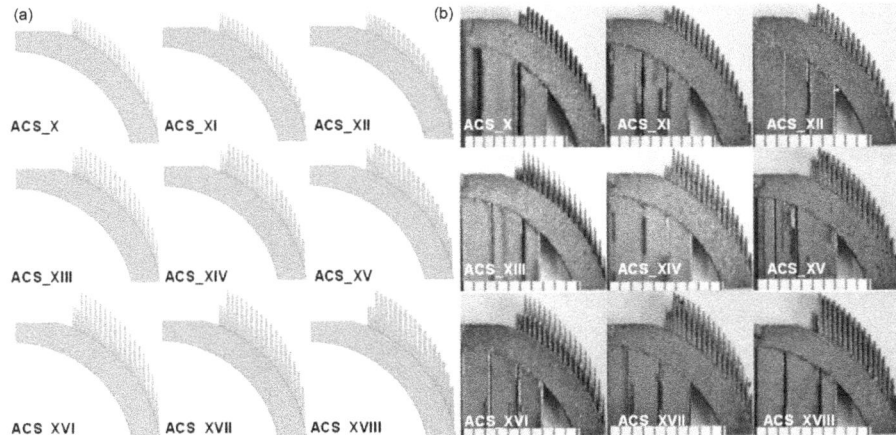

FIGURE 4.6 CAD models (a) and preprototypes (b) manufactured based on these models in SLM technology, representing fragments of the second series of geometric variants of the MSC-Scaffold prototype of the acetabular component of the hip joint resurfacing endoprosthesis.

The effective height H_{ef} of the spikes of the prototype MSC-Scaffold measured on the components of the hip joint resurfacing endoprosthesis prototype manufactured using SLM technology are significantly lower (by 48 ± 9% for the femoral component and by 51 ± 9% for the acetabular component) compared to the corresponding spikes measured on CAD models that were the basis for the manufacturing of these prototypes. It lowers the values of the H_{ef}/R ratio, and consequently significantly reduces the structural pro-osteoconductive functionality of the prototype MSC-Scaffold assumed in the CAD model. Despite the design of spikes with H_{ef}/R

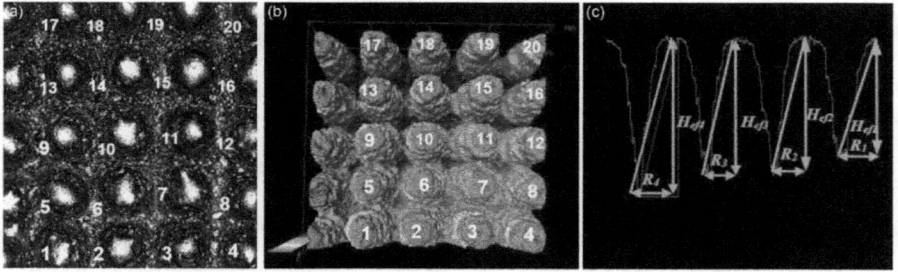

FIGURE 4.7 Confocal microscope image showing a top view of (a) an exemplary area of the MSC-Scaffold on the acetabular component of the hip joint prototype resurfacing endoprosthesis and its three-dimensional digital reconstruction (b); an example of the method of measuring the effective height H_{ef} of the spikes on a profile passing through the tops of the spikes (c).

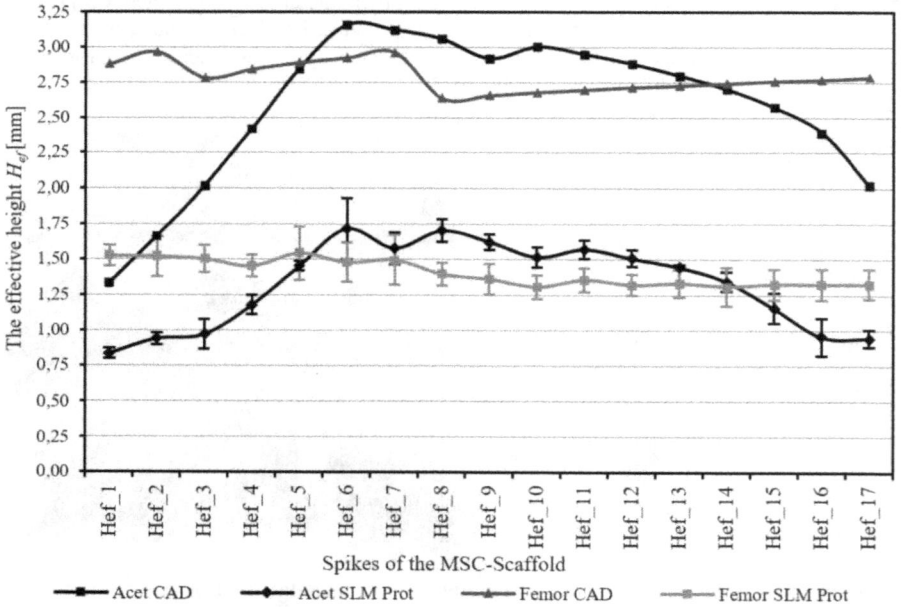

FIGURE 4.8 The effective height H_{ef} of the individual spikes of the prototype MSC-Scaffold measured on the CAD model of the prototype resurfacing endoprosthesis of the hip joint compared to the effective height H_{ef} of the spikes of the prototype MSC-Scaffold measured on both components of this hip joint resurfacing endoprosthesis manufactured in SLM technology.

ratio from 8 to 10 in CAD models, its values below 5 were obtained in prototypes manufactured in the SLM technology.

Figure 4.8 presents the results of measurements of the effective height H_{ef} of the spikes made on the CAD model and the SLM-manufactured prototype of a hip joint resurfacing endoprosthesis with the MSC-Scaffold.

Figures 4.9 and 4.10 show the results of the measurements made on the first series of geometrically modified MSC-Scaffold variants. The curves in the graphs present the measured values of the effective height H_{ef} of consecutive spikes arranged along the arc representing the meridian of the spherical base cap of the femoral component and the acetabular component of the hip joint resurfacing endoprosthesis. Successive concentric circles (parallels) indicating the location of the spikes on the surface of this canopy have been marked with numbers ranging from 1 to 20. The results were related to the nominal height H_n of the spikes adopted in the CAD model as a reference for these design variants of the spikes. In the graphs, they are marked as $H_{n(1-12)}$, $H_{n(13-17)}$, $H_{n(18-20)}$ for the femoral component and $H_{n(1-17)}$ for the acetabular component of the hip joint resurfacing endoprosthesis, respectively. The results for several measurements were averaged and presented as mean values (± standard deviation); however, for better readability of the presented curve sets, error bars have been omitted from the graph.

The effective height H_{ef} of all spikes measured on the CAD models is lower than the nominal height H_n. This difference occurs because the bases of all pyramids (spikes) are located beneath the spherical surface of the base cap. The relative differences between the effective height H_{ef} and the nominal height H_n of the spikes of the MSC-Scaffold vary depending on their position along the arc representing the meridian of the spherical cap and are significant for the spikes closest to the equator

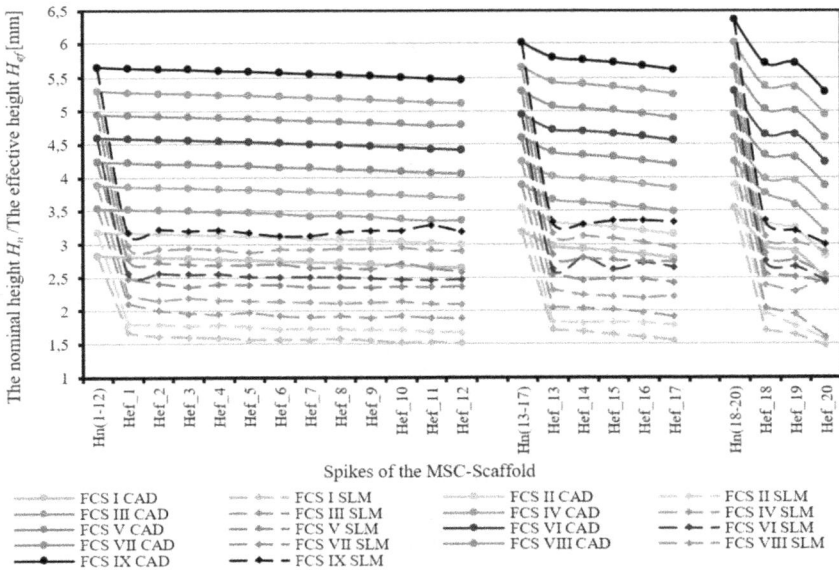

FIGURE 4.9   The effective height H_{ef} of the spikes measured on CAD models and on the preprototypes manufactured based on these CAD models in SLM technology, representing the femoral component of the hip joint resurfacing endoprosthesis in the first series of geometrically modified preprototypes, for which subsequent variants of the prototype MSC-Scaffold were marked as FCS_I-FCS_IX; the effective height H_{ef} was related to the nominal height (H_n) of the spikes adopted in the CAD model as a reference for these design variants of the spikes $H_{n(1-12)}$, $H_{n(13-17)}$, $H_{n(18-20)}$.

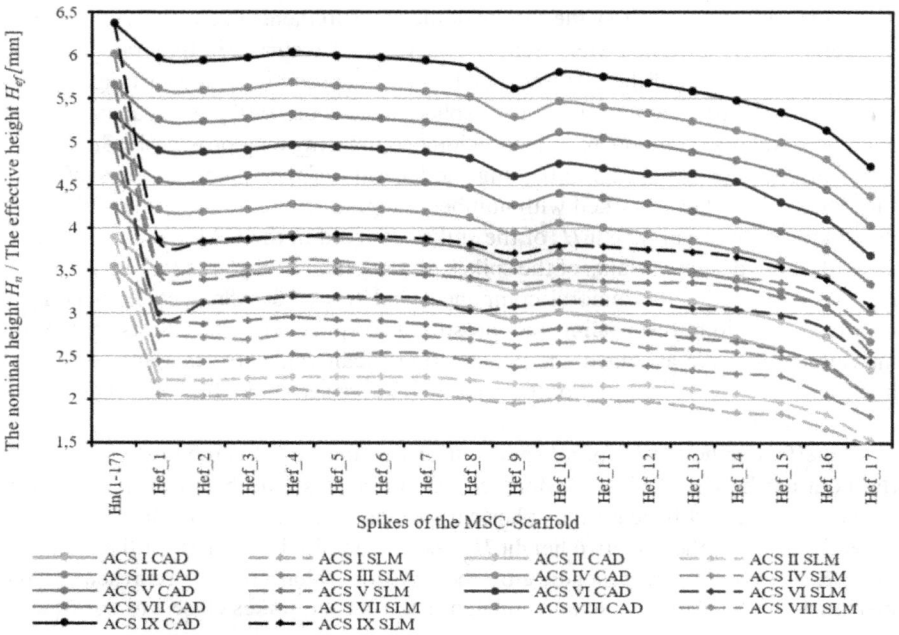

FIGURE 4.10 The effective height H_{ef} of the spikes measured in CAD models and in the preprototypes manufactured based on these CAD models in SLM technology, representing the acetabular component of the hip joint resurfacing endoprosthesis in the first series of geometrically modified preprototypes, for which subsequent variants of the MSC-Scaffold prototype were labelled ACS_I-ACS_IX; the effective height H_{ef} was related to the nominal height (H_n) of the spikes adopted in the CAD model as a reference for these design variants of the spikes $H_{n(1-17)}$.

of this cap. These differences range from 0.4 ± 0.1% to 5.0 ± 1.0% for the first 12 spikes, from 5.0 ± 1.0% to 9.0 ± 2.0% for the next five spikes, and from 12.0 ± 2.0% to 23.0 ± 5.0% for the three spikes farthest from the axis of the cap along the outer arc representing the meridian of the femoral component of the hip joint resurfacing endoprosthesis; in the case of the acetabular component, these differences range from 8 ± 2% to 33 ± 6%. It lowers the structural pro-osteoconductive functionality of the prototype MSC-Scaffold, which is particularly important in the area of its outermost spikes, designed near the equator of the spherical basal cap.

Ensuring structural homogeneity of pro-osteoconductive functionality within the entire interspike space of the MSC-Scaffold of the resurfacing endoprostheses of the hip joint requires differentiation of the effective height H_{ef} of the MSC-Scaffold spikes arranged along the arc constituting the meridian of the spherical base cap.

The difference between the values of the effective height H_{ef} of the prototype MSC-Scaffold spikes, measured in CAD models, and the values of the effective height H_{ef} of the spikes measured in the preprototypes manufactured using SLM technology is 43 ± 2% and 44 ± 1%, respectively. This confirms a significant difference between the microgeometry of the MSC-Scaffold designed in the CAD model and the preprototypes manufactured on the basis of that model using SLM technology. This result corresponds to the measurements made using the confocal profilometry method on the prototypes of both components of the hip joint resurfacing endoprosthesis.

Modification of the geometric structural features of the MSC-Scaffold prototype spikes in the first series of preprototypes assumed a gradual increase in the H_n/R ratio value of the spikes. Figures 4.11 and 4.12 show the curves of the relative increase in the effective height H_{ef} of the spikes in successive geometric variants for a series of nine preprototypes representing the fragments of the femoral component, respectively (Figure 4.11) and a fragment of the acetabular component (Figure 4.12), together with the curves presenting the total difference in the effective height H_{ef} in individual preprototypes manufactured using SLM technology related to the effective height H_{ef} of the spikes in CAD models of the prototype MSC-Scaffold adopted as the base preprototype and related to the nominal height H_n of these spikes.

The relative increase in the effective height H_{ef} estimated for the preprototypes manufactured using SLM technology oscillates around the same values as found in the CAD models of the prototype MSC-Scaffold, while the increased rate drops

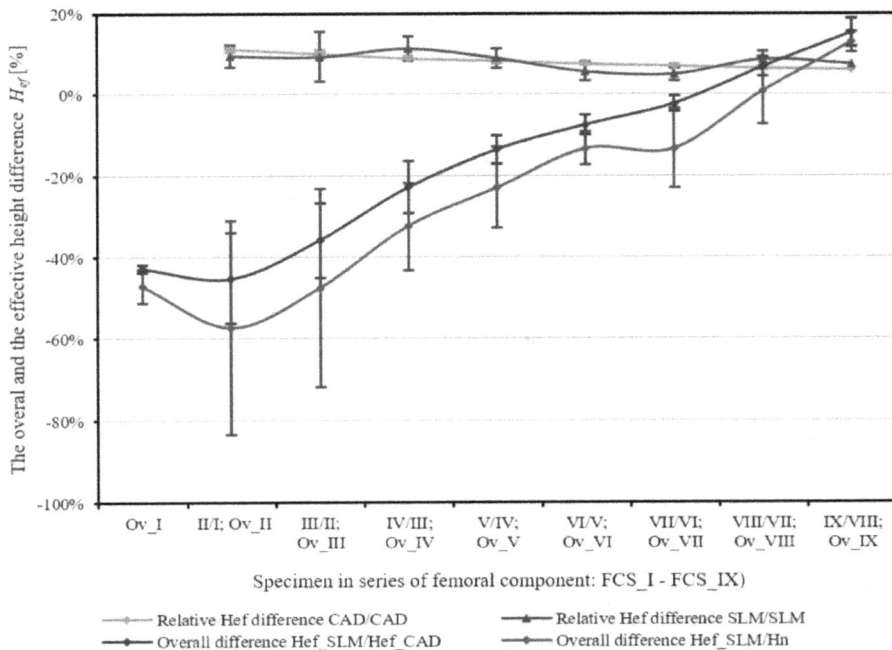

FIGURE 4.11 Curves showing the relative increase in the effective height H_{ef} of the MSC-Scaffold spikes in the consecutive series of nine preprototypes representing the femoral component FCS_I to FCS_IX along with the curves showing the total difference in the effective height H_{ef} in individual SLM-manufactured preprototypes to the effective height H_{ef} in corresponding CAD models of the prototype MSC-Scaffold regarded as the base scaffold (FCS_I) and to the nominal height H_n of these spikes.

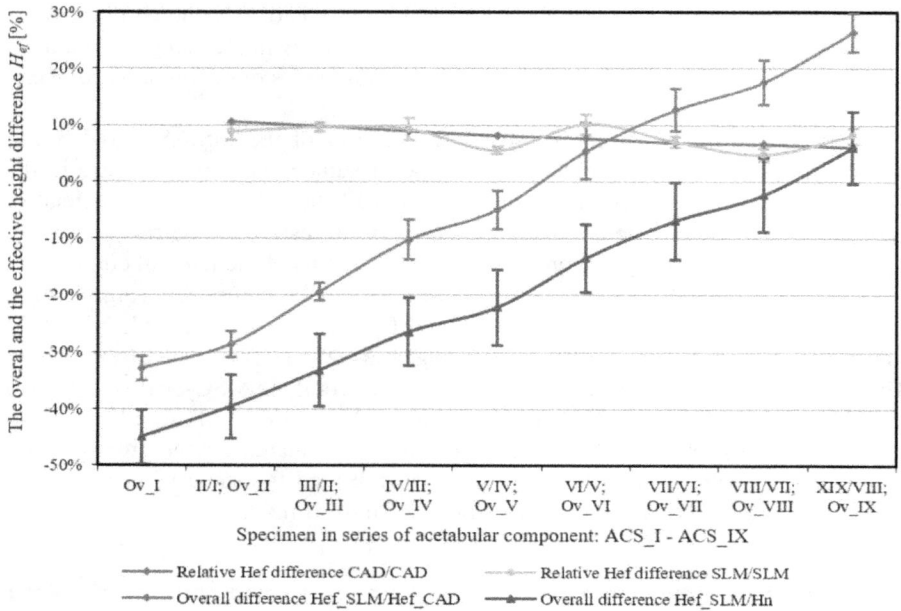

FIGURE 4.12 Curves showing the relative increase in the effective height H_{ef} of the MSC-Scaffold spikes in the following of the series of nine preprototypes representing the acetabular component ACS_I to ACS_IX along with the curves showing the total difference in the effective height H_{ef} in individual SLM preprototypes to the effective height H_{ef} in corresponding CAD models of the prototype MSC-Scaffold regarded as the base scaffold (ACS_I) and to the nominal height H_n of these spikes.

from $11.3 \pm 0.5\%$ to $6.3 \pm 0.2\%$ and $11.0 \pm 1.0\%$ to $6.1 \pm 0.4\%$, respectively, for the preprototypes representing a fragment of the femoral and acetabular components of the resurfacing arthroplasty endoprosthesis. The total relative increase in the effective height H_{ef} of the spikes in the first series of preprototypes is $50 \pm 2\%$ and $49 \pm 3\%$, respectively, for the MSC-Scaffold fragments representing the femoral and acetabular components of the hip joint resurfacing endoprosthesis.

The analysis of the curves presenting the total difference in the effective height H_{ef} of the spikes measured in successive preprototypes manufactured using the SLM technology related to the corresponding curves obtained based on the measurements made in the CAD models of the first series of preprototypes representing fragments of the MSC-Scaffold allowed for an observation that increasing the value of the H_n/R coefficient by at least 7 and 6, respectively, for the femoral and acetabular components, should be recommended for the production of MSC-Scaffold with spikes of the effective height H_{ef} as originally designed in the CAD model. Providing the structural pro-osteoconductive functionality of the prototype MSC-Scaffold connecting the hip joint resurfacing endoprosthesis, as assumed by ensuring the appropriate value of the H_n/R ratio, involves the increase in the effective height H_{ef} of the spikes in the CAD model by at least 7 and 9 for the femoral and acetabular component, respectively.

Figures 4.13 and 4.14 present the results of the measurement of the effective height H_{ef} of the spikes of the prototype MSC-Scaffold manufactured using SLM technology in the second series of nine variants of modifications of the geometric features of the spikes. The results were compared to the effective height H_{ef} of the spikes selected as a reference for each subgroup.

Modification of the geometric features of the MSC-Scaffold spikes, consisting of cutting the top and changing the value of the pyramid vertical angle, increased the effective height H_{ef} of the MSC-Scaffold spikes in the SLM preprototypes (Figure 4.13) from 20 ± 2% to 22 ± 2% to the preprototypes produced in the SLM technology, which are the basis for each subgroup of construction of the spikes. A slight increase of approximately 1% can be observed for the effective height H_{ef} of the spikes generated in subsequent preprototypes within each of the subgroups.

A much smaller increase was observed in the case of the preprototypes representing the MSC-Scaffold fragments of the acetabular component of the hip joint resurfacing endoprosthesis (Figure 4.14). Although the increase for particular spikes reached values of up to 10% in relation to the SLM-manufactured specimens used as the reference for each subgroup, the large discrepancy between the data, especially in case of spikes of the MSC-Scaffold located in the terminal parallels of latitude,

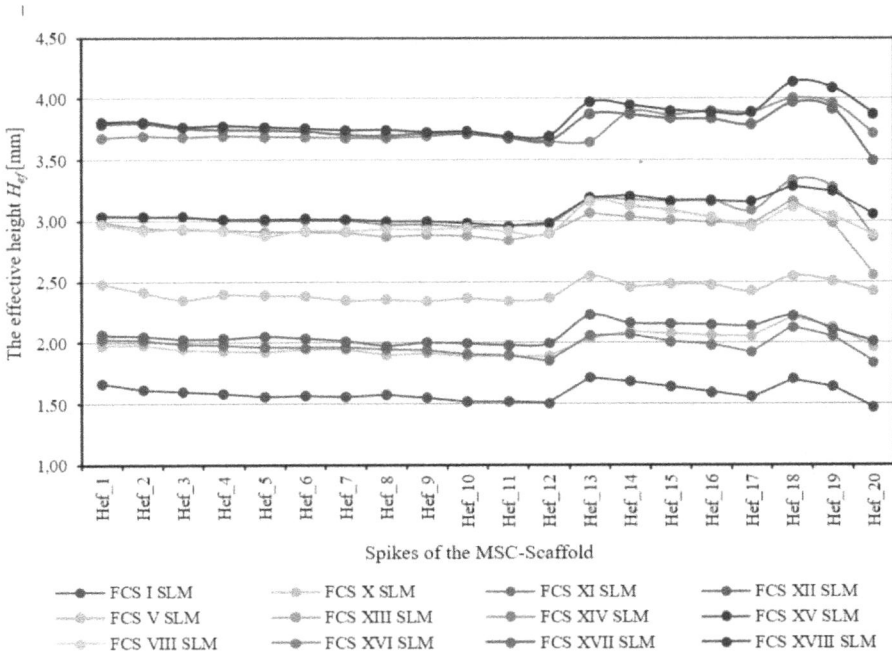

FIGURE 4.13 The effective height H_{ef} of the spikes from the second series of nine variants of the SLM-manufactured preprototypes of the MSC-Scaffold representing fragments of the femoral component (FCS_X-FCS_XVIII) of the hip joint resurfacing endoprosthesis compared to the effective height H_{ef} of the spikes in the samples from the first series taken as reference for each subgroup: FSC_I, FSC_V, and FSC_VIII.

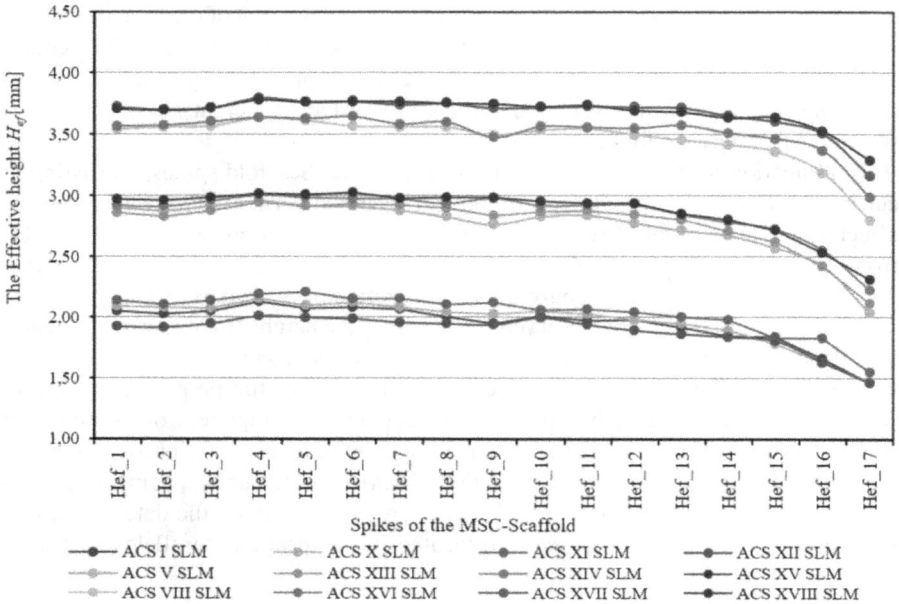

FIGURE 4.14 The effective height H_{ef} of the spikes from the second series of nine variants of the SLM-manufactured preprototypes of the MSC-Scaffold representing fragments of acetabular components (ACS_X-ACS_XVIII) of the hip joint resurfacing endoprosthesis compared to the effective height H_{ef} of the spikes in the preprototypes from the first series adopted as reference for each subgroup: ASC_I, ASC_V, and ASC_VIII.

closest to the equator of the specific spherical cap, produces relatively high values of the standard deviations of the mean values.

Figure 4.15 shows a diagram that presents the comparative possibilities for the formation of the pro-osteoconductive potential of the interspike space of the MSC-Scaffold prototype of arthroplasty endoprostheses built based on the research carried out on the MSC-Scaffold preprototypes, using the example of three geometric variants of the MSC-Scaffold spikes designed on the components of the hip joint resurfacing endoprosthesis. The nominal height H_n of these spikes as designed in the CAD model was 2.828, 3.182, and 3.536 mm.

The spikes of the MSC-Scaffold designed in CAD models along the arc constituting the meridian of the spherical base cap have the effective height H_{ef} of 2.73 ± 0.05, 2.88 ± 0.07, and 2.8 ± 0.3 mm, respectively, and are smaller by 3.3%, 9.4%, and 26.8%, respectively, to their nominal amount (H_n). The effective height H_{ef} of the MSC-Scaffold spikes in the preprototypes manufactured based on these CAD models using SLM technology is 1.57 ± 0.04, 1.64 ± 0.06, and 1.6 ± 0.1 mm, respectively, and is 42.7%, 43.2%, and 42.2% lower compared to the corresponding CAD models.

For the first variant of the simulated structural improvement of pro-osteoconductive functionality, only for the eighth preprototype in the series produced using the SLM technology, we have obtained a satisfactory value of the effective height H_{ef} of the spikes. For the second variant of the simulation of the improvement of

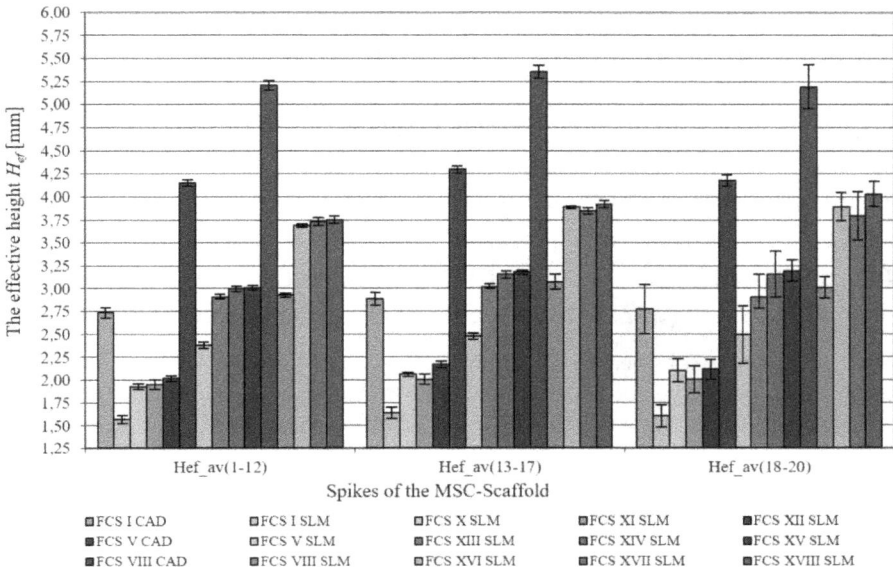

FIGURE 4.15 A diagram presenting the overall effect of the possible enhancement of the interspike structural-geometric pro-osteoconduction potential of the MSC-Scaffold (numbers 1–12, 13–17, and 18–20 represent the particular concentric parallels of latitude of the spikes' location, while the Roman numbers represent the variants of the Scaffold in the first (I-IX) and second (X-XVIII) series).

the structural pro-osteoconductive functionality, it is possible to obtain an improvement in the form of an increase in the value of the effective height H_{ef} of the spikes of approximately 20% to the preprototypes constituting the basis for each subgroup.

The most favourable variant of improving the structural pro-osteoconductive functionality of the MSC-Scaffold can be obtained by jointly modifying the geometry of the MSC-Scaffold spikes in the CAD model (e.g. increasing the nominal height H_n resulting in an increase in the H_n/R ratio by 4 and simultaneous cutting of the pyramid tops in the CAD model so that the square formed in the cross section could have a side length ranging from 0.1 mm to 0.3 mm, which allows the prototype produced using SLM technology to obtain the same effective height H_{ef} of the spikes as designed in the CAD model being the basis of the prototype of the hip joint resurfacing endoprosthesis [10–12]).

The analysis of the geometric structural features of different variants of the prototype MSC-Scaffold for both components (femoral and acetabular) of the hip joint resurfacing endoprosthesis using the confocal profilometry method allowed one to evaluate the possibility of influencing its structural pro-osteoconductive functionality, as defined and specified in this subsection according to [2–4]. We have noted the reduced structural functionality of pro-osteoconduction in the prototypes manufactured using the SLM technology in relation to that assumed in the CAD models, which were the basis of that prototype, and the technological limitations of the production of the MSC-Scaffold in this technology have been quantified. The results allowed for revising the constructional assumptions of the original prototype of the MSC-Scaffold and provided key information on the need to compensate for the identified technological limitations of selective laser beam melting when establishing design directives, i.e. a method of improving structural pro-osteoconductive functionality to properly design subsequent prototypes of resurfacing endoprostheses (partial and complete) of the knee and hip joint with the MSC-Scaffold.

4.3   INITIAL EVALUATION IN CELL CULTURE OF STRUCTURALLY FUNCTIONALIZED MULTI-SPIKED CONNECTING SCAFFOLD

Normal human osteoblasts (NHOst, Lonza, USA) were grown in a professional laboratory on preprototypes of the MSC-Scaffold to assess the initial cell adhesion and proliferation. The cells were grown in 12-well culture plates at an initial seeding density of $5 \cdot 10^4$ cells/well. Cells were seeded in Dulbecco's modified Eagle's Medium (DMEM) (BioWhittaker® Reagents, Lonza, USA) with glucose and L-glutamine (PAA, Austria), 10% foetal bovine serum (PAA, Austria), 10 U/ml penicillin, and 10 U/ml streptomycin (Sigma, Germany), in an atmosphere with 5% CO_2 and 95% air at 37°C (Galaxy 170R, New Brunswick, USA). The medium was changed every 48 hours and the operation was repeated until the cells were confluent (ten days). Fluorescence microscopy images of the MSC-Scaffold after the cultivation of normal human osteoblasts for ten days are presented in Figure 4.16.

Osteoblast cells were found to adhere to the surface of spikes of a prototype MSC-Scaffold and fill the space between them. Cells have the appropriate morphology and, when in contact with the surface of the material, they first attach, adhere, and then spread. Cells spread over the surface of the MSC-Scaffold begin to contact each

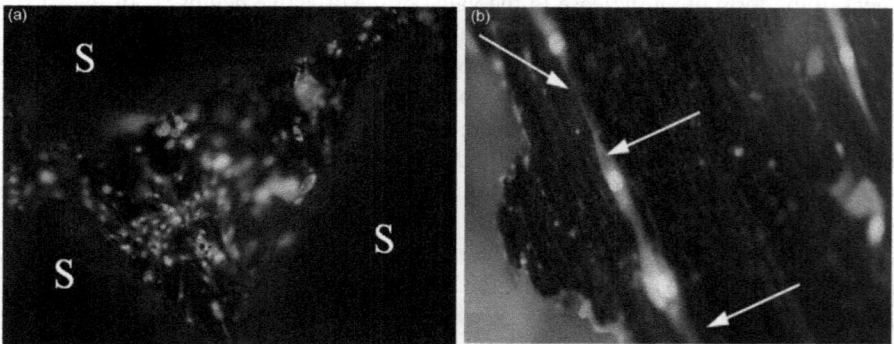

FIGURE 4.16 Fluorescent microscopic images taken after ten days of culturing human osteoblasts (NHOst, Lonza, USA) in the preprototypes of the MSC-Scaffold; acridine orange (AO) staining; the cells adhered to the surface of the MSC-Scaffold spikes (S) filling the space between them (a); the cells spread over the MSC-Scaffold surface and begin to contact each other through cytoplasmic processes (arrows) creating a three-dimensional intercellular network (b). Thus, the MSC-Scaffold spikes (imitating the interdigitations of the periarticular cancellous bone) constitute a scaffold for proliferating and spreading osteoblasts.

other through cytoplasmic processes, creating a three-dimensional intercellular net-work (Figure 4.16b, arrows).

This result shows that adjacent MSC-Scaffold spikes (mimicking the interdig-itations of the cancellous periarticular bone) constitute a scaffold for osteoblasts, which means that the prototype MSC-Scaffold can provide the expected bone tissue ingrowth in its interspike space *in vivo* with the subsequent permanent fixation of the components of the resurfacing arthroplasty endoprosthesis in the surrounding bone tissue. Cells were observed to grow relatively more efficiently between some of the spikes; however, the surface of the MSC-Scaffold material is not conducive to inten-sive cell growth, which means that the spike surfaces in contact with the bone should be subjected to appropriate physicochemical modification to improve the osteoinduc-tive and osseointegration properties.

4.4 PILOT STUDY OF STRUCTURALLY FUNCTIONALIZED MULTI-SPIKED CONNECTING SCAFFOLD IN AN ANIMAL MODEL

To assess the biointegration of the MSC-Scaffold for resurfacing endoprostheses after structural pro-osteoconductive functionalization, pilot implantations of the pre-prototypes of this scaffold were carried out in swine (breed: Polish Large White).

For the initial preclinical orthopaedic evaluation, four MSC-Scaffold preproto-types were implanted under the articular cartilage surface of the medial and lateral femoral condyles of two laboratory swine after opening their knee joints. The first laboratory swine was a 9-month-old boar weighing 85.5 kg, and the second was a 10-month-old boar weighing 91.0 kg. Each of these animals was implanted with two design variants of the MSC-Scaffold preprototypes that differed in the distance between the bases of the spikes (100 µm and 200 µm, circumferentially and radially) and the outer diameter of the base (ø10 mm and ø15 mm) of the preprototype, on which the MSC-Scaffold was manufactured using SLM technology.

Implantation procedures were performed in the operating room of a veterinary clinic with the consent of the Local Ethics Committee in Poznan. General inhalation anaesthesia with endotracheal intubation and anaesthetic monitoring (induction of anaesthesia: Cepetor 0.01-0.04 mg/kg intravenously; anaesthesia was maintained by inhalation using an inhaler) was used during the surgical implantation of the prepro-tototypes of the MSC-Scaffold.

An anteromedial skin incision was made, with a length of approximately 20 cm above the operated joint of the right knee. Approach to the knee joint between the lateral margin of patella and the external side of patellar ligament, and then between vastus lateralis muscle and rectus femoris muscle was applied. The articular capsule was opened on the lateral side of the patella and then the patella was displaced medi-ally. Bleeding was stopped (haemostasis). The patellofemoral area of the knee joint was exposed. Implantation sites in both femoral condyles were prepared using a surgi-cal drill. To be able to insert the implant, cancellous bone cavities were made, which were gradually widened with a milling cutter until the desired size was obtained. During drilling and milling, the bone holes were continuously irrigated with saline. Condyle holes were rinsed with saline and bone debris was removed. The first MSC-Scaffold preprototype was embedded in the medial condyle of the femur and the second preprototype in the lateral condyle of the femur. Implants insertion into the bone holes was performed using surgical mallet.

Figure 4.17a shows two variants of the preprototypes of the MSC-Scaffold (I, II) implanted under the surface of the articular cartilage of both femoral condyles. An anatomical reposition of the patella was performed. A layered wound suture was applied. The wound was covered with a penicillin-soaked mesh and an antiseptic dressing was applied. Then, for three days after the procedure, 1 g of Amikacin (Biodacin) i.v. (or i.m.) was administered twice a day. On the third day after surgery, the operated limbs were fully loaded. The implants remained implanted for six weeks in the first operated animal and nine weeks in the second operated animal.

A control radiographic examination was performed in the fourth week after the implantation procedure. Radiographs (anterior-posterior view) showing two design variants of the MSC-Scaffold preprototypes for resurfacing endoprostheses implanted into the femoral condyles of the knee joint in two swines are presented in Figure 4.18.

Radiographs showed that all four preprototypes were well embedded in both femoral condyles in the operated knee joints. This means that no implant loosening, migration, or other possible early postoperative complications have been observed.

At six and nine weeks post-implantation, the operated animals were euthanized according to the protocol approved by the Local Ethics Committee in Poznan (Morbitan/Pentobarbital natrium/in lethal doses 200 mg/kg BW i.v.), and

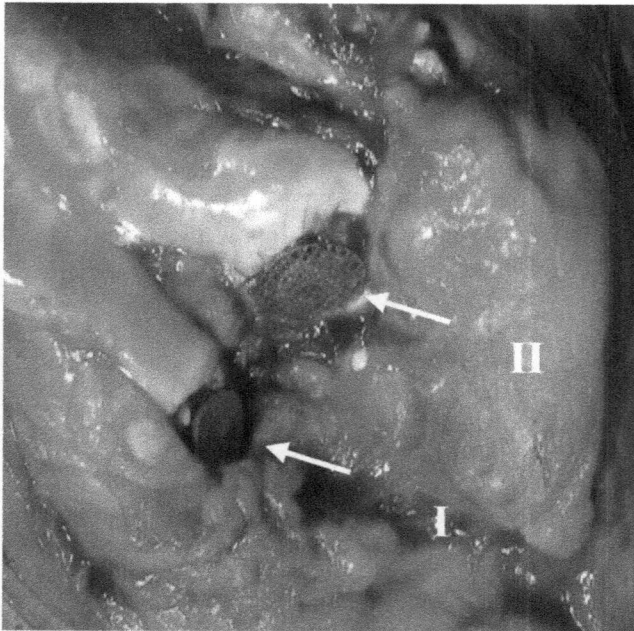

FIGURE 4.17   Two variants of the preprototypes of the MSC-Scaffold (I, II) implanted under the surface of the articular cartilage of both femoral condyles of the operated animals.

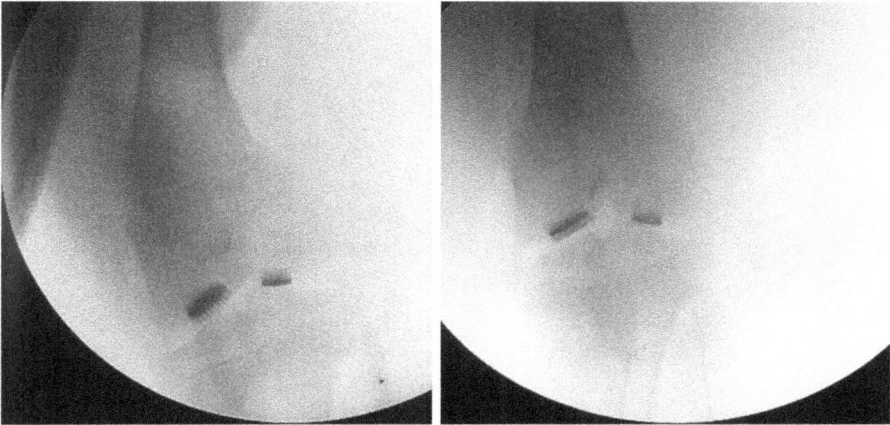

FIGURE 4.18 Anteroposterior radiographs taken at week 4 post-implantation of two vari-ants of MSC-Scaffold preprototypes for non-cemented non-stemmed resurfacing endo-prostheses implanted in the femoral condyles of laboratory swine knee joints; neither the loosening of the implants nor their migration after the procedure was observed.

the two knee joints with the MSC-Scaffold preprototypes were harvested from ani-mals. Fragments of bone-implant slides were excised from the distal epiphysis of the femur and prepared for histopathological analysis. Thin slices 1.5 mm thick were excised from each bone-implant fragment using an IsoMet™ 4000 Linear Precision Saw (Buehler, Esslingen am Neckar, Germany) under continuous water irrigation conditions. The slices were excised in the direction parallel to the central axis of the preprototype spike. Bone-implant slices were fixed in 6% formalin (phosphate-buff-ered formaldehyde) for seven days. In the next step, the bone fragments containing the implant were decalcified with 4% wt. nitric acid (HNO_3) solution for 24 hours. The MSC-Scaffold preprototypes were then separated from the bones and further, the bone sections were dehydrated in a series of ethanol solutions (50 wt.%, 60 wt.%, 70 wt.%, 95 wt.%, 99.8 wt.%) and degreased in a series of acetone solutions (90 wt.% and 99.8 wt.%). A hydrophobic agent (xylene) was then used to remove the alcohol and finally the slides were infiltrated with molten paraffin wax to replace xylene. All steps of the preparation process, starting from dehydration and each of them lasting 2 hours, were performed using a Leica TP1020 automatic tissue carousel proces-sor (Leica Microsystems GmbH, Germany). The bone fragments separated from the implant were embedded in paraffin wax and ground into specimens with a thickness of 4 μm. Following the reverse sequence of process steps, bone sections separated from the implant were stained with haematoxylin-eosin (H&E) and examined under an Olympus CX41 light microscope (Olympus, Tokyo, Japan).

An exemplary microscopic and histopathological (H&E) documentation of the peri-implant bone tissue after the removal of the MSC-Scaffold prototype is pre-sented in Figure 4.19. It was found that the contact surfaces of the bone with the implant were smooth, and the mechanical separation of the implant from the bone did not tear the peri-implant bone tissue.

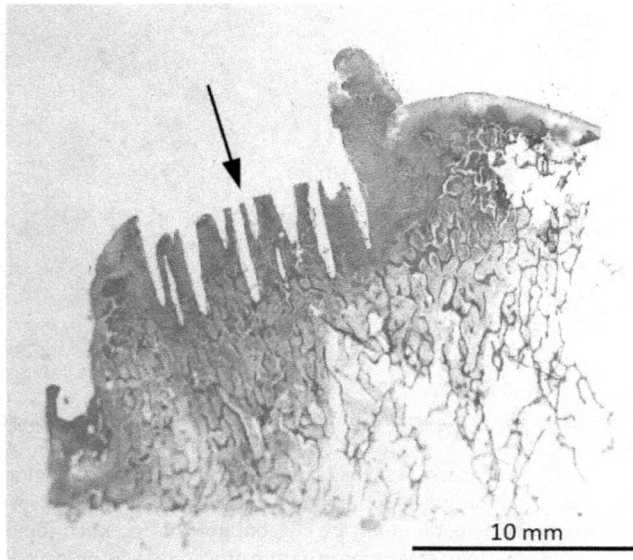

FIGURE 4.19 Exemplary histological section (H&E) of the peri-implant bone tissue after removing the MSC-Scaffold preprototype from the bone-implant slices after their decalcification showed smooth contact surfaces between the bone and the implant (arrow), suggesting insufficient osteointegration.

This means that osseointegration with the surface of the spikes was most likely not sufficient, as the adsorption of bone proteins to the surface of the MSC-Scaffold spikes during the proper osseointegration would tear out fragments of peri-implant bone tissue along with the removed implant.

No morphological markers of inflammation were found in the examined histopathological slides collected six weeks after implantation, while relatively numerous osteoblasts were observed on the surface of the bone trabeculae near the contact between the bone and the MSC-Scaffold, which means that the osteogenesis process was still taking place at that point (Figure 4.20).

In the case of histological sections obtained from bone-implant specimens harvested in the ninth week after the implantation procedure, practically the entire interspike space of the prototype MSC-Scaffold was occupied with mature bone tissue (Figure 4.21a) without morphological markers of the osteogenesis process. There were no necrotic bone fragments formed during the first stage of surgical implantation. The bone trabeculae of the periarticular bone in these histological slides are viewed as mature and equal in age. This is evidenced by clearly visible interlamellar cement lines of bone tissue and osteocytes (mature bone cells) in bone trabeculae (Figure 4.21b).

In histological sections obtained from bone fragments containing the implant, both those collected at the sixth and ninth week after implantation, we have found numerous metallic microparticles in bone tissue at the surface of its contact with the MSC-Scaffold, in particular, located in the interspike space proximal to the base of the spikes (Figure 4.22a, arrows) which are residues remaining after blasting the

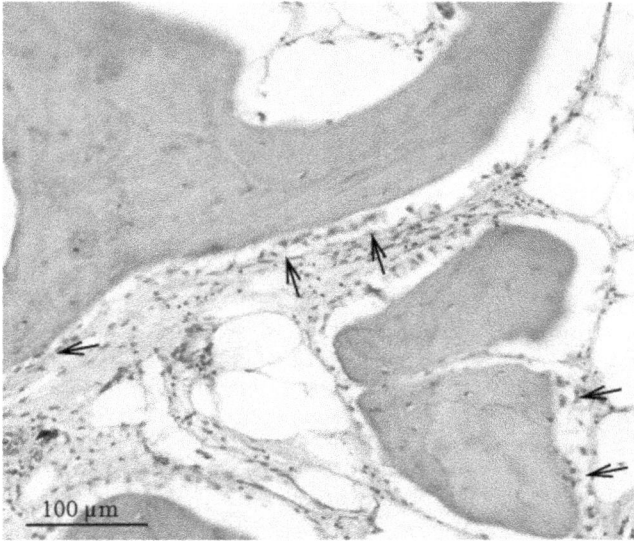

FIGURE 4.20   Relatively numerous osteoblasts (arrows) on bone trabeculae surfaces in peri-scaffold bone tissue histological sections (H&E) obtained from bone fragments containing implants harvested in the sixth week after the surgery.

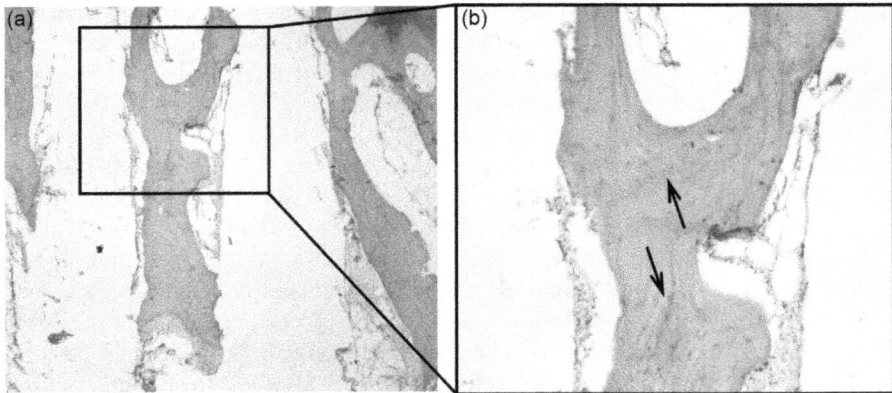

FIGURE 4.21   Histopathological sections (H&E) obtained from bone specimens containing implants collected in the ninth week post-implantation, showing a fragment of the interspike space of the MSC-Scaffold preprototypes occupied with cancellous bone tissue (a): the trabeculae of the periarticular bone look equal; it is indicated by clearly visible interlamellar cement lines and osteocytes in the bone trabeculae (b).

surface of the spikes of MSC-Scaffold preprototypes manufactured in the SLM technology (cf. Figure 3.38d). In histological sections obtained from bone-implant fragments harvested in the ninth week after implantation, presented in Figures 4.22b and 4.22c, we have shown an exemplary area of the MSC-Scaffold interspike space,

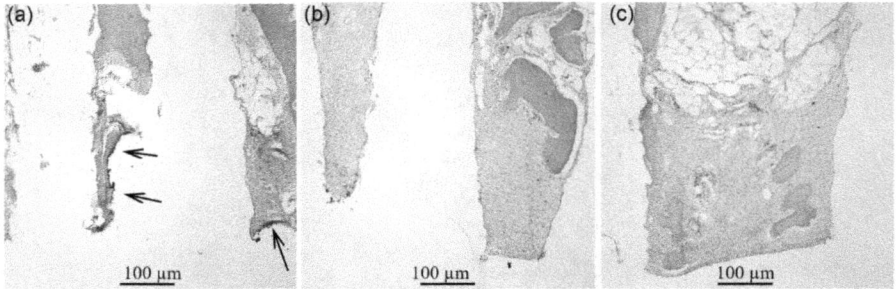

FIGURE 4.22 Histopathological sections (H&E) obtained from bone specimens containing implants harvested in the ninth week after implantation (H&E) showing: (a) numerous metallic particles (arrows) being the remains after blasting the surface of the spikes of the prototype MSC-Scaffold manufactured in SLM technology; (b) and (c) areas of the interspike space of the MSC-Scaffold preprototype near the edge of the base of the spikes (distance between the base of the spikes: (b) 100 μm and (c) 200 μm) almost entirely filled with fibrous connective tissue.

located directly near the edge of the spike bases, almost entirely filled with fibrous connective tissue.

Based on the analysis of microscopic and histological documentation obtained from bone-implant specimens harvested in the ninth week after implantation (Figure 4.21), it can be concluded that the surfaces of the spikes in contact with the bone constitute a scaffold for bone tissue that allows it to grow into and fill the interspike space of the prototype MSC-Scaffold, which allows biological fixation of the implant (a component of the resurfacing arthroplasty endoprosthesis) in the periarticular bone.

The absence of bone tissue in the interspike space of the MSC-Scaffold preprototypes within the edges of the spike bases indicates that due to the small distance between these edges (100 μm – Figure 4.22b and 200 μm – Figure 4.22c) both of these areas are not sufficiently capacious to allow the formation of bone tissue in them. Moreover, bone formation in this area can be inhibited by the inflammatory process associated with the immune response to the metallic particles that remain adhered on the surface of the spikes after the SLM process to produce a prototype MSC-Scaffold. Pilot implantations indicate the need to increase the distance between the edges of the spike bases in the prototype MSC-Scaffold for resurfacing arthroplasty endoprostheses. Moreover, increasing the space between the spikes near the edge of their bases will increase the efficiency of blasting the surface of the spikes, improving the conditions for cleaning this area from metallic particles remained after the SLM manufacturing process of the prototype MSC-Scaffold.

REFERENCES

1. Uklejewski, R.; Winiecki, M.; Rogala, P. On the structural-adaptive compatibility of bone with porous coated implants on the base of the traditional one-phase and the modern two phase poroelastic biomechanical model of bone tissue. *Eng Biomater.* 2006; 9(54–55): 1–13.

2. Winiecki, M. The investigation on the microgeometrical constructional properties of porous intraosseous implants and the influence of these properties on the strength of the boneimplant model fixation (In Polish: Badanie mikrogeometrycznych cech konstrukcyjnych porowatych implantów dokostnych i ocena wpływu tych cech na wytrzymałość modelowego połączenia implant-kość). PhD Thesis, Poznan University of Technology, Poznań, 2006.

3. Uklejewski, R.; Winiecki, M.; Rogala, P.; Mielniczuk, J.; Auguściński, A.; Stryła, W. Structural and biomechanical biocompatibility in bone-porous implant fixation region – on the basis of two-phase poroelastic biomechanical model of bone tissue. *Eng Biomater.* 2007; 10(69–72): 93–5.

4. Uklejewski, R.; Winiecki, M.; Mielniczuk, J.; Rogala, P.; Auguściński, A. The poroaccessibility parameters for three-dimensional characterization of orthopaedic implants porous coatings. *Metrol Meas Syst.* 2008; 15(2): 215–26.

5. Uklejewski, R.; Winiecki, M.; Rogala, P. Computer aided stereometric evaluation of porostructural-osteoconductive properties of intra-osseous implants porous coatings. *Metrol Meas Syst.* 2013; 20(3): 427–38. doi:10.2478/mms-2013-0037

6. Rogala, P. Endoprosthesis. EU Patent No. EP072418 B1, 22 December 1999.

7. Rogala, P. Acetabulum Endoprosthesis and Head. U.S. Patent US5,911,759 A, 15 June 1999.

8. Rogala, P. Method and Endoprosthesis to Apply This Implantation. Canadian Patent No. 2,200,064, 1 April 2002.

9. Mielniczuk, J.; Rogala, P.; Uklejewski, R.; Winiecki, M.; Jokś, G.; Auguściński, A.; Berdychowski, M. Modelling of the needle-palisade fixation system for the total hip resurfacing arthroplasty endoprosthesis. *Trans VŠB-TU Ostrava, Metallurgical Series.* 2008; 51(1): 160–6.

10. Uklejewski, R.; Rogala, P.; Winiecki, M.; Mielniczuk, J. Prototype of innovating bone tissue preserving THRA endoprosthesis with multi-spiked connecting scaffold manufactured in selective laser melting technology. *Eng Biomater.* 2009; 12(87): 2–6.

11. Uklejewski, R.; Rogala, P.; Winiecki, M.; Mielniczuk, J. Prototype of minimally invasive hip resurfacing endoprosthesis – bioengineering design and manufacturing. *Acta Bioeng Biomech.* 2009; 11(2): 65–70.

12. Uklejewski, R.; Winiecki, M.; Rogala, P.; Mielniczuk, J. Selective laser melted prototype of original minimally invasive hip endoprosthesis. *Rapid Prototyp J.* 2011; 17(1): 76–85. doi:10.1108/13552541111098653

5 Formation of osteoinductive and osseointegrative properties of the bone-contacting surface of the multi-spiked connecting scaffold prototype by the electrochemical cathodic deposition of calcium phosphates*

5.1 INITIAL ATTEMPTS TO MODIFY THE SURFACE OF THE MULTI-SPIKED CONNECTING SCAFFOLD PREPROTOTYPES

Unmodified bone-contacting surface of components of resurfacing endoprostheses made of titanium alloys exhibit poor osteoinductive behaviour; therefore, modification of such surface is usually necessary to improve the functionality of implants in this respect [4]. The commonly used materials to modify the bone-contacting surface of implants that improve their osteoinductive properties, used both in orthopaedics and dentistry, are calcium phosphate-based bioceramics, among which the most common and characterized by excellent bioactivity is hydroxyapatite $(Ca_{10}(PO_4)_6(OH)_2$,

---

* The research works described in this chapter were carried out at the Institute of Chemical Technology and Engineering of the Faculty of Chemical Technology of the Poznan University of Technology as part of the research project of the National Science Centre Poland No. NN518412638, and then continued in the doctoral dissertation [1], the supervisor of which was the principal investigator of the research project mentioned above, and published in papers [2,3].

DOI: 10.1201/9781003364498-5
85

HA) – a biomineral that naturally occurs in bones [4–10]. Calcium phosphates (CaP) are of particular importance in this regard, because they are the most important inorganic components of hard tissues in vertebrates [5–10].

Synthetic CaP coatings can be prepared using a variety of processes. In general, commonly used methods can be divided into two groups, physical deposition techniques and wet-chemical techniques [11]. Physical methods include plasma spraying [12], pulsed laser deposition [13], low-temperature high-speed collision [14], radio frequency magnetron sputtering [15], gas-detonation deposition [16], and ion implantation [17]. Chemical methods include chemical vapour deposition [18], biomimetic deposition [19–22], hydrothermal treatment [23], sol-gel deposition [24,25], and electrochemical methods [20,26–34].

CaP coating deposition on flat substrates has been widely investigated, while CaP deposition on the bone-contacting surface of complex geometric shapes, for example, porous implants or additively manufactured scaffolds, has only been studied relatively rarely and quite recently [35–37]. Most CaP deposition methods have a line-of-sight requirement, which greatly limits the choices in coating with complex shapes [32]. Only a few methods can be applied to complex-shaped or porous materials and scaffolds. Therefore, to improve the osteoinductive and osseointegrative behaviour of the bone-contacting surface of the MSC-Scaffold, electrochemical methods are preferred because of their shape complexity. The technologies commonly used for this purpose are electrophoretic deposition (EPD) and electrochemical deposition (ECD) [26].

The ECD process can be carried out at room temperature and allows the CaP surface modification of complex-shaped Ti-alloy implants with control of the adhesive strength of the coating [38], resulting in a non-delaminating CaP coating of approximately 1 μm thickness characterized by relatively high adhesive strength compared to the EPD process, where the hydroxyapatite (HA) coating is obtained from a suspension containing HA particles. Without applying thermal post-processing by subsequent sintering, the EPD-deposited HA coating delaminates [14,17,26,27].

In the ECD process, CaP coatings are formed from an electrolyte containing calcium nitrate, $Ca(NO_3)_2$, and ammonium dihydrogen phosphate, $NH_4H_2PO_4$, where the molar ratio of calcium to phosphorus is approximately 1.67 and is the same as the ratio of Ca/P in native osseous CaPs [28,39–43]. This method enables control of the properties of the deposited coatings by appropriately choosing the electric parameters of the ECD process, such as current density [44] or electric potential [24], and by adjusting the processing time [16]. The subsequent immersion of the modified substrates in simulated body fluid (SBF) leads to the transformation of the amorphous CaP coating into a crystalline CaP coating [24,27]. The coatings obtained in this way are characterized by layers made of different phases of Ca-P, which depends on the composition of the SBF where the surface-modified biomaterial is immersed and the initial preparation of its surface [36]. The advantage here is the possibility of conducting the process of transforming the CaP coating at a relatively low temperature, and this process consists of the heterogeneous nucleation of CaP from the SBF solution [22]. The application of chemical pretreatment, such as acid, alkaline, or acid-alkaline treatment (AAT), may advantageously influence the outcome of the ECD process [45–50].

Initial attempts to modify the bone-contacting surface of the MSC-Scaffold preprototypes for resurfacing arthroplasty endoprostheses were carried out using the method of electrochemical cathodic deposition of CaPs at constant current density values. Before the actual modification process, the lateral spike surfaces was chemically cleaned each time successively: in distilled water, ethanol, acetone, and then three times in distilled water; each stage lasted 15 minutes. The modification process using Autolab PGSTAT302N potentiostat/galvanostat (Metrohm Autolab B.V., The Netherlands) was carried out in a dual-electrode system at current densities of 1.25, 5, and 10 mA/cm^2, in a solution containing 0.042 M Ca(NO$_3$)$_2$ – and 0.025 M NH$_4$H$_2$PO$_4$, at pH = 6, at room temperature, for 1 hour. The preprototypes acted as a working electrode, and the gold electrode was used as an anode. Subsequently, the preprototypes were incubated (part for 24 h and part for 48 h) in SBF of the composition of: 6.8 g/l NaCl, 0.4 g/l KCl, 0.2 g/l CaCl$_2$, 0.2048 g/l MgSO$_4$·7H$_2$O, 0.1438 g/l NaH$_2$PO$_4$·H$_2$O, and 1.0 g/l NaHCO$_3$.

Qualitative analysis of surface morphology and microanalysis of the chemical composition using the X-ray energy-dispersive spectroscopy (EDS) of the modified microstructure of the preprototype MSC-Scaffold was performed using the Hitachi TM-3030 scanning electron microscope (Hitachi High-Tech Technologies Europe GmbH, Krefeld, Germany) equipped with the EDS system (Oxford Instruments, Oxfordshire, United Kingdom) and the Vega 5135 scanning electron microscope (Tescan, Brno-Kohoutovice, Czech Republic) equipped with the EDS system (Princeton Gamma-Tech, Inc., Princeton, NJ, USA). Surface mapping on three randomly selected subareas of the modified lateral surface of the spikes of each prototype MSC-Scaffold was performed using a specialized software analyser available in the EDS system. On the basis of the mapping of the lateral surface of the spikes, the average degree of coverage with a CaP layer was determined. In each of the analysed subareas, ten-point measurements of the chemical composition were made and molar Ca/P ratios were calculated. The analysis of the degree of coverage of the lateral surface of the spikes and the homogeneity of the deposited coating was performed using a professional ImageJ software tool (National Institutes of Health, Bethesda, MD, USA).

Due to the complex shape of the MSC-Scaffold, it was not possible to apply the commonly used method to determine the adhesion of the coatings in the scratch test [51]. Therefore, a proprietary ultrasonic method was developed to assess the adhesive strength of the coatings deposited on the bone-contacting surface of the MSC-Scaffold. Surface-modified preprototypes were placed in a glass vessel filled with experimentally selected abrasives (glass microspheres with granulation of 30–50 μm) and placed in an ultrasonic cleaner (Sonic 3, Polsonic, Poland). The preprototypes were weighted at equal time intervals and the surface of the spikes was observed using a scanning electron microscope. The criterion for completion of the test was the lack of mass loss in three consecutive measurements.

Figure 5.1 presents the SEM documentation of the surface of the spikes of the MSC-Scaffold preprototypes after the modification process at different current densities and different immersion times in the SBF. Figure 5.2 presents the SEM documentation of the surface of the spikes of the preprototype MSC-Scaffold after the adhesive strength test. Figure 5.3 presents examples of adhesive strength test results for applied coatings. Table 5.1 gives examples of the results of the test of the chemical composition of the coatings obtained as a result of the modification by electrochemical cathodic deposition of CaP carried out at a constant current density of 5 mA/cm^2.

An electrochemical cathodic deposition allows the formation of CaP coating on the surface of MSC-Scaffold spikes in a short time. On the basis of the SEM documentation of the surface of the preprototype MSC-Scaffold for resurfacing arthroplasty endoprostheses subjected to electrochemical modification, it can be noted that as the density of the current used for deposition increases, the degree of coverage of the lateral surface of spikes with a CaP layer increases. For the modification carried out at the current density of 5 mA/cm^2, no cracks were observed on the surface of

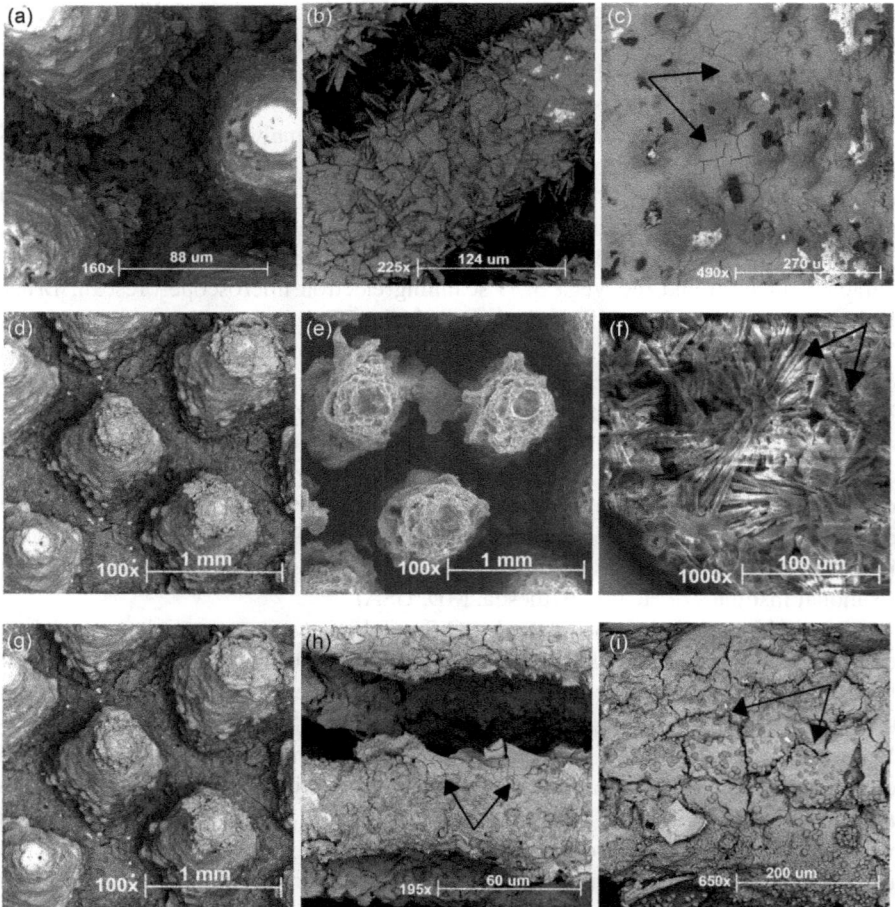

FIGURE 5.1 SEM documentation of the lateral spike surfaces of the preprototype MSC-Scaffold for resurfacing arthroplasty endoprostheses subjected to electrochemical treatment at a current density of: (a) 1.25 mA/cm^2 and after 24 h immersion in SBF, (b) and (c) 1.25 mA/cm^2 and 48 h immersion in SBF, (d) and (f) 5 mA/cm^2 and 24 h immersion in SBF, (e) 5 mA/cm^2 and 48 h immersion in SBF, (g) 10 mA/cm^2 and 24 h immersion in SBF and (h) and (i) 10 mA/cm^2 and 48 h immersion in SBF.

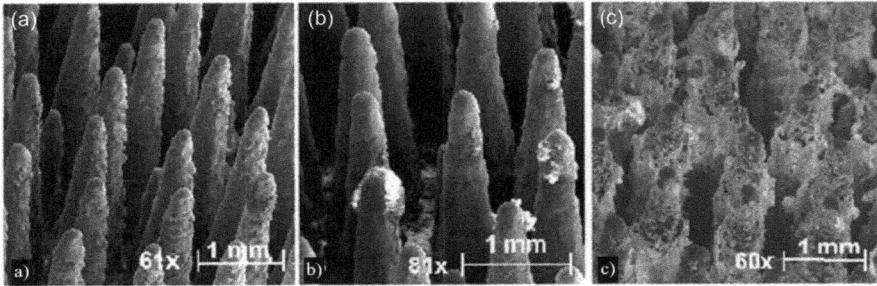

FIGURE 5.2 SEM documentation after testing the adhesive strength of the CaP-modified surface of the MSC-Scaffold for resurfacing endoprostheses subjected to electrochemical modification at the current density: (a) 1.25 mA/cm^2, (b) 5 mA/cm^2, and (c) 10 mA/cm^2.

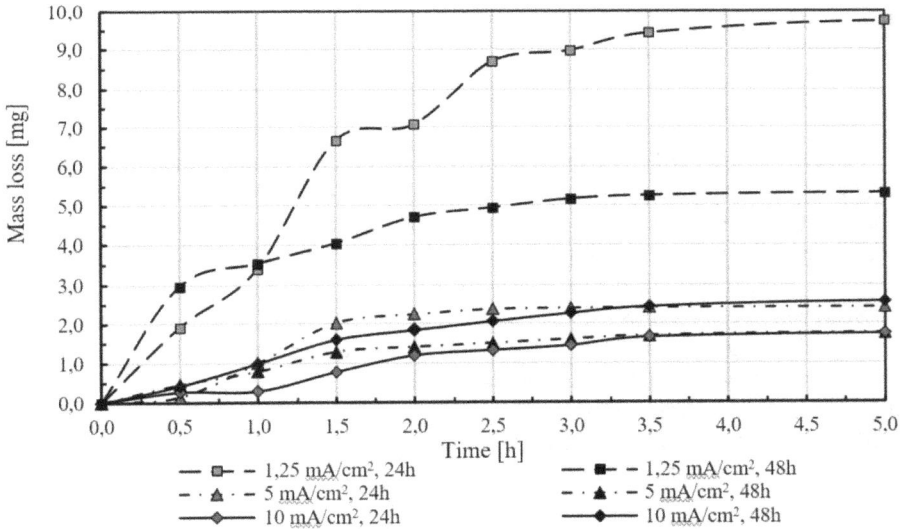

FIGURE 5.3 The mean mass loss of the surface layer is a function of the duration of ultrasonic abrasion of the surface of the MSC-Scaffold preprototypes.

the deposited layer, while at the current density of 1.25 and 10 mA/cm^2 (Figures 5.2c and Figure 5.2i), cracks were observed on the surface of the formed layer, where for the current density of 10 mA/cm^2, the number of surface cracks is greater than for the preprototypes modified at the current density of 1.25 mA/cm^2. In the deposited coating, we can also see crystalline forms of CaPs (Figure 5.2f).

X-ray analysis (EDS) showed that both calcium and phosphorus are present on the titanium surface of the spikes subjected to the modification process. The example results of the chemical composition analysis presented in Table 5.1 indicate that the molar ratio of these two elements is approximately 1.67, which corresponds to the value occurring in native bone hydroxyapatite. For other preprototypes, this ratio is similar.

TABLE 5.1

Example results of EDS analysis of the chemical composition of the produced coating

Incubation Time in SBF Solution

Element	24 h		48 h	
	Mass Contribution (%)	Molar Contribution (%)	Mass Contribution (%)	Molar Contribution (%)
O	56.93	75.09	44.24	65.68
Al	–	–	1.32	1.16
Si	–	–	0.24	0.20
Ti	3.34	1.47	16.86	8.36
P	16.30	11.11	14.44	11.07
Ca	23.43	12.34	22.45	13.30
Total	100	100	100	100

Analysis of the SEM documentation of preprototypes subjected to the adhesive strength test using an experimentally developed ultrasonic method (Figure 5.3) allows the observation of coating defects on all preprototypes. A smaller loss of coating of CaP deposited at higher current densities was found; however, this result required confirmation in further research.

SEM images in Figures 5.4a and 5.4b show the surface of the spikes of the preprototype subjected to electrochemical cathodic deposition at a current density of 5 mA/cm^2, followed by 24 hour incubation in SBF. The arrows show the CaP plate crystals deposited on the lateral surface of the spikes of the MSC-Scaffold preprototypes, as well as near the edge of their base. Figure 5.4c shows an example of SEM microphotography and Figure 5.4d presents corresponding surface EDS mapping images; the darker grey colour corresponds to calcium atoms and the lighter grey to phosphorus atoms. Figure 5.4e presents an example EDS spectrogram of the example area of the lateral surface of the spikes in Figure 5.4c.

According to the EDS spectrum presented in Figure 5.4e, the main elements detected on the lateral surface of the MSC-Scaffold were the following: Ca, P, and O, which indicates the deposition of CaP coating on their surface. Elements such as Ti, Al, and V found in the EDS analysis come from the Ti-6Al-4V substrate, because, as can be seen in Figure 5.4d, only part of the lateral surface of the spikes of the MSC-Scaffold has been covered with a CaP layer, i.e. this coating is not homogeneous. Elements such as Si and partial Al elements shown in the EDS spectra can be derived from an abrasive mixture used to jet clean the surface of the MSC-Scaffold spikes, consisting mainly of alumina (Al$_2$O$_3$) and glass microspheres (70% SiO$_2$). The determined values of the molar ratio Ca/P (1.56 | 1.74) on the lateral surface of the preprototype spikes correspond to the values of native bone CaP, which allows us to conclude that as a result of the modification a layer of CaP with microcracks was formed.

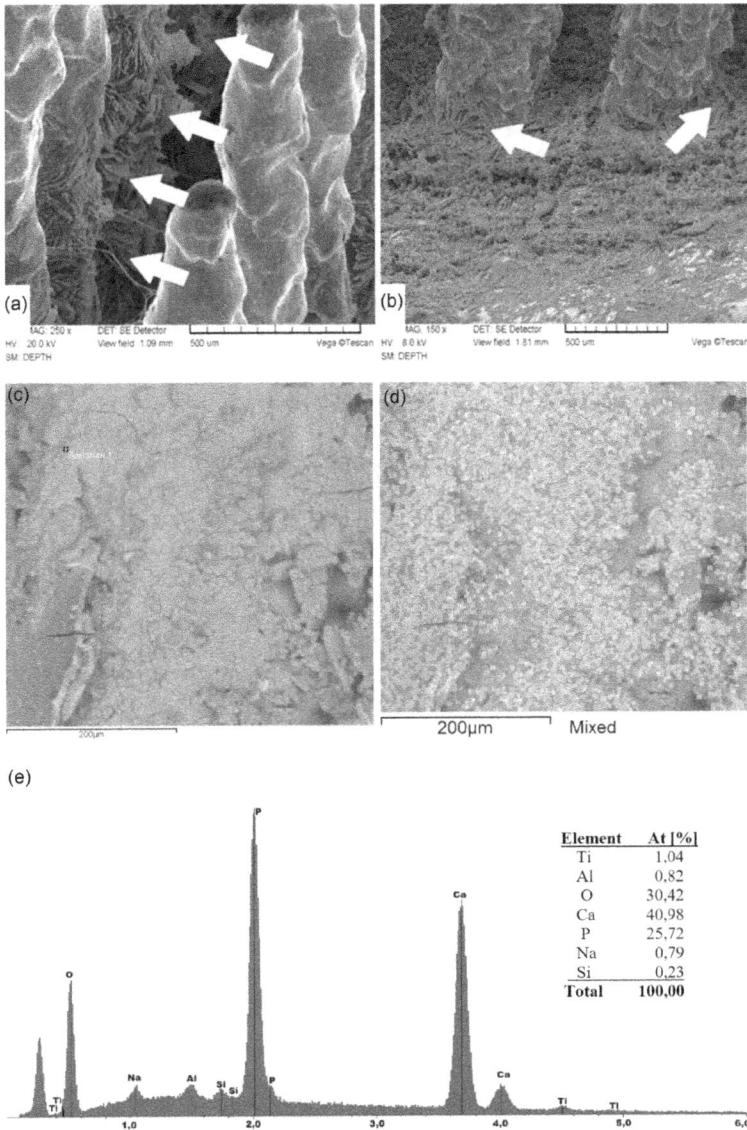

FIGURE 5.4   SEM documentation of the bone-contacting surface of the MSC-Scaffold pre-prototype subjected to electrochemical modification at a current density of 5 mA/cm^2, followed by a 24-hour incubation in SBF (a, b); arrows show lamellar CaP crystals deposited on the lateral surface of the spikes of the MSC-Scaffold preprototype (a) and also at the base of the MSC-Scaffold preprototype near the edge of the spikes (b); SEM microphotograph of an example area on the lateral surface of the spike and an image showing the same area with the mapping made using specialized software included in the EDS system (c, d); dark grey corresponds to calcium atoms, and light grey correspond to phosphorus atoms, and the example EDS spectrogram (e) for the area on the lateral surface of the spikes with the corresponding chemical composition shows that the Ca/P molar ratio here is 1.59.

5.2   RESEARCH ON THE PROCESS OF CALCIUM PHOSPHATE POTENTIOSTATIC ELECTROCHEMICAL CATHODIC DEPOSITION ON THE SURFACE OF THE SPIKES WITH THE SUBSEQUENT IMMERSION OF THE PREPROTOTYPES OF THE MULTI-SPIKED CONNECTING SCAFFOLD IN A SIMULATED BODY FLUID

As a result of the preliminary attempts of modifying the bone-contacting surface of preprototypes of the MSC-Scaffold by electrochemical cathodic deposition of CaPs carried out at constant current density values and subsequent immersion of the pre-prototypes of the MSC-Scaffold in SBF, it was observed that the deposition of CaPs can be controlled by regulating the current density. During further pilot tests also carried out using the potentiostatic process, significantly higher repeatability of this type of process was observed in comparison to that of the galvanostatic process. Therefore, it was decided to continue the research of the CaP modification of the lateral spike surfaces of the MSC-Scaffold using an ECD process carried out at constant electric potential values.

A few works devoted to the modification of the substrates with complex geometric shapes using the above method (e.g. in the case of bone scaffolds), as well as the unsatisfactory effects of tests of the use of parameters of the CaP modification process with the ECD method, recommended for flat substrates in the case of MSC-Scaffold, justified the need to undertake an experimental search for an suitable range of conditions for conducting this process at constant electric potential values.

The research aimed to experimentally determine the proper range of conditions for the process of potentiostatic electrochemical deposition of CaPs on the bone-contacting surface of the spikes of MSC-Scaffold preprototypes, leading to the deposition of a biomineral coating with the values of the molar Ca/P ratio occurring in the native bone hydroxyapatite, which is of great importance for the good biocompatibility of the implant *in vivo*.

Following the conclusions drawn from our research presented in Chapter 4, the design of the MSC-Scaffold has been modified in the area of its interspike space near the edge of the spike bases. Two new variants of preprototypes, differing in the distance between the bases of the spikes: 200 μm (P_{Sc200}) and 350 μm (P_{Sc350}), both peripherally and radially, were designed to test the modification of the bone-contacting surface of the MSC-Scaffold by ECD of CaPs (carried out at constant electric potential values). The research was performed on the MSC-Scaffold prepro-totypes designed as fragments of the middle part of the femoral component of the total hip resurfacing arthroplasty endoprosthesis. The prototype hip joint resurfac-ing endoprosthesis with MSC-Scaffold manufactured in the SLM technology from Ti-6Al-4V powder is shown in Figure 5.5a. Figure 5.5b presents the CAD models of the MSC-Scaffold preprototypes developed for these tests, and Figure 5.5c presents the preprototypes produced on their basis using SLM technology.

A total of 56 preprototypes have been used to determine the most suitable electric potential range for CaP modification process using the ECD method (28 for each variant).

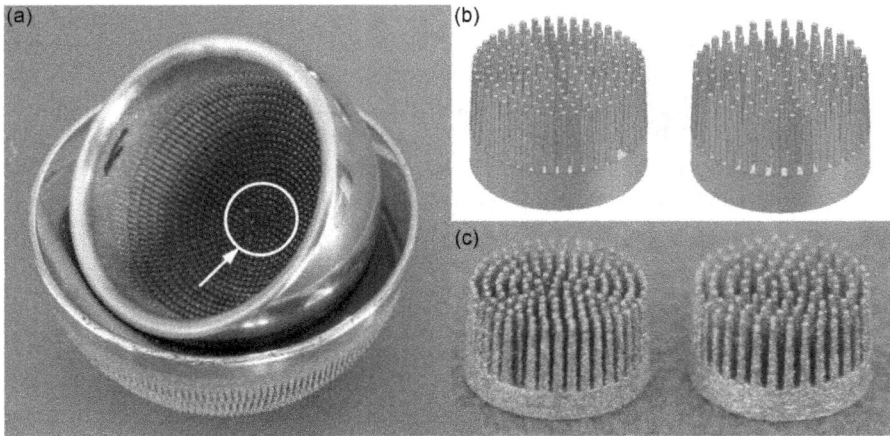

FIGURE 5.5 A prototype of an entirely cementless resurfacing hip joint endoprosthesis with MSC-Scaffold manufactured in the SLM technology from Ti-6Al-4V powder (a). CAD models of the MSC-Scaffold preprototypes for resurfacing endoprostheses designed in two variants of geometric configuration, which differ in the distance between the bases of the spikes, 200 μm (P_{Sc200}) and 350 μm (P_{Sc350}), both circumferentially and radially (b), and the preprototypes produced based on these CAD models in the SLM technology (c).

The preprototypes were weighed using an analytical balance AS 110/X (Radwag, Poland) and then modified with Autolab PGSTAT302N (Metrohm Autolab B.V., The Netherlands). Electric potential values in the range of −9 to −3 V have been examined. The composition of the solution used in the ECD process was identical to that presented in Section 5.1. The composition of the SBF was also not changed. After incubation in SBF, the MSC-Scaffold preprototypes were dried at room temperature and weighed again. The mass growth caused by the deposition of CaP layer preprototypes on the surface of the spikes was calculated as the difference between the initial mass (before modification) and the final mass (after modification). Analysis of the chemical composition of the coating deposited on the lateral surface of preprototype spikes was carried out using the Hitachi TM-3030 scanning electron microscope (Hitachi High-Tech Technologies Europe GmbH, Krefeld, Germany) equipped with EDS spectrometer (Oxford Instruments, Abingdon, United Kingdom).

Subsequently, electric potential values, for which the largest increase in the mass of the preprototypes was recorded with the molar Ca/P ratio in the coating corresponding to the native bone hydroxyapatite, were used during the cathodic deposition process to modify the new series of MSC-Scaffold preprototypes. A total of 36 MSC-Scaffold preprototypes were modified, 12 for each selected electric potential value considered preferred.

To investigate the effect of pretreatment on the final surface modification effect for half of the preprototypes, an acid-alkali treatment (AAT) was applied in a 40% sulphuric acid (H_2SO_4) solution for 40 minutes at 60°C and then in a 1 mol/l sodium hydroxide solution (NaOH) for 40 minutes at 80°C.

To create elemental maps showing the distribution of elements on the lateral surface of the spikes, an EDS mapping of the surface composition was performed on three randomly selected lateral subareas of the lateral spike surfaces of each of the modified preprototypes. Based on the analysis of the mapping results, we have indicated the regions with a CaP coating deposited on the lateral surface of the spikes, as well as the degree of coverage of the lateral surface of the spikes. In each of the analysed subareas, we made 10-point measurements of the chemical composition and calculated the molar Ca/P ratios. The analysis of the degree of coverage of the lateral surface of the spikes and the homogeneity of the deposited coating was performed using a professional ImageJ software tool (National Institutes of Health, Bethesda, MD, USA).

The X-ray Powder Diffraction (XRD) test was performed on the PANalytical EMPYREAN diffractometer (Malvern, UK) at a scanning speed of 0.02/s in the Cu Kα radiation ($\lambda = 0.15405$ nm, 40 mA, 40 kV) in the range of 2θ 30–70. Because it was not technically possible to directly analyse the surface of the MSC-Scaffold preprototypes, it was necessary to use mechanically separated micro-fragments of the coating from the surface of the spikes as a powder sample to perform the test.

Figure 5.6 presents a graph of the increase in mass caused by the deposition of a CaP layer on the lateral surface of the spikes of the MSC-Scaffold preprototypes for both modified variants of the spike configuration in P_{Sc200} and P_{Sc350} MSC-Scaffold preprototypes, depending on the electric potential values used in the ECD process.

In the case of the P_{Sc200} MSC-Scaffold preprototypes modified using electric potential values in the range of −9 to −5.25 V, mass growth was approximately 3 mg

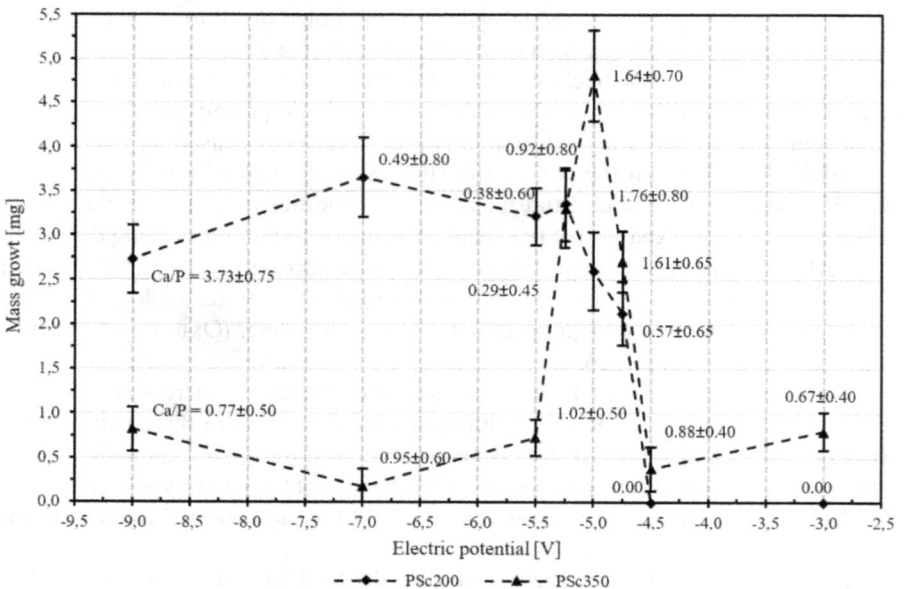

FIGURE 5.6 Graphs of the increase in mass caused by the deposition of the CaP layer on the lateral surface of the spikes of the P_{Sc200} and P_{Sc350} MSC-Scaffold preprototypes, depending on the electric potential values used in the ECD process.

(from 2.75 mg for a potential equal to −9 V to 3.65 mg for a potential equal to −7 V). An increase in the electric potential value above −5.25 V resulted in a decrease in the mass growth of the deposited coating to 2 mg (for a potential equal to −4.75 V), while for a potential equal to −4.5 V and a potential equal to −3 V, no mass growth was recorded. An EDS analysis of the chemical composition has proven the absence of Ca and P on the lateral surface of spikes of the MSC-Scaffold preprototypes modified with the applied electric potential values of −4.5 V and −3 V. SEM analysis has indicated that in the case of the P_{Sc200} MSC-Scaffold preprototypes, for which mass growth was observed, the CaP layer was deposited only in the upper areas of the spikes. In this case, a significant amount of CaP deposit was found, which was located in the interspike space of the MSC-Scaffold preprototypes. This phenomenon was considered unfavourable. An example of SEM documentation showing this effect is presented in Figure 5.7. None of the molar ratios of Ca/P determined for the lateral surface of the spikes in the P_{Sc200} MSC-Scaffold preprototypes corresponds to the molar ratio of Ca/P in the native bone hydroxyapatite. The EDS analysis indicates that the molar Ca/P ratios reached values below 1.00 and 3.73, so in this case, it was not possible to detect any deposition of a CaP coating on the surface of the spikes, but we have detected only Ca and P ions accidentally deposited on the surface of the spikes. In the first case, almost only Ca was found on the surface of the spikes, while in the second case almost all surface sediments were identified as P. With an electric potential of −4.5 V, no mass growth was observed in the preprototypes.

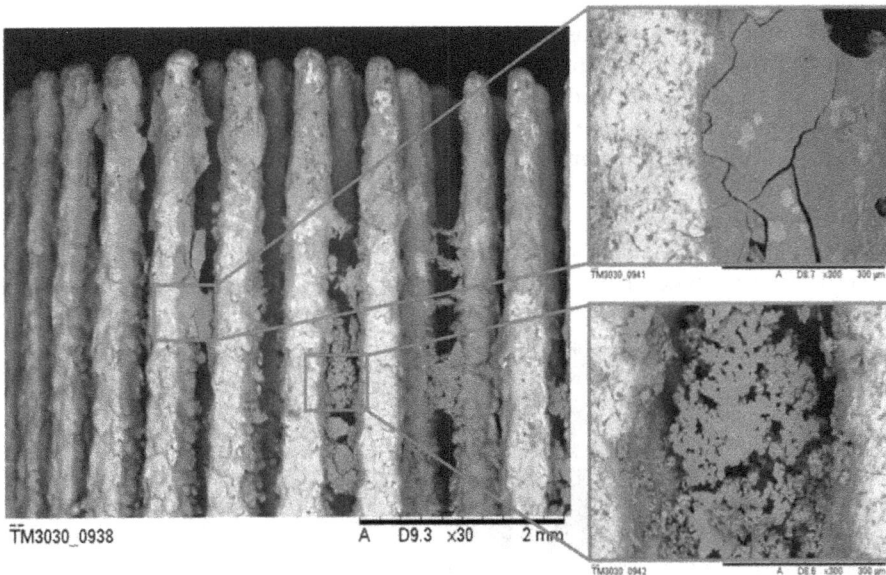

FIGURE 5.7 Sample SEM images showing the undesirable effect of CaP deposit formation in the space between the spikes of the P_{Sc200} MSC-Scaffold preprototypes; magnification: 30× and 300×.

Example elemental maps of the two areas of the MSC-Scaffold enlarged in Figure 5.7 are shown in Figure 5.8. According to the presented elemental maps, the colours reflecting elements derived from the preprototype material, such as Ti, V, and Al, are located on the lateral surface of the spikes (similarly to O, which is not shown), while Ca and P are arranged only as deposits in the space between the spikes. This phenomenon can be explained by referring to the interspike distance. The MSC-Scaffold preprototypes designed in this variant, characterized by a distance between the spike bases equal to approximately 200 μm, do not provide sufficient space between the spikes to lead to the deposition of a CaP coating on the surface of the MSC-Scaffold spikes during the potentiostatic ECD process. The unwanted result of the modification of the surface of the P_{Sc200} MSC-Scaffold preprototypes led us to decide to discontinue further research using this geometric variant of the MSC-Scaffold preprototype.

For the MSC-Scaffold preprototypes designed in the P_{Sc350} MSC-Scaffold preprototype variant modified using electric potential in the range of −9 to −5.50 V, the mass growth of the deposited coating was small (less than 1 mg), and the values of the molar Ca/P ratios determined by the EDS method for these coatings do not correspond to the values of the molar Ca/P ratio characteristic for native bone CaP. A significant increase in the mass of the deposited coatings (approximately 5 mg) was found using electric potential values in the range from −5.25 to −4.75 V. In the case of the ECD process carried out at electric potential values above −4.50 V, a slight increase in mass was observed (approximately 0.50–0.75 mg). Unfortunately, the values of the Ca/P molar ratios in the deposited CaP coating did not correspond to the characteristic values of the Ca/P molar ratio for the CaP of native bone. EDS analysis of the surface composition of all MSC-Scaffold preprototypes in the modified P_{Sc350} MSC-Scaffold preprototype variant using the electric potential of −5.25, −5.00, and −4.75 V confirmed the presence of CaP with Ca/P molar ratios consistent with Ca/P for native bone HA. Therefore, electric potential values ranging from −5.25 to −4.75 V may be recommended as the most suitable conditions for CaP modification of the P_{Sc350} MSC-Scaffold preprototypes using ECD carried out at constant electric potential values.

Figure 5.9 shows the dependence of the average mass growth of the P_{Sc350} MSC-Scaffold preprototypes modified at a constant electric potential value of −5.25,

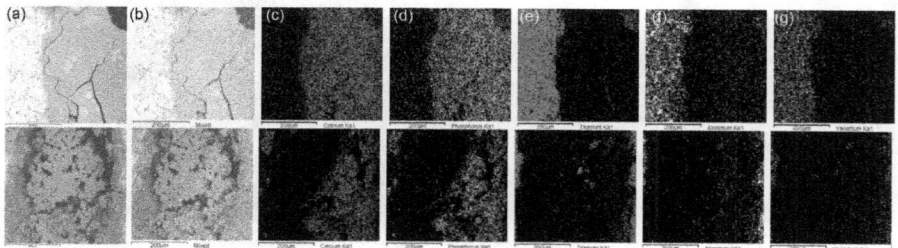

FIGURE 5.8 Documentation of EDS mapping of the surface of the two enlarged areas of the MSC-Scaffold P_{Sc200} in Figure 5.7: (a) SEM images, (b) CaP maps, (c) Ca maps, (d) P maps, (e) Ti maps, (f) Al maps, and (g) V maps.

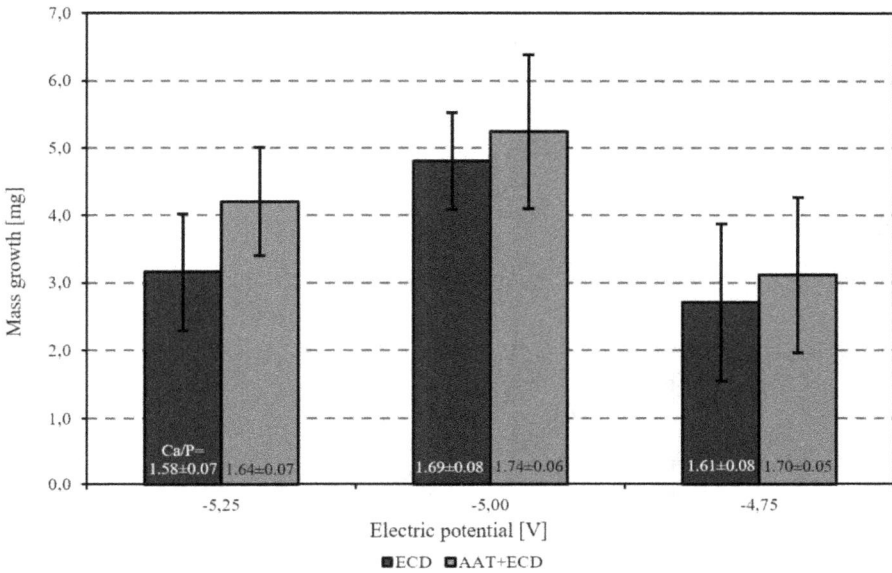

FIGURE 5.9   The mean mass growth of the P_{Sc350} MSC-Scaffold preprototypes depends on the applied electric potential values of the modification performed by electrochemical cathodic deposition with acid-alkali treatment (ECD + AAT) and without such treatment (ECD).

−5.00, and −4.75 V. The mass growth was determined for both preprototypes subjected to AAT and those that were not subjected to such treatment.

In both tested cases, the largest average mass growth of the modified P_{Sc350} MSC-Scaffold preprototypes was obtained for the electric potential of −5.00 V. The diagram presented in Figure 5.9 shows that the initial AAT affects the mass increase of the deposited CaP coating (by 44% for the electric potential of −5.25 V, by 9% for the electric potential of −5.00 V, and by 15% for the electric potential of −4.75 V).

Figure 5.10 shows the SEM documentation of the lateral surface of the P_{Sc350} MSC-Scaffold spike preprototypes modified by a 1-hour ECD process carried out at constant electric potential values of −5.25, −5.00, and −4.75 V and subsequent incubation for 48 hours in SBF, without initial AAT (Figures 5.10a–c) and with initial AAT (Figures 5.10d–f).

The SEM analysis of the lateral surface of the spikes showed that the CaP coating obtained during the modification not preceded by the initial AAT is heterogeneous and seems to be unstable (with reduced adhesion strength). In the case of the MSC-Scaffold preprototypes, whose lateral spike surfaces was modified with the electric potential value of −5.25 V, most of the lateral surface of the spikes in their central part remained uncovered. The cover was deposited mainly on the upper part of the spikes. In the case of other preprototypes (modified using an electric potential of −5.00 and −4.75 V), the entire lateral surface of the spikes was coated with CaP, but numerous microcracks were observed, especially for the modification process carried out with an electric potential of −5.00 V.

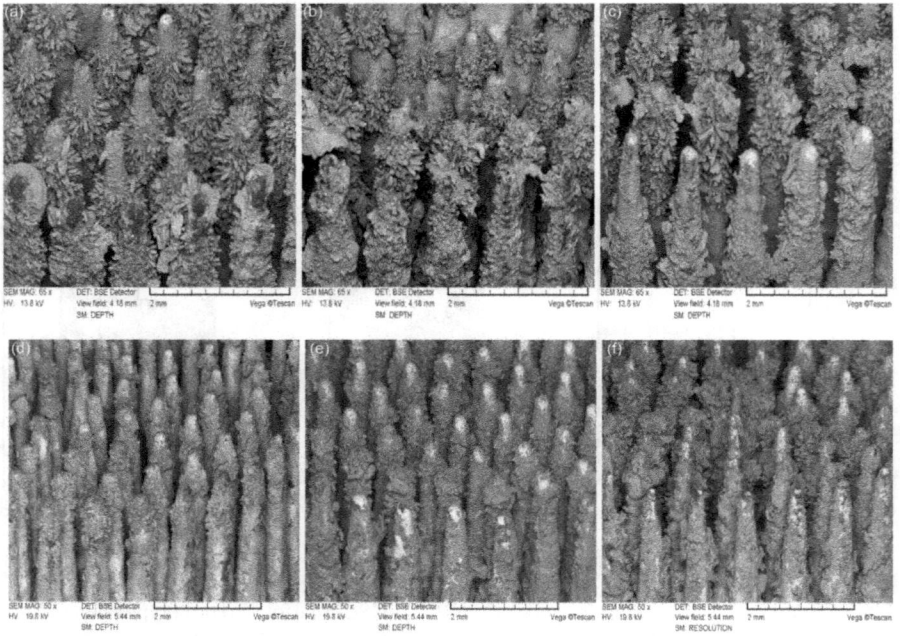

FIGURE 5.10   SEM documentation of the lateral surface of the spikes of the MSC-Scaffold preprototypes modified in a 1-hour ECD process conducted at constant electric potential values of: (a) −5.25 V, (b) −5.00 V, and (c) −4.75 V, and after 48 h of incubation in SBF without AAT and, respectively (d–f), with AAT.

As can be seen in the SEM images shown in Figures 5.10d–f, the application of the initial AAT increased homogeneity (no microcracks on the surface of the spikes) and the degree of covering the surface of the spikes with a CaP coating deposited with all tested electric potential values of the potentiostatic ECD process. Needle and plate crystals of CaP appear on the lateral surface of the preprototypes of the MSC-Scaffold.

In particular, a significant accumulation of such crystals can be observed in the upper part of the MSC-Scaffold spikes (Figures 5.10a–c).

The EDS analysis shows that the Ca/P molar ratios on the lateral surface of the spikes ranged from 1.58 to 1.74, which is consistent with the values of the Ca/P molar ratio of native bone hydroxyapatite. The graph in Figure 5.11 presents the dependence of the degree of coverage of the lateral spike surfaces of the P_{Sc350} preprototypes of the MSC-Scaffold with the CaP layer deposited after a 1-hour ECD process carried out at constant electric potential values of −5.25, −5.00, and −4.75 V and subsequent immersion in SBF for 48 h, with and without pretreatment, on the applied values of electric potential during the ECD process. Figure 5.12 shows examples of elemental maps of lateral spike surfaces in preprototypes of the MSC-Scaffold. Examples of elemental maps relate to the preprototypes presented in Figure 5.10.

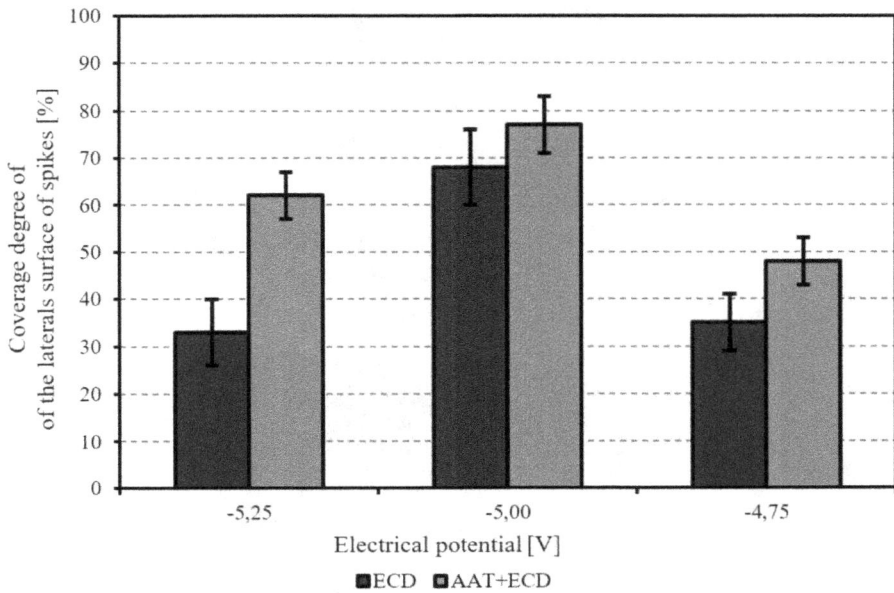

FIGURE 5.11 The degree of coverage of the lateral surface of the MSC-Scaffold P_{Sc350} preprototypes with CaP coating deposited after 1-hour of modification by ECD at constant electric potential values of −5.25, −5.00, and −4.75 V and subsequent 48 h of incubation in SBF, with acid-alkali treatment (ECD + AAT) and without acid-alkali treatment (ECD), depending on the electric potential value used.

The results of EDS mapping for the modified lateral surface of the MSC-Scaffold spikes and the quantitative analysis of the chemical composition carried out based on the obtained elemental maps show that the greatest degree of coverage of the lateral surface of spikes with the CaP layer was obtained for the P_{Sc350} MSC-Scaffold preprototypes modified with the electric potential of −5.00 V (on average 68 ± 6%). For other electric potential values, the degree of coverage of the lateral surface of the spikes was half (33 ± 5% to 35 ± 5%). The use of AAT increases the degree of coverage of the lateral surface of the spikes (40% for the electric potential of −5.25 V, 14% for the electric potential of −5.00 V, and 100% for the electric potential of −4.75 V).

To confirm that the CaP layer deposited on the lateral surface of the spikes obtained in the process of modification with a constant electric potential value of −5.00 V is in crystalline form, we have carried out an analysis of the crystalline structure and phase composition of the surface using the X-ray diffraction (XRD) method. The results are shown in Figure 5.13.

As can be seen from the diffractogram presented in Figure 5.13, the CaP coating obtained is multiphase. Angular positions of diffraction reflections assigned to such phases as octa-calcium phosphate – $Ca_8H_2(PO_4)_6 \cdot 5H_2O$ (according to PDF2 #00–026–1056), calcium metaphosphate – $Ca(PO_3)_2$ (according to PDF2 #00–003–0348), and hydrated calcium dihydrogen phosphate – $Ca(H_2PO_4)_2 \cdot H_2O$ (according

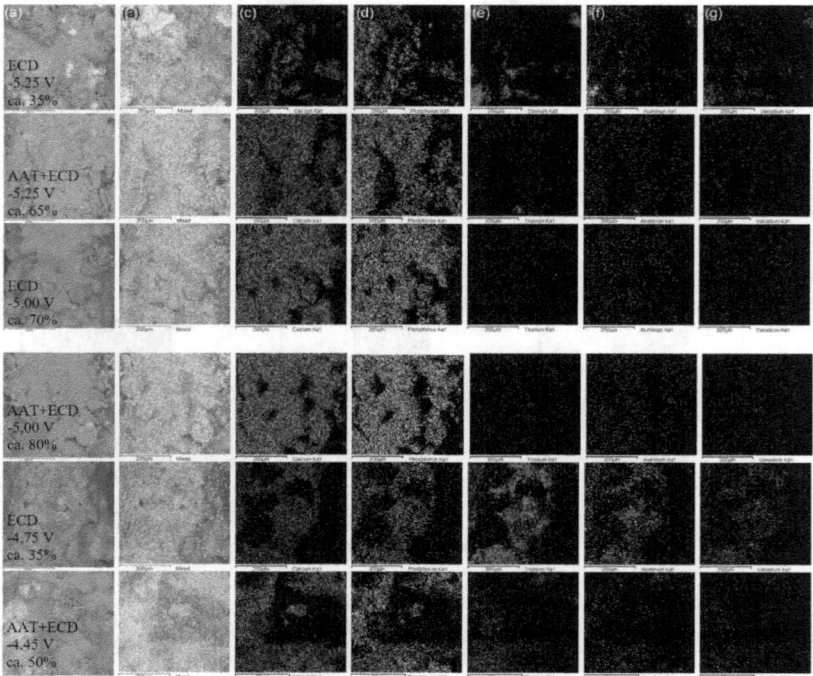

FIGURE 5.12 Example results of EDS mapping of the lateral surface of the spikes of the MSC-Scaffold preprototypes corresponding to the variants of the modification carried out presented in Figure 5.10: (a) SEM pictures, (b) CaP maps, (c) Ca maps, (d) P maps, (e) Ti maps, (f) Al maps, and (g) V maps.

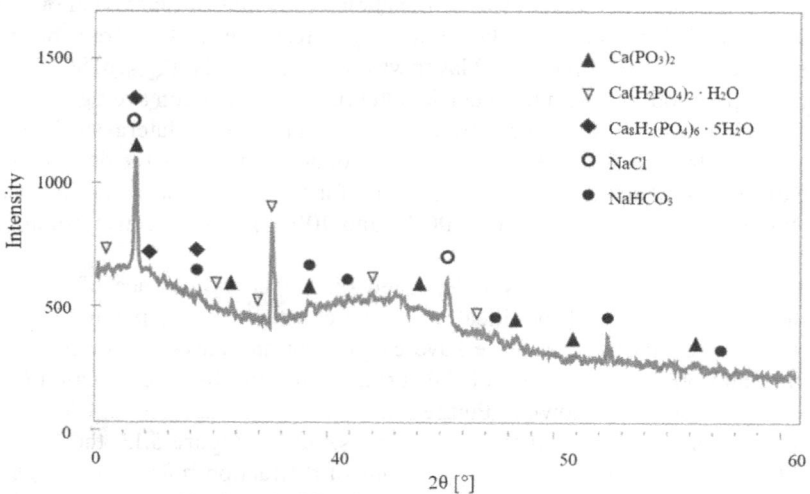

FIGURE 5.13 XRD diffractogram of the lateral surface of the spikes of the MSC-Scaffold preprototype coated with a CaP layer in the ECD process carried out at a constant electric potential of −5.00 V, followed by immersion for 48 h in SBF.

to PDF2 #00–003–0284) were identified. In addition, impurities from the SBF solution in the form of sodium chloride – NaCl (according to PDF2 #01–077–2064) and sodium bicarbonate – $NaHCO_3$ (according to PDF2 #00–021–119) were found on the surface. The results of XRD tests showed that during the ECD process combined with subsequent incubation in SBF carried out under certain conditions, a multi-phase biomineral CaP coating is formed on the lateral surface of the spikes of the MSC-Scaffold.

5.3   EVALUATION IN HUMAN OSTEOBLASTS CULTURE OF THE PROTOTYPE MULTI-SPIKED CONNECTING SCAFFOLD WITH CALCIUM PHOSPHATE-MODIFIED BONE-CONTACTING SURFACE

Study in human osteoblasts cultures of the MSC-Scaffold preprototypes (unmodi-fied and with a CaP-modified surface) evaluated the proliferation of cells around the spikes and the enzymatic activity of alkaline phosphatase (ALP). The alkaline phosphatase enzyme is considered one of the first key factors in the osteogenesis and mineralization of bone tissue, as one of the molecular parameters of osteoblasts dif-ferentiation is the collagen synthesis process and the alkaline phosphatase activity.

Human osteoblasts (U-2 OS cell line) were purchased from American Type Cell Culture (ATCC, Manassas, MA, USA) and cultured in modified McCoy 5A medium (Sigma-Aldrich, St. Louis, MO, USA) supplemented with 10% foetal calf serum (FCS; Sigma, St. Louis, MO, USA), 2 mmol/l L-glutamine (Cambrex, Charles City, IA, USA), 100 IU/ml penicillin, and streptomycin solution (Sigma, St. Louis, MO, USA) in a humidified atmosphere of 5% CO_2 at 37°C. 2×10^4 cells were seeded on an unmodified and CaP-modified surface of the P_{Sc350} MSC-Scaffold preprototypes placed in 12-well culture plates and incubated for up to five days in a humid culture medium (37°C, 5% CO_2) to allow cells to attach to the surface. Subsequently, U-2 OS cells were stained with 0.1 µg/ml Hoechst 33342 and 0.125 µg/ml propidine iodide solution (Sigma-Aldrich, St. Louis, MO, USA). The presence of intact (live), apop-totic, and/or necrotic cells was evaluated using the Zeiss LSM 780 confocal micro-scope (Jena, Germany). Excitation signals with wavelengths of 345 and 543 nm were used and fluorescence emission was selected using 460 and 560 nm bandpass filters.

The human bone cell line (MG63) was provided by ATCC (USA), and cells were cultured for ten days in Eagle's minimal essential medium (EMEM) (Sigma-Aldrich, St. Louis, MO, USA) with the addition of 10% foetal bovine serum (FBS, Sigma-Aldrich, St. Louis, MO, USA) and solutions of 1% streptomycin and penicillin. The activity of alkaline phosphatase (ALP) was then measured using a colorimetric test (Alkaline Phosphatase Assay Kit, Abcam, Cambridge, UK). First, the EMEM medium was removed from the culture and the washed cells (1×10^5) were homogenized in the test buffer and centrifuged for three min. Then, all samples of the MSC-Scaffold prototype (unmodified P_{Sc200}, P_{Sc350}, and surface-modified with the CaP layer P_{Sc350}) were placed in a 48-well microplate with the addition of 80 µl of test buffer. Then 50 µl of 5 mM p-nitrophenyl phosphate (pNPP) was added to each well containing the test samples and to the control wells (reference wells) as an enzyme-substrate solution. The plates were then stirred in an orbital shaker for five minutes and incubated for 60 minutes at 25°C, protecting them from daylight. 10 µl of the ALP enzyme solution was added to each well containing the pNPP standard and mixed. The main reaction between the enzyme and the substrate was stopped by adding 20 µl of retention solution to each test and well containing the standard. The whole plate was gently shaken and then alkaline phosphatase activity was measured at 405 nm in a Tecan microplate colorimetric reader (Tecan Group Ltd., Männedorf, Switzerland).

Figure 5.14 shows the results of the five-day osteoblasts culture on an unmodified surface and a CaP-modified surface of the P_{Sc350} preprototypes of the MSC-Scaffold. Numerous proliferating osteoblast cells are visible in the space between spikes of the PSc350 MSC-Scaffold with CaP-modified spikes.

As demonstrated in Figure 5.14, a few cells attached to the unmodified surface of the P_{Sc350} preprototype of the MSC-Scaffold were observed (Figure 5.14a). On the surface of the MSC-Scaffold modified with a CaP layer, bone cells focused around the spikes, creating a large cellular network (Figure 5.14b). Due to the use of higher magnification, a large number of cells attached to the surface were observed to be intact (blue colour, Figure 5.14c), with no signs of DNA fragmentation (no apoptotic cells were detected). However, necrotic cells were also observed (red, Figure 5.14c).

The diagram in Figure 5.15 shows the activity of the enzyme alkaline phosphatase as a function of the incubation time in the culture of human bone cell lines for the variants tested from the MSC-Scaffold preprototypes.

For all variants of MSC-Scaffold preprototypes subject to testing, in the culture of human bone cell lines, the measured alkaline phosphatase activity increases in proportion to the incubation time of the sample. The alkaline phosphatase activity values for the P_{Sc200} MSC-Scaffold preprototypes with densely spaced spikes (approximately 200 µm) are significantly lower than the alkaline phosphatase activity values for the P_{Sc350} preprototypes with less densely spaced spikes (approximately 350 µm). For the CaP-modified surface of the MSC-Scaffold preprototypes, alkaline phosphatase activity increases more rapidly over time compared to the preprototypes with an unmodified surface, and after 48 hours of incubation, the alkaline phosphatase

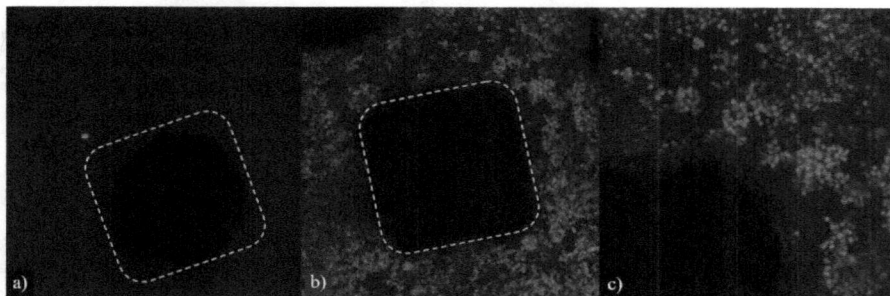

FIGURE 5.14 Microphotographs showing a fragment of the interspike space of the P_{Sc350} MSC-Scaffold after five days of osteoblasts cultivation, after staining with Hoechst 33342 dye and propidium iodide. Fragment of the unmodified surface (a) and surface modified with CaP layer P_{Sc350} shown from the perspective of the spike tips; a magnification of 10× (b) and a magnification of 20× (c); the dashed line shows the contour of the spike base of the tested MSC-Scaffold preprototypes.

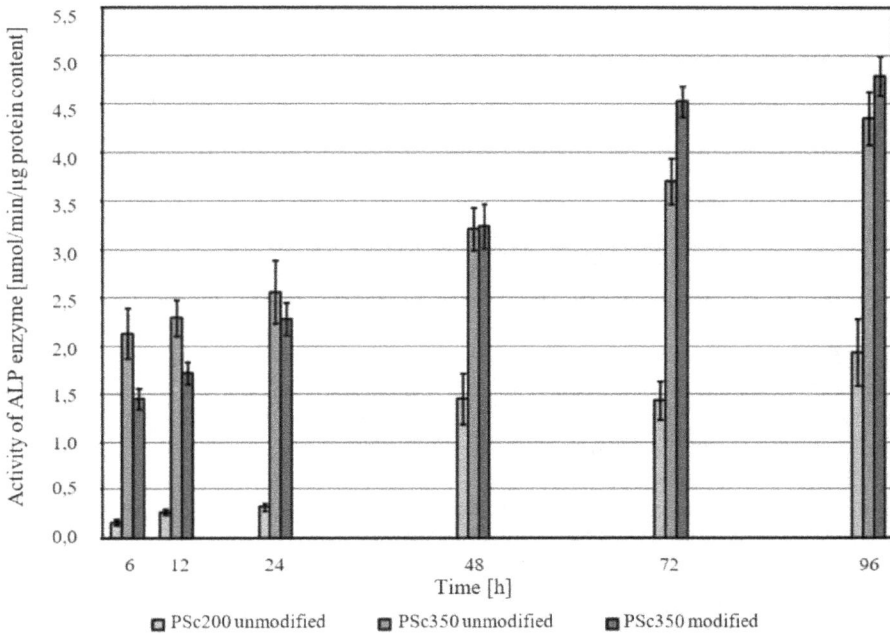

FIGURE 5.15   The activity of the enzyme alkaline phosphatase as a function of incubation time in the culture of human bone cell lines for the tested variants of the preprototypes of the MSC-Scaffold: P_{Sc200} with an unmodified lateral spike surfaces, P_{Sc350} with an unmodified lateral spike surfaces, and P_{Sc350} with a CaP-modified lateral spike surfaces.

activity for the CaP-modified surface of the MSC-Scaffold preprototypes exceeds the alkaline phosphatase activity for the unmodified preprototypes. Furthermore, modification of the lateral spike surfaces with a CaP layer did not show cytotoxicity to the MG63 cell line used in the study.

The research conducted shows that the factor that has a large impact on the activity of alkaline phosphatase (and thus on mineralization) is the appropriate distance between the spikes of the MSC-Scaffold. Modification with a CaP layer on the surface of the spikes is beneficial for bone cell proliferation and alkaline phosphatase activity, and thus for the bioprocess of mineralization of the organic bone matrix.

A biological study in human osteoblasts culture was carried out on structural variants of the MSC-Scaffold preprototypes, where the distances between the bases of the spikes were differentiated: 200 μm (P_{Sc200}) and 350 μm (P_{Sc350}), both radially and circumferentially, indicate the need to verify the construction guidelines for the MSC-Scaffold in the areas of its interspike space within the edges of the bases of the spikes. It is necessary to provide more space for the new bone ingrowth into the interspike region of the MSC-Scaffold.

The low activity of alkaline phosphatase for the P_{Sc200} preprototypes observed in the culture of human bone cells together with the previous negative result of the CaP modification of the lateral spike surfaces of these MSC-Scaffold preprototypes by ECD carried out at constant electric potential values disqualifies this structural variant of the MSC-Scaffold preprototype from further research. Thus, it has been proven that the rational justification is to increase the distance between the edges of the spikes to 350 μm, both peripherally and radially, in the prototype MSC-Scaffold for resurfacing arthroplasty endoprostheses.

5.4 BIOINTEGRATION OF THE PROTOTYPE MULTI-SPIKED CONNECTING SCAFFOLD WITH CALCIUM PHOSPHATE COATING IMPLANTED IN SWINE KNEE *IN VIVO*

In order to comparatively test the effects of biointegration between bone and surface of the MSC-Scaffold preprototypes with the unmodified surface of spikes and with CaP-modified surface of spikes, we have carried out pilot implantations of the above-mentioned preprototypes in swine (Polish Large White breed). The preprototypes were implanted (in a veterinary clinic with the consent of the Local Ethics Committee in Poznan) in the knee joints of experimental animals. Biointegration of MSC-Scaffold preprototypes with bone tissue was evaluated eight weeks after implantation.

The animals for the treatment were selected by a certified butcher 8–12 weeks before the planned slaughter by the breeder; 24 hours before treatment, the swines were starved by restricting access to food, but access to water was free. Access to water was restricted 12 hours before the procedure. In the operating block of the veterinary clinic, the animals operated received premedication: atropine sulphate (0.2 mg/kg intramuscularly) and xylazine hydrochloride (0.25 mg/kg i.v.). Then, the animals were shaved locally and the operated area was prepared. In the operating room, the animal skin was also anaesthetized in the operating area with 2% lidocaine.

During surgical implantation of the MSC-Scaffold preprototypes, inhaled general anaesthesia with endotracheal intubation and anaesthetic monitoring was used – induction of anaesthesia: Cepetor (0.01–0.04 mg/kg b.w.); anaesthesia was maintained by inhalation using an inhaler using Isoflurane with pulse oximetric control and cardiac monitoring with the Dräger AT-1 cardio monitor (Drägerwerk AG & Co. KGaA, Lubeck, Germany); premedication, administered once intramuscularly (in the same syringe): Cepetor (0.02–0.04 mg/kg b.w., i.m.) and Levomethadone (0.25–0.5 mg/kg b.w., i.m.). General anaesthesia was induced by ketamine hydrochloride (30 mg/kg b.w., i.v.). Sodium metamizole (30 mg/kg b.w., i.v.) and infusion fluids were also administered as painkillers.

A medial peripatellar approach was used to the knee joint of the swine. An anteromedial skin incision was made, with a length of approximately 20 cm above the operated joint of the right knee. We have used an approach to the knee joint going between the lateral edge of the patella and the outer edge of the patellar ligament, and then between the vastus lateralis and the rectus femoris. The joint capsule was opened on the side of the patella, and then the patella was displaced centrally. The bleeding was stopped (haemostasis). The patellofemoral area of the knee joint was exposed. Implantation sites in both femoral condyles were prepared using a surgical drill. The holes in the subchondral bone in which the implant was placed were gradually widened with a cutter to the final size. During drilling and milling, the bone holes were continuously irrigated with saline. The holes in the femoral condyles were flushed with saline and the bone chips were removed. Two preprototypes (i.e. unmodified and modified with a CaP layer) of the MSC-Scaffold for entirely non-cemented resurfacing arthroplasty endoprostheses were placed under the surface of the articular cartilage of the medial and lateral femoral condyle of the knee joint of the swine. Implants embedded in the bone holes of the femoral condyle were performed with a surgical mallet. The patella was replicated to the anatomical position. A layered wound suture was applied. After implantation, an antibiotic regimen was introduced: at the end of the procedure, penicillin powder was applied to the subcutaneous layer, the wound was covered with a penicillin-saturated mesh, and an antiseptic dressing was applied. After the procedure: Amikacin (Biodacin) 1 g two times a day was administered i.v. (or i.m.) for three days. On the third day after the operation, the swine was allowed to fully load the operated limb.

Eight weeks after implantation in the operating room of the veterinary clinic (following the protocol approved by the Local Ethics Committee in Poznan), surgical collection of operated joints with implants (premedication and general anaesthesia as during implantation) was performed. Treatment was completed with euthanasia of animals using Morbital (Pentobarbital sodium) at lethal doses of 200 mg/kg b.w., i.v., following a protocol approved by the Local Ethics Committee in Poznan. The explanted knee joints were subjected to radiological examinations (2D Digital Specimen Radiography System, XPERT 40, Kubtec, Milford, CT, USA).

Microtomographic examination of the harvested knee joints was carried out using the SkyScan 1173 high-energy microtomographic scanner (Bruker, Kontich, Belgium). The specimens of the knee joints harvested immersed in formalin were placed on a rotating table and scanned entirely according to the following parameters: source voltage 130 keV, source current: 61 μA, resolution: 9.92 μm, filter: brass 0.25 mm, exposure time: 4,000 ms, rotation: 360°, every 0.2°, scan time: about 6 hours. 3D visualization and 2D image analysis of digitally reconstructed knee microtomography and implants were performed using SkyScan CT-Analyzer software (Bruker, Kontich, Belgium). Radiographic density 3D images of bone-implant specimens have been reconstructed using microcomputed tomography to highlight areas that have been identified as implants (the MSC-Scaffold made of a titanium alloy), bone tissue (bone trabeculae), and soft tissues, including bone marrow. On the eight reference planes designated perpendicular to the axis of the MSC-Scaffold spikes below the tops of these spikes, spaced 0.5 mm apart in the area between the MSC-Scaffold spikes, the shares of bone beams around the unmodified and modified MSC-Scaffold spikes with a CaP layer were calculated and compared.

After explantation, the specimens of the harvested knee joints of the operated swine were fixed for seven days in 10% formalin (formaldehyde in phosphate buffer) at pH 7.25, and then dehydrated in various concentrations of ethanol (70%, 80%, 90%, 99%, 99.8%, and 99.8% v/v) for two days at each concentration and then immersed in resin. Thick slices (200 μm) were cut using the IsoMet™ 4000 Linear Precision Saw (Buehler, Esslingen am Neckar, Germany) and then hand sanded to a thickness of 20 μm using the MetaServ 250 grinder polisher (Buehler, Esslingen am Neckar,

Germany). The sections were stained with haematoxylin and eosin and examined under the Olympus CX41 light microscope (Olympus, Tokyo, Japan).

Figures 5.16–5.18 show example results of an experimental study of biointegration of a non-modified and CaP-modified surface of the P_{Sc350} MSC-Scaffold preprototypes carried out on an animal model. Figure 5.16a shows a specimen of the operated knee joint of a swine with two MSC-Scaffold preprototypes implanted surgically eight weeks after implantation. There was no damage to the femoral condyle in the surgically removed knee joint. Two implanted preprototypes showed good fixation without any signs of loosening. Figures 5.16b and 5.16c show 2D digital radiographs (XPERT 40, Kubtec, Milford, CT, USA) of the side and anteroposterior resected knee joint of the swine, respectively.

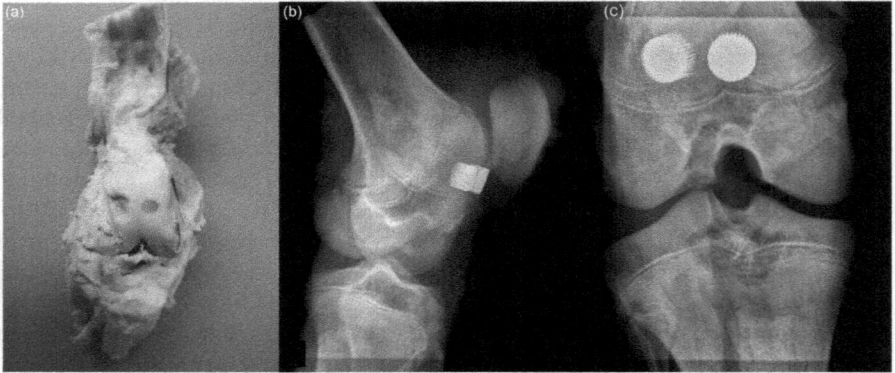

FIGURE 5.16　Swine knee specimen implanted with two MSC-Scaffold preprototypes surgically explanted eight weeks after implantation (a); lateral (b) and anteroposterior (c) digital 2D X-ray of the harvested knee joint of the operated swine.

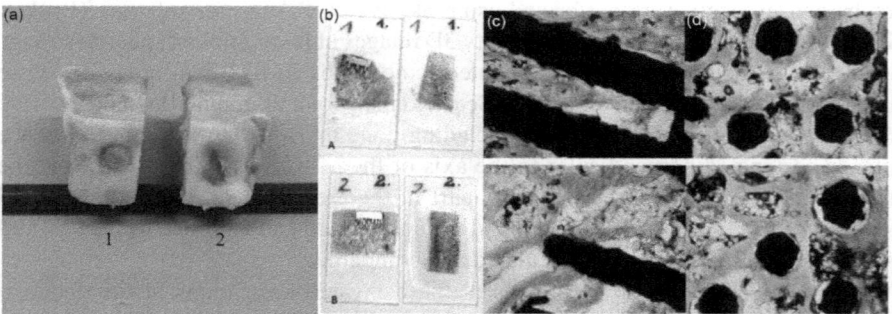

FIGURE 5.17　Specimens harvested eight weeks after implantation into the knee joint containing intraosseous implants with (a) an unmodified surface (1) and a CaP-modified surface of (2) the MSC-Scaffold preprototypes; example thin sections mounted on a microscope slide before staining (b); example histological images (H&E); cross sections for two in the longitudinal (c) and transverse (d) directions to the axis of the spikes.

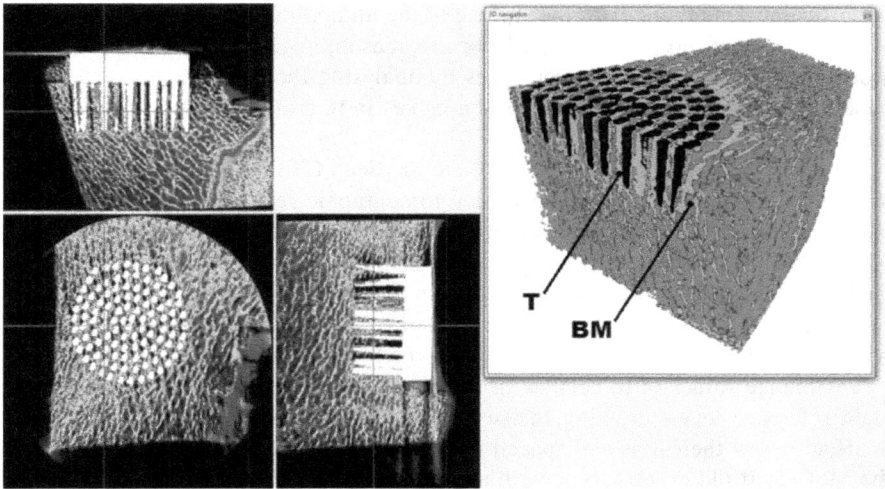

FIGURE 5.18   View of the window showing the 3D micro-CT reconstruction of the bone-implant specimen in projections on three perpendicular planes and an example 3D view of the MSC-Scaffold with the unmodified surface of the spikes, distinguishing between elements such as: implant (black), trabeculae (T), and bone marrow (BM).

Clinical and radiological examination confirmed the very good stability of the knee joint and the lack of implant migration and showed that the spaces between the spikes of both implanted MSC-Scaffold preprototypes are occupied with the ingrown bone tissue.

Figure 5.17a shows excised specimens containing intraosseous implants with an unmodified surface (1) and a CaP-modified surface (2) of the MSC-Scaffold pre-prototypes eight weeks after implantation into the knee joint, for example, thin sections (Figure 5.17b) mounted on a microscope slide before staining. Figures 5.17c and 5.17d show example histological images (H&E) taken eight weeks post-implantation surgery; cross sections for the two types of sections were made in the longitudinal and transverse direction to the axis of the spikes, respectively.

Based on the microscopic and histological assessment of bone-implant specimens excised from knee joint specimens harvested in operated swines eight weeks post-implantation, it was found that in the case of preprototypes of the MSC-Scaffold both unmodified (1) and modified with CaP layer (2), biointegration with bone occurred, as evidenced by the presence of bone trabeculae in the interspike spaces of the MSC-Scaffold in both the longitudinal and transverse sections of the bone-implant specimen (Figure 5.17).

Histological images (Figures 5.17c and 5.17d) showed trabecular bone tissue (purple) between the MSC-Scaffold spikes and soft tissue (connective tissue and bone marrow; white colour). Artefacts in the form of metal particles in the area of peri-implant tissue introduced during the process of grinding scraps are also visible. The microscopic observation of histological specimens in cross section does not allow for a satisfactory assessment of the differences between the osteointegration of periarticular bone tissue with the surface of the unmodified and modified CaP layer of the MSC-Scaffold preprototypes. For this reason, it was decided to quantify the osseointegration of these preprototypes by analysing the percentage of cancellous bone trabeculae in the area between the spikes in microtomographic bone-implant reconstructions.

Figure 5.18 shows a window view of the SkyScan CT analyser software (Bruker, Kontich, Belgium) with sample 3D microtomographic reconstruction sections of a bone-implant specimen harvested eight weeks after implantation into the knee joint of the MSC-Scaffold preprototypes. Figure 5.18 also shows an example 3D view of the bone-implant specimen that distinguishes areas identified by radiological density such as the titanium alloy MSC-Scaffold (marked in black), bone trabeculae (marked with the letter T), and the bone marrow (marked with the letters BM).

Percentage values of trabeculae in the area between the spikes at the designated eight reference levels crossing the perpendicular axes of the spikes of the MSC-Scaffold below their tops and spaced 0.5 mm apart for bone specimens containing the MSC-Scaffold preprototype with an unmodified surface and CaP-modified surface are given in Table 5.2.

Based on the results presented in Table 5.2 a higher percentage of bone trabeculae can be found in the space between the spikes of the MSC-Scaffold with the CaP-modified bone-contacting surface. The average increase in the percentage of bone trabeculae between the spikes as a result of the modification of the surface of the spikes with the CaP layer is $12.0 \pm 2.0\%$, which indicates the possibility of improving

---

TABLE 5.2

Percentage of bone trabeculae in the interspike space of explanted bone specimens containing the preprototype of the MSC-Scaffold on the unmodified surface and the modified CaP coating on the bone-contacting surface of the MSC-Scaffold

Reference Level	Trabeculae (%) (Non-modified)	Trabeculae (%) (Ca-P Modified)	The Relative Difference (%)
Level 1	61.99	68.66	10.8
Level 2	60.37	68.79	13.9
Level 3	61.41	66.56	8.4
Level 4	56.82	64.02	12.7
Level 5	55.51	62.32	12.3
Level 6	52.77	59.83	13.4
Level 7	50.97	57.41	12.6
Level 8	53.70	58.75	9.4
		Mean ± SD	12 ± 2

The eight reference levels are eight planes perpendicularly crossing the axes of the MSC-Scaffold spikes below their tops, spaced 0.5 mm apart from the top of the tops to the base of the spikes.

the osteoinduction and osseointegration potential of the prototype MSC-Scaffold by modifying the lateral surface of its spikes with the CaP coating.

REFERENCES

1. Tokłowicz, R. Calcium-phosphate thermo-electrochemical surface modification of Multi-Spiked Connecting Scaffold for prototype RA endoprosthesis. (In Polish: Wapniowo-fosforanowa modyfikacja termiczno-elektrochemiczna wieloszpilkowej powierzchni dokostnej skafoldu łączącego dla prototypowej endoprotezy typu RA stawu biodrowego). PhD Thesis, Poznan University of Technology, Poznan 2018.
2. Uklejewski, R.; Rogala, P.; Winiecki, M.; Tokłowicz, R.; Ruszkowski, P.; Wołuń-Cholewa, M. Biomimetic multispiked connecting Ti-alloy scaffold prototype for entirely cementless resurfacing arthroplasty endoprostheses – exemplary results of implantation of the Ca-P surface modified scaffold prototypes in animal model and osteoblast culture evaluation. *Materials.* 2016; 9(7): 532. doi:10.3390/ma9070532
3. Uklejewski, R.; Winiecki, M.; Krawczyk, P.; Tokłowicz, R. Native Osseous CaP Biomineral coating on a biomimetic multi-spiked connecting scaffold prototype for cementless resurfacing arthroplasty achieved by combined electrochemical deposition. *Materials.* 2019; 12(23): 3994. doi:10.3390/ma12233994
4. Liu, X.; Chu, P.K.; Ding, C. Surface modification of titanium, titanium alloys, and related materials for biomedical applications. *Mater Sci Eng R Rep.* 2004; 7(3–4): 49–121. doi:10.1016/j.mser.2004.11.001
5. Eliaz, N.; Metoki, N. Calcium phosphate bioceramics: a review of their history, structure, properties, coating technologies and biomedical applications. *Materials.* 2017; 10(4): 334. doi:10.3390/ma10040334
6. Habraken, W.; Habibovic, P.; Epple, M.; Bohner, M. Calcium phosphates in biomedical applications: materials for the future? *Mater Today.* 2016; 19(2): 69–87. doi:10.1016/j.mattod.2015.10.008
7. Xie, C.; Lu, H.; Li, W.; Chen, F.M.; Zhao, Y.M. The use of calcium phosphate-based biomaterials in implant dentistry. *J Mater Sci Mater Med.* 2012; 23(3): 853–62. doi:10.1007/s10856-011-4535-9
8. Surmenev, R.A.; Surmeneva, M.A.; Ivanova, A.A. Significance of calcium phosphate coatings for the enhancement of new bone osteogenesis – a review. *Acta Biomater.* 2014; 10(2): 557–79. doi:10.1016/j.actbio.2013.10.036
9. Junker, R.; Dimakis, A.; Thoneick, M.; Jansen, J.A. Effects of implant surface coatings and composition on bone integration: a systematic review. *Clin Oral Implants Res.* 2009; 20 Suppl 4: 185–206. doi:10.1111/j.1600-0501.2009.01777.x
10. Shepperd, J.A.; Apthorp, H. A contemporary snapshot of the use of hydroxyapatite coating in orthopaedic surgery. *J Bone Joint Surg Br.* 2005; 87(8): 1046–9. doi:10.1302/0301-620X.87B8.16692
11. Dorozhkin, S.V. Calcium orthophosphate deposits: Preparation, properties and biomedical applications. *Mater Sci Eng C Mater Biol Appl.* 2015; 55: 272–326. doi: 10.1016/j.msec.2015.05.033
12. Sun, L.; Berndt, C.C.; Gross, K.A.; Kucuk, A. Material fundamentals and clinical performance of plasma-sprayed hydroxyapatite coatings: a review. *J Biomed Mater Res.* 2001; 58(5): 570–92. doi:10.1002/jbm.1056
13. Arias, J.L.; Mayor, M.B.; Pou, J.; Leng, Y.; León, B.; Pérez-Amor, M. Micro- and nano-testing of calcium phosphate coatings produced by pulsed laser deposition. *Biomaterials.* 2003; 24(20): 3403–8. doi:10.1016/s0142-9612(03)00202-3
14. Lee, K.W.; Bae, C.M.; Jung, J.Y.; Sim, G.B.; Rautray, T.R.; Lee, H.J.; Kwon, T.Y.; Kim, K.H. Surface characteristics and biological studies of hydroxyapatite coating by a new method. *J Biomed Mater Res B Appl Biomater.* 2011; 98(2): 395–407. doi:10.1002/jbm.b.31864

15. López, E.O.; Mello, A.; Sendão, H.; Costa, L.T.; Rossi, A.L.; Ospina, R.O.; Borghi, F.F.; Silva Filho, J.G.; Rossi, A.M. Growth of crystalline hydroxyapatite thin films at room temperature by tuning the energy of the RF-magnetron sputtering plasma. *ACS Appl Mater Interfaces.* 2013; 5(19): 9435–45. doi:10.1021/am4020007

16. Klyui, N.I.; Temchenko, V.P.; Gryshkov, A.P.; Dubok, V.A.; Shynkaruk, A.V.; Lyashenko, B.A.; Barynov, S.M. Properties of the hydroxyapatite coatings, obtained by gas-detonation deposition onto titanium substrates. *Funct Mater.* 2011; 18: 285–92.

17. Krupa, D.; Baszkiewicz, J.; Kozubowski, J.A.; Barcz, A.; Sobczak, J.W.; Biliński, A.; Lewandowska-Szumieł, M.; Rajchel, B. Effect of dual ion implantation of calcium and phosphorus on the properties of titanium. *Biomaterials.* 2005; 26(16): 2847–56. doi:10.1016/j.biomaterials.2004.08.015

18. Avila, I.; Pantchev, K.; Holopainen, J.; Ritala, M.; Tuukkanen, J. Adhesion and mechanical properties of nanocrystalline hydroxyapatite coating obtained by conversion of atomic layer-deposited calcium carbonate on titanium substrate. *J Mater Sci Mater Med.* 2018; 29(8): 111. doi:10.1007/s10856-018-6121-x

19. Zhao, J.M.; Park, W.U.; Hwang, K.H.; Lee, J.K.; Yoon, S.Y. Biomimetic deposition of hydroxyapatite by mixed acid treatment of titanium surface. *J Nanosci Nanotechnol.* 2015; 15(3): 2552–5. doi:10.1166/jnn.2015.10266

20. Duarte, L.T.; Biaggio, S.R.; Rocha-Filho, R.C.; Bocchi, N. Preparation and characterization of biomimetically and electrochemically deposited hydroxyapatite coatings on micro-arc oxidized Ti-13Nb-13Zr. *J Mater Sci Mater Med.* 2011; 22(7): 1663–70. doi:10.1007/s10856-011-4338-z

21. Bharati, S.; Sinha, M.K.; Basu, D. Hydroxyapatite coating by biomimetic method on titanium alloy using concentrated SBF. *Bull Mater Sci.* 2005; 28: 617–21.

22. Reiner, T.; Gotman, I. Biomimetic calcium phosphate coating on Ti wires versus flat substrates: structure and mechanism of formation. *J Mater Sci Mater Med.* 2010; 21(2): 515–23. doi:10.1007/s10856-009-3906-y

23. Valanezhad, A.; Tsuru, K.; Ishikawa, K. Fabrication of strongly attached hydroxyapatite coating on titanium by hydrothermal treatment of Ti-Zn-PO_4 coated titanium in CaCl2 solution. *J Mater Sci Mater Med.* 2015; 26(7): 212. doi:10.1007/s10856-015-5548-6

24. Wang, D.; Chen, C.; He, T.; Lei, T. Hydroxyapatite coating on Ti6Al4V alloy by a sol-gel method. *J Mater Sci Mater Med.* 2008; 19(6): 2281–6. doi:10.1007/s10856-007-3338-5

25. Hirai, S.; Nashinaka, K.; Shimakage, K. Hydroxyapatite coating on titanium substrate by the sol-gel process. *J Am Ceram Soc.* 2004; 87(1): 29–34. doi:10.1111/j.1151-2916.2004.tb19940.x

26. Zhang, Y.-Y.; Tao, J.; Pang, Y.-C.; Wang, W.; Wang, T. Electrochemical deposition of hydroxyapatite coatings on titanium. *Trans Nonferrous Met Soc China.* 2006; 16(3): 633–7. doi:10.1111/j.1151-2916.2004.tb19940.x

27. Lee, K.; Jeong, Y.-H.; Brantley, W.A.; Choe, H.-C. Surface characteristic of hydroxyapatite films deposited on anodized titanium by an electrochemical method. *Thin Solid Films.* 2013; 546: 185–8. doi:10.1016/j.tsf.2013.04.077

28. Vasilescu, C.; Drob, P.; Vasilescu, E.; Demetrescu, I.; Ionita, D.; Prodana, M.; Drob, S.I. Characterisation and corrosion resistance of the electrodeposited hydroxyapatite and bovine serum albumin/hydroxyapatite films on Ti-6Al-4V-1Zr alloy surface. *Corros Sci.* 2011; 53: 992–9. doi:10.1016/j.corsci.2010.11.033

29. Sridhar, T.M.; Eliaz, N.; Kamachi Mudali, U.; Baldev, R. Electrophoretic deposition of hydroxyapatite coatings and corrosion aspects of metallic implants. *Corros Rev.* 2002; 20(4–5): 255–93. doi:10.1515/CORRREV.2002.20.4-5.255

30. Eliaz, N.; Sridhar, T.M.; Kamachi Mudali, U.; Baldev, R. Electrochemical and electrophoretic deposition of hydroxyapatite for orthopaedic applications. *Surf Eng.* 2005; 21(3): 238–42. doi:10.1179/174329405X50091

31. Oriňáková, R.; Orinak, A.; Kupková, M.; Hrubovčáková, M.; Škantárová, L.; Morovská Turoňová, A.; Markušová Bučková, L.; Muhmann, C.; Arlinghaus, H.F. Study of electrochemical deposition and degradation of hydroxyapatite coated iron biomaterials. *Int J Electrochem Sci.* 2015; 10(1): 659–70.

32. Blackwood, D.J.; Seah, K.H.W. Electrochemical cathodic deposition of hydroxyapatite: Improvements in adhesion and crystallinity. *Mater Sci Eng C Mater Biol Appl.* 2009; 29: 1233–8. doi:10.1016/j.msec.2008.10.015

33. Geuli, O.; Metoki, N.; Eliaz, N.; Mandler, D. Electrochemically driven hydroxyapatite nanoparticles coating of medical implants. *Adv Funct Mater.* 2016; 26: 8003–10. doi:10.1002/adfm.201603575

34. He, D.-H.; Wang, P.; Liu, P.; Liu, X.-K.; Ma, F.-C.; Zhao, J. HA coating fabricated by electrochemical deposition on modified Ti6Al4V alloy. *Surf Coat Tech.* 2016; 277: 203–9. doi:10.1016/j.surfcoat.2015.07.038

35. Lindahl, C.; Xia, W.; Engqvist, H.; Snis, A.; Lausmaa, J.; Palmquist, A. Biomimetic calcium phosphate coating of additively manufactured porous CoCr implants. *Appl Surf Sci.* 2015; 353: 40–7. doi:10.1016/j.apsusc.2015.06.056

36. Zhang, Q.; Leng, Y.; Xin, R. A comparative study of electrochemical deposition and biomimetic deposition of calcium phosphate on porous titanium. *Biomaterials.* 2005; 26(16): 2857–65. doi:10.1016/j.biomaterials.2004.08.016

37. Trybuś, B.; Zieliński, A.; Beutner, R.; Seramak, T.; Scharnweber, D. Deposition of phosphate coatings on titanium within scaffold structure. *Acta Bioeng Biomech.* 2017; 19(2): 65–72. doi:10.5277/abb-00631-2016-03

38. Kim, K.H.; Ramaswamy, N. Electrochemical surface modification of titanium in dentistry. *Dent Mater J.* 2009; 28(1): 20–36. doi:10.4012/dmj.28.20

39. Djošić, M.S.; Panić, V.; Stojanović, J.; Mitrić, M.; Mišković-Stanković, V.B. The effect of applied current density on the surface morphology of deposited calcium phosphate coatings on titanium. *Colloids Surf A Physicochem Eng Asp.* 2012; 400: 36–43. doi:10.1016/j.colsurfa.2012.02.040

40. Chen, J.S.; Juang, H.Y.; Hon, M.H. Calcium phosphate coating on titanium substrate by a modified electrocrystallization process. *J Mater Sci Mater Med.* 1998; 9(5): 297–300. doi:10.1023/A:1008825926440

41. Hsu, H.C.; Wu, S.C.; Lin, C.H.; Ho, W.F. Electrolytic deposition of hydroxyapatite coating on thermal treated Ti-40Zr. *J Mater Sci Mater Med.* 2009; 20(9): 1825–30. doi:10.1007/s10856-009-3757-6

42. Wang, J.; Chao, Y.; Wan, Q.; Yan, K.; Meng, Y. Fluoridated hydroxyapatite/titanium dioxide nanocomposite coating fabricated by a modified electrochemical deposition. *J Mater Sci Mater Med.* 2009; 20(5): 1047–55. doi:10.1007/s10856-008-3673-1

43. Popa, C.; Simon, V.; Vida-Simiti, I.; Batin, G.; Candea, V.; Simon, S. Titanium—hydroxyapatite porous structures for endosseous applications. *J Mater Sci Mater Med.* 2005; 16(12): 1165–71. doi:10.1007/s10856-005-4724-5

44. Wen, H.B.; Wolke, J.G.; de Wijn, J.R.; Liu, Q.; Cui, F.Z.; de Groot, K. Fast precipitation of calcium phosphate layers on titanium induced by simple chemical treatments. *Biomaterials.* 1997; 18(22): 1471–8. doi:10.1016/s0142-9612(97)82297-1

45. Łukaszewska-Kuska, M.; Krawczyk, P.; Martyła, A.; Hędzelek, W.; Dorocka-Bobkowska, B. Hydroxyapatite coating on titanium endosseous implants for improved osseointegration: Physical and chemical considerations. *Adv Clin Exp Med.* 2018; 27(8): 1055–9. doi:10.17219/acem/69084

46. Jonásová, L.; Müller, F.A.; Helebrant, A.; Strnad, J.; Greil, P. Hydroxyapatite formation on alkali-treated titanium with different content of Na+ in the surface layer. *Biomaterials.* 2002; 23(15): 3095–101. doi:10.1016/s0142-9612(02)00043-1

47. Yanovska, A.; Kuznetsov, V.; Stanislavov, A.; Danilchenko, S.; Sukhodub, L. Synthesis and characterization of hydroxyapatite-based coatings for medical implants obtained on

chemically modified Ti6Al4V substrates. *Surf Coat Tech.* 2011; 205(23–24): 5324–29 doi:10.1016/j.surfcoat.2011.05.040

48. Ou, S.-F.; Chou, H.-H.; Lin, C.-S.; Shih, C.-J.; Wang, K.-K.; Pan, Y.-N. Effects of anodic oxidation and hydrothermal treatment on surface characteristics and biocompatibility of Ti-30Nb-1Fe-1Hf alloy. *Appl Surf Sci.* 2012; 258(17): 6190–8. doi:10.1016/j.apsusc.2012.02.109

49. Iwai-Yoshida, M.; Shibata, Y.; Wurihan; Suzuki, D.; Fujisawa, N.; Tanimoto, Y.; Kamijo, R.; Maki, K.; Miyazaki, T. Antioxidant and osteogenic properties of anodically oxidized titanium. *J Mech Behav Biomed Mater.* 2012; 13: 230–6. doi:10.1016/j.jmbbm.2012.01.016

50. Szesz, E.M.; Pereira, B.L.; Kuromoto, N.K.; Marino, C.E.B.; de Souza, G.B.; Soares, P. Electrochemical and morphological analyses on the titanium surface modified by shot blasting and anodic oxidation processes. *Thin Solid Films.* 2013; 528: 163–6. doi:10.1016/j.tsf.2012.09.096

51. ISO 20502:2005 Fine ceramics (advanced ceramics, advanced technical ceramics) – Determination of adhesion of ceramic coatings by scratch testing.

6 Research on the system of bone and the prototype multi-spiked connecting scaffold in order to design the structural and biomechanical properties of this system[*]

6.1 NUMERICAL STUDY OF THE INFLUENCE OF GEOMETRIC FEATURES OF THE MULTI-SPIKED CONNECTING SCAFFOLD ON THE MECHANICAL STRESS DISTRIBUTION IN THE PERI-IMPLANT BONE

To determine the key geometric structural features of the MSC-Scaffold, significantly determining the distribution of elastic stress and strain in the peri-implant bone, a simulation analysis of the stress and strain state in the peri-implant bone was performed. For the study, a numerical model of a prototype MSC-Scaffold manufactured of a titanium alloy embedded in simulated bone material was built, which was assumed to be a transversely isotropic linear elastic material. This assumption is often made for both cortical and trabecular bone [4,5]. Among structural-geometric features of the MSC-Scaffold, the distance between the bases of adjacent spikes a, the vertical angle of spikes β, and the height of the spherical cap h were taken into account. Huber-von Mises-Hencky (HMH) reduced stress and strain in the peri-implant bone were determined. This enabled in subsequent stages the determination

---

[*] The research works described in this chapter were carried out at the Institute of Chemical Technology and Engineering of the Faculty of Chemical Technology of the Poznan University of Technology as part of the research project of the National Science Centre Poland No. NN518412638, and then continued in the doctoral dissertation in the field of biomedical engineering [1], the supervisor of which was the principal investigator of the above-mentioned research project, and published in papers [2,3].

DOI: 10.1201/9781003364498-6

113

of the most advantageous geometric design variants of the MSC-Scaffold for the transfer of loads in the bone-implant system.

Mechanical property values of the Ti-6Al-4V alloy [6–8] (Table 6.1) were adopted for analysis. The assumed values of the mechanical properties of the simulated bone material, that is, cancellous bone, are presented in Table 6.2 [5,9–14].

CAD models of the MSC-Scaffold fragments were designed based on photographic documentation of the MSC-Scaffold preprototypes manufactured in SLM technology. In the CAD models based on which these prototypes were manufactured, the spikes were modelled with regular quadrilateral pyramids. Since it was found that in the produced preprototypes, the spikes have the shape of irregular pyramids passing above half of their height into the shape of a truncated cone with an apical canopy, in the CAD models of the fragments of the MSC-Scaffold, it was assumed for the sake of simplicity that they had the shape of a truncated cone ended with an apical canopy.

Spikes of height of 4.5 mm (without taking into account the apex) are arranged concentrically around the central spike in three circles. The diameter of the upper surface (top) of the spikes was 0.25 mm and the diameter of their base was the resulting value, depending on the variant angle of the top of the MSC-Scaffold spikes.

The simulated bone material was modelled in the shape of a cylinder fragment, which is a matrix for the MSC-Scaffold prototype. The so-called bone sockets reflect the state of plastic deformation caused by initial intraoperative embedding by an orthopaedic surgeon of a prototype MSC-Scaffold in the bone up to about half the height of the spikes.

A simulation analysis of the stress and strain state in the bone near the MSC-Scaffold was performed for seven of its variants with the following geometric

---

TABLE 6.1

Mechanical properties of Ti-6Al-4V titanium alloy [6–8]

Young's Modulus (GPa)	Tensile Strength (MPa)	Yield Strength (MPa)	Elongation at Rupture (%)	Poisson's Ratio
116.0	1,150.0	1,010.0	25.0	0.34

TABLE 6.2

Mechanical properties of bone material used in computational studies (based on the mechanical properties of cancellous bone) [5,9–14]

E_1 (MPa)	E_2 (MPa)	G_1 (MPa)	G_2 (MPa)	ν_1	ν_2	σ_c (MPa)
608	771	260	269	0.17	0.15	25

E_1 – transverse Young's modulus, E_2 – longitudinal Young's modulus, G_1 – transverse shear modulus, G_2 – longitudinal shear modulus, ν_1 – transverse Poisson ratio, ν_2 – longitudinal Poisson ratio, σ_c – ultimate compressive strength.

features: (1) the distance between the bases of adjacent spikes a (equivalent for D_{is-rep}, see Section 4.1) – 0.2, 0.35, and 0.5 mm. The distance between the bases of adjacent spikes was kept accurate in the radial direction, with an accuracy of ±0.03 mm in the circumferential direction; (2) the vertical angle of spikes β (equivalent for Ω_{rep-is}, see Section 4.1) – 2°, 3°, and 4°; and (3) the height of the spherical cap h – 0.08 mm, 0.12 mm, and 0.15 mm.

Due to the symmetry of the CAD model, numerical tests were carried out for one-fourth of the model. Figure 6.1 shows one-fourth of the CAD sketch of the MSC-Scaffold.

The base of the bone material cylinder was assumed to be fixed support (i.e. the translations of the bone cylinder base were constrained in all directions). On the symmetry planes of the model, translations of the lateral surface in the normal directions were excluded.

The uniformly distributed load of a constant value of 50 N was applied to the top surface of the MSC-Scaffold prototype model. The assumed load value was determined in preliminary simulations which took into account the results of Bergmann et al. obtained with a telemetric endoprosthesis [15–18] and the loading conditions defined in ISO 14242 [19]. It allowed assuming that the average maximum load in the hip joint is 3,000 N. This value divided by the average number of spikes in the MSC-Scaffold of the femoral component of the hip resurfacing endoprosthesis (i.e. 600 spikes) produces the limit load of 5 N per spike.

The contact area of the MSC-Scaffold and bone material was defined as the contact of the front and lateral surfaces of the spikes with the surface of the cavities of the body that simulate the bone. As a type of contact, the "slide without separation" was adopted, which is characterized by all rotations and translations in the normal direction of the contact plane being blocked between the contact elements. Then advanced options for the definition of the contact area were applied, such as penetration tolerance and the update of the stiffness. It was found that the Augmented Lagrangian Method would be used on contact surface – contact penetration was present but controlled to some degree [20]. This method of contact formulation is applicable for any type of contact behaviour and is commonly used for symmetric and asymmetric contacts, which are recommended for general frictionless or frictional contacts [21–23].

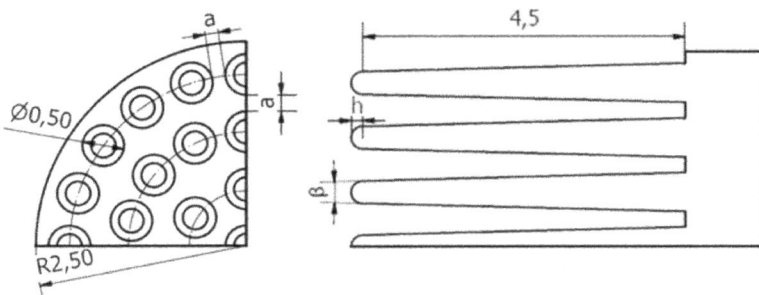

FIGURE 6.1   Sketch of one-fourth of the prototype MSC-Scaffold model.

Hexahedral finite elements, i.e. solid elements of cube shape, have been used because they provide more accurate results than other elements [24,25]. The average size of the mesh element was set at about 0.2 mm. To maintain consistency between the two contact elements of the simulation model near the contact surface, the mesh was densified and its compatibility between the two objects of the simulation model was ensured. The local reduction in mesh size in the critical implant contact area was 0.04 mm [26–28]. Under boundary conditions, the nodes of the simulated bone material on one surface were immobilized. The simulation model of the MSC-Scaffold partially embedded in the cancellous bone material with the finite element mesh generated is shown in Figure 6.2.

Three simulation analysis scenarios were developed in which one of the variants of the geometric construction features of the MSC-Scaffold was variable and the others were constant. The total number of nodes of the finite element mesh of the simulation model was approximately 300,000. The boundary conditions described above were determined after comparing the stress distribution in the peri-implant area of the simulated geometric bone model created as a cylindrical bone segment with a diameter of 20 mm and a height of 7 mm.

The results are presented in the form of maximum values of the HMH reduced stress in the simulated material of the periarticular bone near the MSC-Scaffold partially embedded in the bone (given in Table 6.3) and representative maps of the HMH reduced stress distribution in the simulated material of the periarticular bone

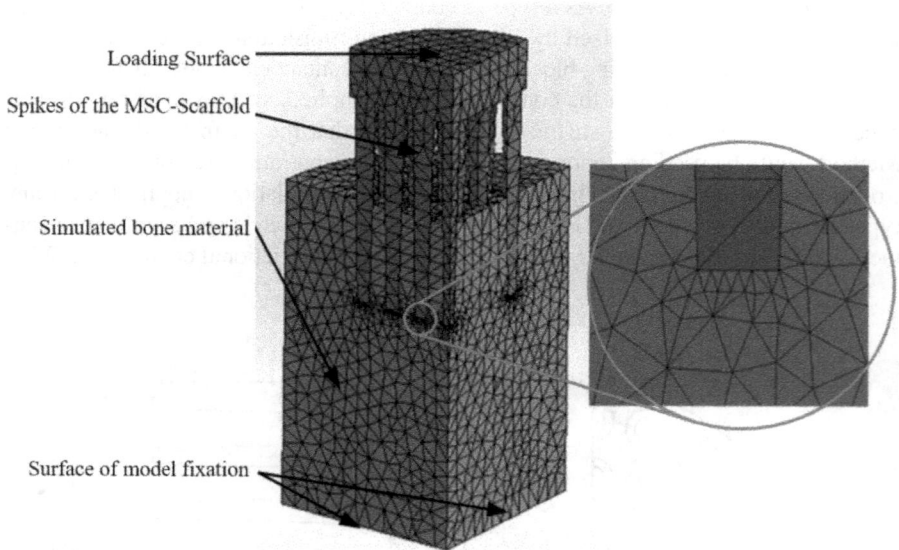

FIGURE 6.2 A simulation model of the MSC-Scaffold partially embedded in the periarticular bone was made with the generated mesh of finite hexahedral elements, which is compacted near the contact surface, and the compatibility between the contact elements of the simulation model was ensured.

in the region of the MSC-Scaffold, respectively for the variant geometric features of this scaffold: the distance between the bases of adjacent spikes a in Figure 6.3, the vertical angle of spikes β of the spikes in Figure 6.4, and the height of the spherical cap h in Figure 6.5.

The highest values of HMH stress in the cancellous bone around the MSC-Scaffold were observed in the periapical zone of the scaffold. The maximum value of HMH stress increases with increasing the distance between the bases of adjacent spikes of the MSC-Scaffold. Changing the distance in the range from 0.20 to 0.50 mm results in an increase of the HMH stress in the range from 15.2 to 20.0 MPa, that is, by 32%. As the distance between the bases of the spikes increases, the HMH stress distribution around the individual spikes becomes more concentric. For the model tested, with a distance between the bases of adjacent spikes a = 0.35 mm, the application of MSC-Scaffold penetration load of 50 N caused the maximum HMH stress of 18.4 MPa, which is 74% of the ultimate strength of the cancellous bone subjected

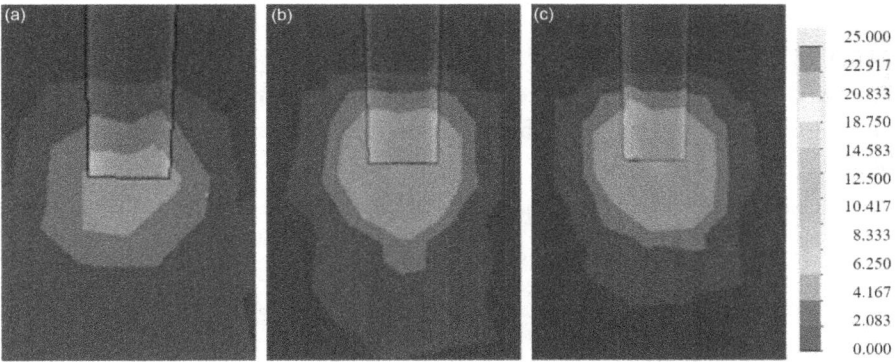

FIGURE 6.3 Maps of the HMH stress distribution in the area around the apex of the MSC-Scaffold spikes for the value of the distance between the bases of adjacent spikes a: (a) 0.2 mm, (b) 0.35 mm, (c) 0.5 mm.

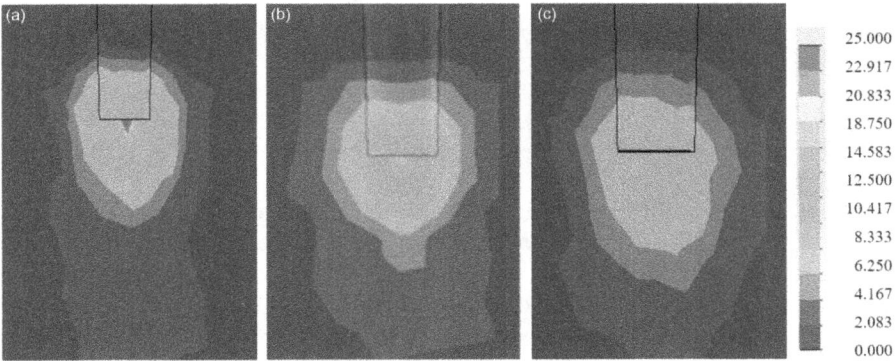

FIGURE 6.4 Maps of the HMH stress distribution in the periapical area of the MSC-Scaffold spikes for the value of the vertical angle of spikes β: (a) 2°, (b) 3°, (c) 4°.

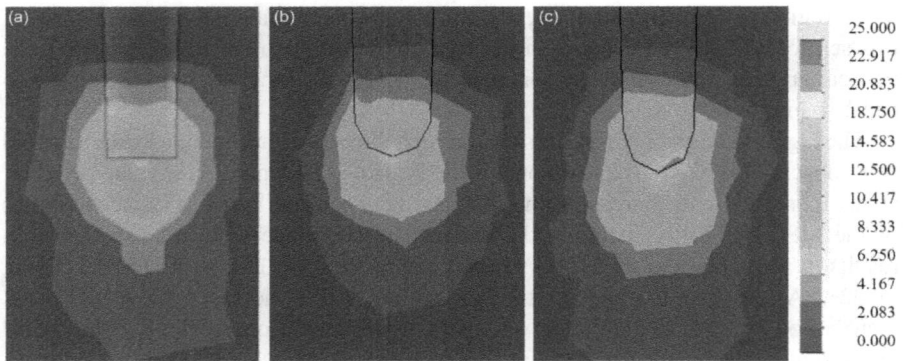

FIGURE 6.5 Maps of the stress distribution in the periapical area of the MSC-Scaffold spikes for the height of the spherical cap *h*: (a) 0 mm, (b) 0.08 mm, (c) 0.12 mm.

TABLE 6.3
The maximum values of HMH reduced stress in the simulated bone material of the periarticular bone near the MSC-Scaffold, partially embedded in the bone

The Distance between the Bases of Adjacent Spikes *a* (mm)	The Maximum HMH Stress in Simulated Bone Material (MPa)
0.20	15.2
0.35	18.4
0.50	20.0
The Vertical angle of Spikes *β* (°)	**The Maximum HMH Stress in Simulated Bone Material (MPa)**
2.0	24.5
3.0	18.4
4.0	14.6
The Height of the Spherical Cap *h* (mm)	**The Maximum HMH Stress in Simulated Bone Material (MPa)**
0.00	18.4
0.08	20.5
0.12	22.8

to compression. For the other design variants, these values were: for $a = 0.20$ mm, the maximum HMH stress = 15.2 MPa, which is 61% of the assumed strength of the cancellous bone; for $a = 0.50$ mm, the maximum HMH stress = 20.0 MPa, which is 80% of the assumed strength of the cancellous bone.

Changing the value of the vertical angle of the spikes of the MSC-Scaffold spikes β from 2.0° to 4.0° results in a decrease in the value of the maximum HMH stress. The change of the vertical angle of the spike value in the considered range reduces the maximum HMH stress from 14.6 to 24.1 MPa, that is, by 39%. For the model tested, at the vertical angle of the spikes $\beta = 3.0°$, under the MSC-Scaffold penetrating the load of 50 N, the maximum HMH stress was 18.4 MPa, which is 74% of the final strength of the cancellous bone subjected to compression. For the remaining design variants, these values were as follows: the variant with the vertical angle of spikes $\beta = 2.0°$ – the maximum HMH stress = 24.5 MPa, which is 98% of the assumed strength of the cancellous bone; the variant with the vertical angle of spikes $\beta = 4.0°$ – the maximum HMH stress = 14.6 MPa, which is 58% of the assumed strength of the cancellous bone.

The maximum values of the HMH reduced stress and the strain of the periarticular bone material increased with the increase of the height of the spherical cap h of the spikes of the MSC-Scaffold. The change in height h in the range from 0 to 0.12 mm resulted in a change in the maximum HMH stress values from 18.6 to 22.8 MPa, i.e. an increase by 24%. In Figure 6.5, a change in the HMH stress distribution can be observed between the model without the apex cap (height value $h = 0$ mm) and the model with the apex cap $h = 0.012$ mm, which is caused by the redistribution of internal forces accompanying this change. The maximum values of the HMH stress are concentrated directly in the area of the spikes of the MSC-Scaffold. This is due to a change in the geometry of the spikes, as in the case of a flat peak of the spikes of the MSC-Scaffold the maximum HMH stress values are concentrated around the edge of the peak.

For the model tested, at the height of the spherical cap $h = 0.08$ mm, under the MSC-Scaffold penetrating the load of 50 N, the HMH stress was 20.5 MPa, which is 82% of the maximum strength of the cancellous bone subjected to compression. For the remaining design variants, respectively: variant with the height of the spherical cap $h = 0.12$ mm – stress HMH = 22.8 MPa, which is 91% of the assumed strength of the cancellous bone; variant without apical cap h – stress HMH = 18.4 MPa, which is 74% of the ultimate strength of the cancellous bone.

The aim of the numerical simulations carried out, in which the MSC-Scaffold partially embedded in the periarticular bone was loaded, was to determine its most important geometric features to ensure a physiological load transfer from the MSC-Scaffold to the bone in the vicinity of the implant. The obtained results showed that the following geometric structural features of the MSC-Scaffold had a significant impact on the state of stress in the bone around the spikes: (a) the distance between the bases of adjacent spikes a, (b) the vertical angle of spikes β, and (c) the height of the spherical cap h. Based on the analysis of the maximum values and distribution of HMH reduced stress in the area around the implant, it was found that the vertical angle of spikes β (changes from 2.0° to 4.0° reduce the HMH stress in the bone material by 39%) and the distance between the bases of adjacent spikes a (changes from 0.20 to 0.50 mm cause an increase in HMH stress in the bone material by 32%) are the key geometric features that determine the correct design of a suitable prototype of the MSC-Scaffold for cementless resurfacing endoprostheses. The influence of the height of the spherical cap h of the MSC-Scaffold (changes from 0.00 to 0.12 mm increase HMH stress in bone material by 24%) is of secondary importance.

6.2 VALIDATION OF THE NUMERICAL MODEL REFLECTING THE EMBEDMENT OF THE PROTOTYPE MULTI-SPIKED CONNECTING SCAFFOLD IN THE PERIARTICULAR BONE

Numerical study of the influence of geometric features of the MSC-Scaffold initially embedded in the bone on the distribution of mechanical stress in the periprosthetic bone allowed to select those features that significantly determine its proper design. Before the planned experimental implantation in an orthopaedic clinic of a new type of endoprosthesis in humans, it is crucial to develop a validated numerical model necessary for the bioengineering design of this new type of biomimetic fixation of the components of resurfacing endoprostheses in the bone.

Combining laboratory mechanical research with numerical simulation analysis based on numerical models, especially finite element models, is a widely used approach to studying the mechanics of the bone-implant system. For example, Enns-Bray et al. [29] used experimental data to validate anisotropic FEM models of the proximal femur. Affes et al. [30] showed that the experimental attempt to extract the implant in the form of a screw from the tibia (implant pull-out test) is useful for the validation of the numerical models developed for the tested system. Huang et al. [31] used finite element analysis and tomography imaging to study the stress in the bone around a dental implant. Du et al. [32] embedded dental implants in the mandibular bone of humans, then using microtomographic imaging visualized the microgeometry of the trabecular structures around the implant, calculated the stress and strain distributions in the bone resulting from implant loading, and compared the results of previous laboratory study. The advantage of microtomographic examination is that it does not damage the bone sample, so it is possible to accurately visualize changes in the structure of the peri-implant bone [33,34].

To build a validated numerical model for the design of a new type of biomimetic fixation of resurfacing endoprostheses, X-ray computed microtomography was used to monitor and evaluate changes in the density of the periarticular bone structure during the process of mechanical embedding of the prototype MSC-Scaffold in it. A schematic description of the experimental validation of the numerical model considered is shown in Figure 6.6.

The FE model of the MSC-Scaffold prototypes for resurfacing arthroplasty endoprostheses embedded in periarticular bone was validated in two experimental steps preceded by preparation tasks, including computer aided design (CAD) modelling, selective laser melting (SLM) manufacturing, and bone sample preparation.

In the first stage, the transfer of mechanical load from the MSC-Scaffold to the periarticular bone was investigated for different levels of embedding of the MSC-Scaffold, using the initial numerical model used to study the influence of the geometric structural features of this scaffold on the distribution of mechanical stress in the periarticular bone (see Figure 6.2). As in the previous case, the values of material properties for the MSC-Scaffold [35,36] and simulated bone material [5,9,37] were adopted, respectively, in Tables 6.1 and 6.2. Then, mechanical tests were carried out to embed the MSC-Scaffold in the periarticular bone samples of fresh swine femoral heads.

In the second stage, to quantify the density distribution of the bone material before and during the mechanical deposition of the prototype MSC-Scaffold,

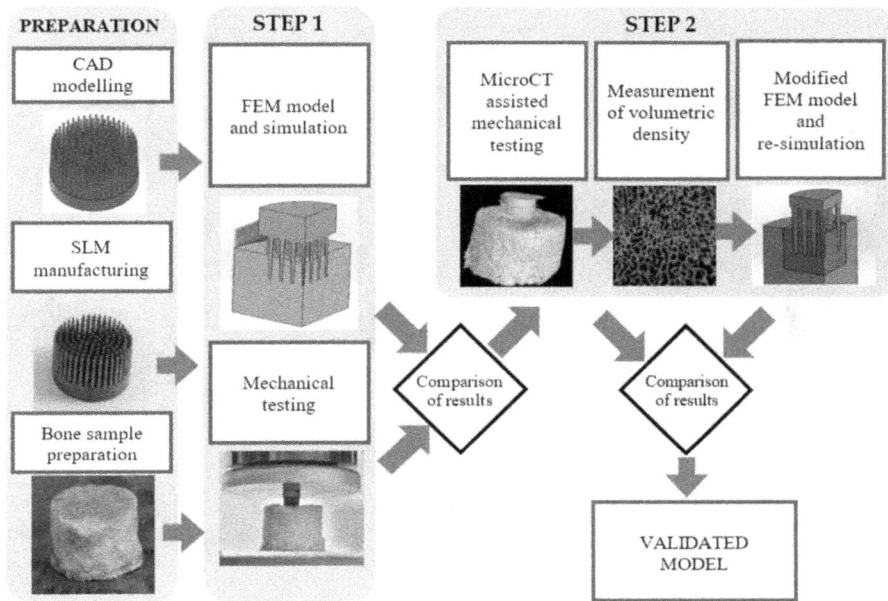

FIGURE 6.6 A schematic description of the experimental validation of the finite element (FE) model of the MSC-Scaffold prototype embedded in periarticular bone.

a microtomographic examination of the periarticular bone samples was performed and the embedding test with the prototype MSC-Scaffold was performed under microtomographic control.

The obtained data from microtomographic imaging were used to modify the numerical model and to conduct further simulation study. The convergence between the experimental and numerical results was analysed for both stages.

The design guidelines developed by our team and published in [2,38] were taken into account in the CAD models. MSC-Scaffold spikes in the shape of a truncated cone with a base diameter of 0.5 mm and a height of 5 mm are placed on concentric circles around a central spike coaxial with the axis of the cylindrical base. The distance between the bases of the adjacent spikes was 0.35 mm, which corresponds to the thickness of the cancellous bone trabeculae, in the radial direction it was kept exactly and in the circumferential direction it was kept with an accuracy of ±0.03 mm.

The CAD model of the prototype MSC-Scaffold used in this study is shown in Figure 6.7a. The manufacturing of this prototype scaffold of the Ti-6Al-4V powder in SLM technology according to the developed CAD model was subcontracted to the Center for New Materials and Technologies of the West Pomeranian University of Technology in Szczecin, and the specialized post-production processing of the manufactured prototype MSC-Scaffold was made according to the procedures described in Section 3.5. The preprototype of the MSC-Scaffold after blasting is shown in Figure 6.7b.

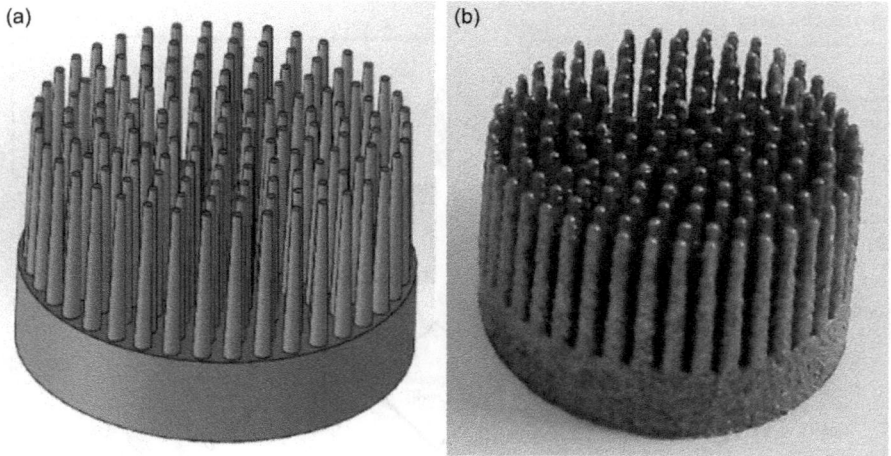

FIGURE 6.7 (a) CAD model of the prototype MSC-Scaffold; (b) a preprototype of the MSC-Scaffold produced based on the CAD model in SLM technology, after specialized abrasive blasting.

The hip joints of a swine of the Polish Large White breed aged 8–10 months were purchased from a local slaughterhouse. Swine bone was used in the investigation as it is a recognized good animal model for human bone. Its mechanical properties are similar to those of human bone [39]. The heads of the femurs were mechanically cleaned of soft tissues, protected (against drying) with a dressing soaked in Ringer's solution, sealed in a plastic bag, and stored at 4°C. The research was carried out on fresh bone (i.e. up to 5 hours after slaughter). Cylinder-shaped samples (ø26 mm × 20 mm) were cut with a saw hole cutter. An IsoMet™ 4000 Linear Precision Saw (Buehler, Esslingen am Neckar, Germany) was used to remove the cartilage sections, i.e. to expose the subcartilage bone with unbroken trabeculae.

To analyse the force required to embed the MSC-Scaffold into the periarticular bone, numerical simulations were performed at five different levels of embedding.

It was assumed that the force required to embed the MSC-Scaffold in the periarticular bone caused the limit stress value determined as the mean of the internodal stresses of the maximum values on the surface contacting with the spike apexes. The HMH reduced stress distribution was determined in the peri-implant area of the bone material with properties corresponding to the periarticular bone.

Mechanical tests of the MSC-Scaffold prototype quasi-static embedding in the swine periarticular bone samples were performed with a universal testing machine (Instron, Norwood, MA, USA). A 120-grit sandpaper was attached to the lower handle of the testing machine, which stabilized the bone sample placed on it, preventing it from sliding. The MSC-Scaffold preprototype was placed on the bone sample and preloaded with the upper handle of the testing machine to reach the point of contact and apply a recordable load. A quasi-static embedding was performed by loading the MSC-Scaffold preprototype with a crosshead speed of 0.1 mm/s until the spikes reached a value of 3.0 mm embedment in bone. Quasi-static loading of

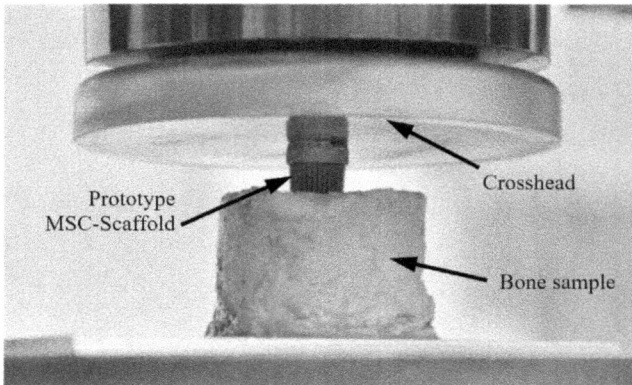

FIGURE 6.8   An experimental stand with a bone sample placed on the bottom plate attached to the base of a testing machine and a prototype MSC-Scaffold (implant-bone system) mounted on this bone sample. The clamping plate of the measuring head attached to the moving traverse causes the initial load and then embedding of the MSC-Scaffold spikes into the bone.

the MSC-Scaffold with a speed of 0.1 mm/s corresponds to the speed of elastic bone strain induced during calm gradual loading of the limb operated during postoperative rehabilitation [40,41]. During the tests, the penetration force and the displacement of the traverse corresponding to the depth of the embedment were measured. Figure 6.8 shows the experimental stand with a bone sample on which the MSC-Scaffold preprototype was mounted.

Figure 6.9 shows the exemplary results of the mechanical tests of the embedding of the MSC-Scaffold in the periarticular bone in the form of the force-displacement curves, i.e. the embedding force of the MSC-Scaffold in the bone on the displacement of the embedded spikes (embedment depth) for ten representative repetitions. The embedding force is the force that causes the crosshead of the testing machine to move and, consequently, to embed the spikes of the MSC-Scaffold preprototypes into the periarticular bone.

Based on the embedding force-distance curves, three phases were distinguished. Phase I, the initial phase of embedding the MSC-Scaffold in the periarticular bone, was characterized by a slight increase in the embedding force. Spikes of the MSC-Scaffold penetrated the intertrabecular space of the periarticular bone, and the embedding force increased as the spikes gradually made contact with the trabeculae. Phase II showed the linear increase in the embedding force from the partially embedded MSC-Scaffold in the periarticular bone and the spikes in contact with the trabeculae. During this phase, the load was transferred from the spikes of the MSC-Scaffold prototype to the trabeculae of the cancellous bone, a phenomenon that caused elastic deformation of this bone. Phase III was characterized by changes in embedding force due to the destruction of particular trabeculae and the densification of the trabecular bone (cf. [42]).

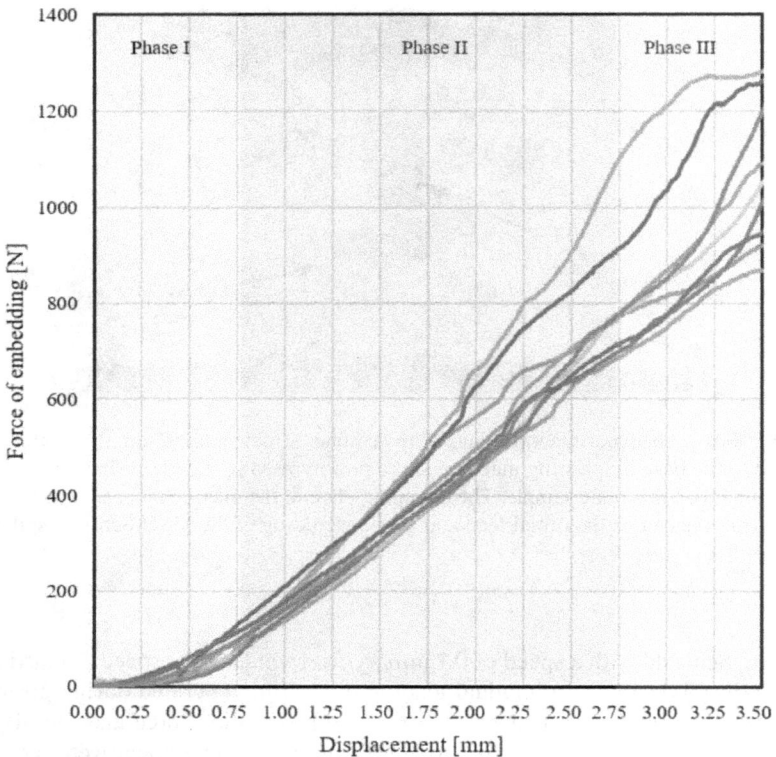

FIGURE 6.9 The embedding force-distance curves for ten representative tests of the MSC-Scaffold prototype embedding in the periarticular bone.

Figure 6.10 shows the section of the force-displacement characteristics of the MSC-Scaffold spikes embedded in the bone corresponding to phase II of the process of embedding the MSC-Scaffold in the periarticular bone, which was averaged based on the data obtained from ten experimental measurements. This section of the experimental characteristic was compared with the results of numerical simulations in the form of points reflecting the value of the embedding force for a specific embedment depth. For certain levels of embedding, representative maps of the HMH reduced stress distribution in the peri-implant bone, calculated for the system under consideration, are presented.

In each case analysed, for different levels of embedding, the stress concentration areas in the periarticular bone were located around the apex of the spikes (i.e. in the periapical area). A submaximal force was reached for each case. These data indicate that the stress is concentrated around the spike apex of the MSC-Scaffold. This results in reduced storage of elastic energy in the periarticular bone in the interstitial spaces and below the spikes.

The linear regression model was used to analyse and compare experimental and simulation results. The fraction of variance unexplained (*FVU*) statistical test was performed to determine what part of the explanatory variable variation observed in

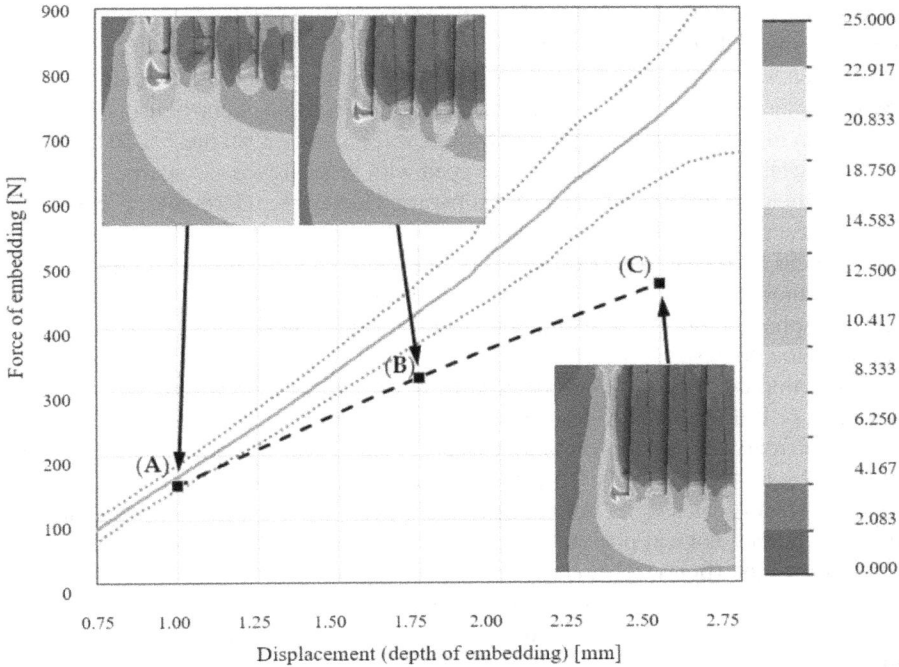

FIGURE 6.10 Phase II of the force-distance curves obtained from experimental measurements (the mean line is presented as the solid grey line, and dotted grey lines are ± standard deviations) and from numerical simulations. The dashed black line represents the results of the numerical simulation of the problem. The insets show representative maps of the Huber-von Mises-Hencky (HMH) stress distributions calculated for the considered system containing the MSC-Scaffold prototype and periarticular bone material with the embedding load applied to the top surface of the MSC-Scaffold prototype. (A) 1 mm embedding displacement and 153 N force of embedding; (B) 1.75 mm embedding displacement and 322 N force of embedding; (C) 2.5 mm embedding displacement and 469 N force of embedding.

the sample does not match the model [43–45]. The *FVU* takes values from the interval {0, 1}. The better the convergence of the model, the closer the *FVU* is to zero. It is expressed by Equation (6.1) [43–45] as follows:

$$FVU = \sum_{i-1}^{n} \frac{(y_i - \hat{y}_i)^2}{\sum_{i-1}^{n}(y_i - \hat{y}_i)^2} \tag{6.1}$$

where y_i represents the empirical value of the dependent variable y at the i-th value; $\hat{y}_i$ represents the theoretical value of the dependent variable y for the i-th value, and $\hat{y}_i$ represents the arithmetic means of the empirical values of the variable.

When the results of the mechanical tests of the embedding of the MSC-Scaffold were compared with the results of numerical simulations of the analogous problem using the initial numerical model, a discrepancy between these results was found.

The value of the *FVU* index was 0.33, indicating an insufficient convergence between the experimental and numerical data.

Mechanical tests of the embedding process of the prototype MSC-Scaffold in the periarticular bone were carried out under microtomographic control using the high-resolution microcomputed tomography scanner GE phoenix vItomelx s240 (Waygate Technologies, Wunstorf, Germany) equipped with software for reconstructing tomographic images (Volume Graphics 2.2 software, Heidelberg, Germany). For this purpose, a specialized device was designed and built, with which it was possible to carry out a mechanical test of embedding inside the measuring chamber of a microtomography scanner. The CAD model of this device is shown in Figure 6.11a; Figure 6.11b shows a photograph of the examined bone-implant system on a bench inside the microtomography scanner chamber.

The samples of the implant-bone system were placed on a rotating table and scanned in full with the following parameters: radiation source energy 130 keV, source current: 125 mA, resolution: 17.5 µm, filter: brass 1.5 mm, irradiation time: 300 ms, rotation: 180°, every 0.5°, scanning time, 20 minutes.

In the reconstructed 3D images of implant-bone samples, based on radiological density, the radiological phases identified as implant (titanium alloy MSC-Scaffold) and bone tissue (bone trabeculae) were distinguished. An area with a radiological density equal to that of soft tissues, including the bone marrow, has been hidden. The digital reconstruction of the implant-bone sample obtained based on the microtomographic examination is shown in Figure 6.12.

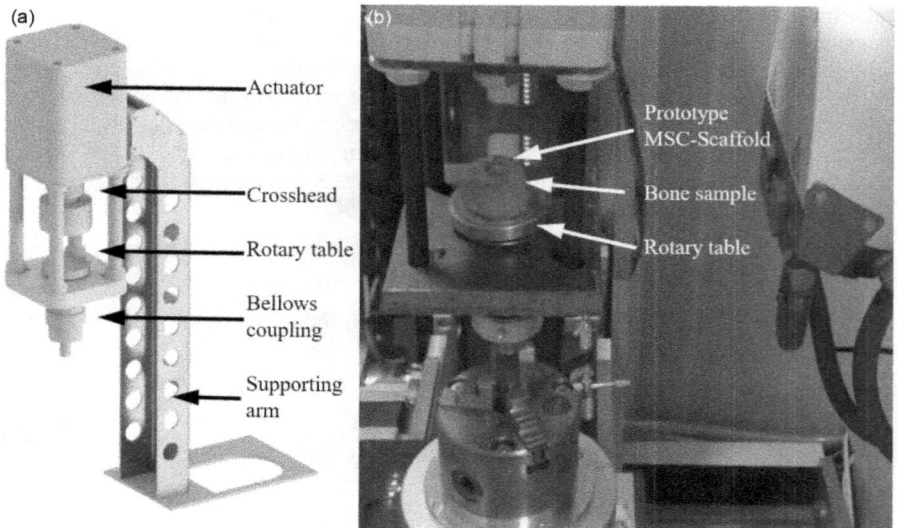

FIGURE 6.11 CAD model of a specialized device that enables the test of embedding the MSC-Scaffold inside the microtomography chamber into the sample (a); a sample of the implant-bone system during the embedding test performed in the microtomography scanner chamber (b).

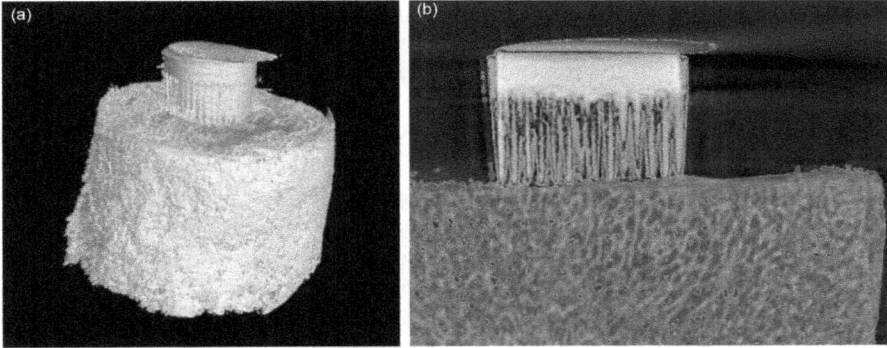

FIGURE 6.12   Three-dimensional digital reconstruction of the research sample of the implant-bone system (a); a representative cross section of a reconstructed sample of the implant-bone system before the embedding test (b).

To observe changes in the microstructure of the periarticular bone as a result of the MSC-Scaffold embedding, sections below the tops of the MSC-Scaffold spikes were selected in the reconstructed images, for which the fractions of individual phases were estimated. Vascular channels and osteocyte pits were digitally extracted from the test volume using VG Studio Max software and were not further analysed. Compartments representing the mineralized phase of the trabecular bone were created by selecting voxels with a radiological density value lower (inverse segmentation) than the threshold values determined by the Hounsfield scale and using threshold methods. The 1-voxel noises were removed by applying two basic morphological operations to process binary images – dilatation and erosion. To prevent the addition or removal of voxels at the edges and boundaries of all segmentations, voxel-based operations were limited to the surface of the original threshold images. Furthermore, to prevent edge effects, the first and last images of the volume of the fragment analysed were discarded.

The volume density of the trabecular bone (ρ_b) was determined based on the formula (6.2) [46–47]:

$$\rho_b = \alpha \cdot \rho_T + (1-\alpha) \cdot \rho_w \qquad (6.2)$$

where: ρ_T – bone trabecular volume density (comparable to the cortical bone density, 1.85 g/cm^3 was assumed) [48–51], ρ_w – bone marrow and soft tissue density (similar to water density, i.e. 1.00 g/cm^3), α – volume fraction of the radiological phase of mineralized trabecular bone, $1-\alpha$ – volume fraction of intercellular soft tissues.

Knowing the density of the trabecular bone density ρ_b, Young's modulus of elasticity E_2 of the periarticular bone can be estimated based on the empirical relationship:

$$E_2 = 315 \cdot \rho_b^3. \qquad (6.3)$$

Figure 6.13 shows representative cross sections of a digital microtomographic reconstruction of a bone sample, which was used to determine the density of the

128   Prototype of a Biomimetic Multi-spiked Connecting Scaffold

periarticular trabecular bone and then calculate Young's modulus E_2. Along with the increase in the embedment of the MSC-Scaffold spikes, the degree of densification of bone material caused by this embedment increased. This entails a reduction in the proportion of soft tissues, including bone marrow, and an increase in Young's modulus. The values of the fractions of marrow and soft tissues depend on the depth of the spikes as a result of embedding the MSC-Scaffold in the bone material and the corresponding values of the trabecular bone density and bone elastic modulus E_2 are presented in Table 6.4.

Based on the observed changes in the density of the periarticular bone within the area of the embedded MSC-Scaffold, an insert that simulates densified bone material was introduced in the numerical model of the problem under consideration. The mechanical properties of this insert were calculated based on the bone area/total area ratio (BA/TA) obtained from microtomographic imaging. The modified numerical model of the preprototype of the MSC-Scaffold embedded in the simulated periarticular bone, into which an insert simulating densified bone material has been inserted, is shown in Figure 6.14.

Figure 6.15 shows a digitally reconstructed test sample of the mechanically embedded MSC-Scaffold preprototype system in the periarticular bone. The area of

TABLE 6.4

The fraction values of the marrow and soft tissues depended on the embedment depth of the MSC-Scaffold in the bone material and the corresponding values of the trabecular bone density and Young's modulus of bone elasticity

Embedding Displacement (mm)	Fraction of Marrow and Soft Tissue (%)	Trabecular Bone Density (g/cm³)	Bone Longitudinal Elastic Modulus (MPa)
1.5	58.2	1.37	821
2.0	49.1	1.46	976
2.5	40.3	1.55	1,173

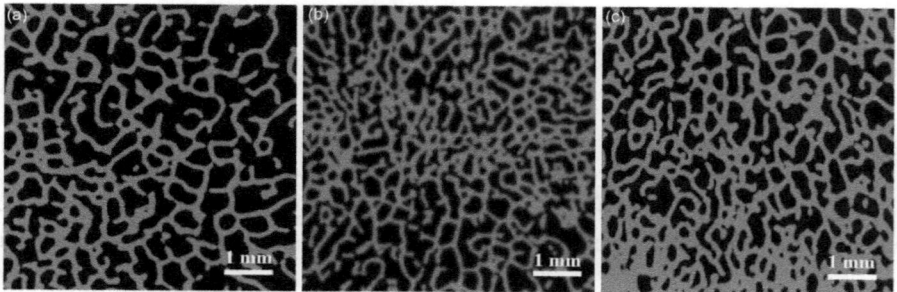

FIGURE 6.13 Representative cross sections of microtomographic digital reconstruction of a sample of bone material below the top of the MSC-Scaffold spikes at different levels of its embedding in the periarticular bone: (a) 1.5 mm; (b) 2.0 mm; (c) 2.5 mm.

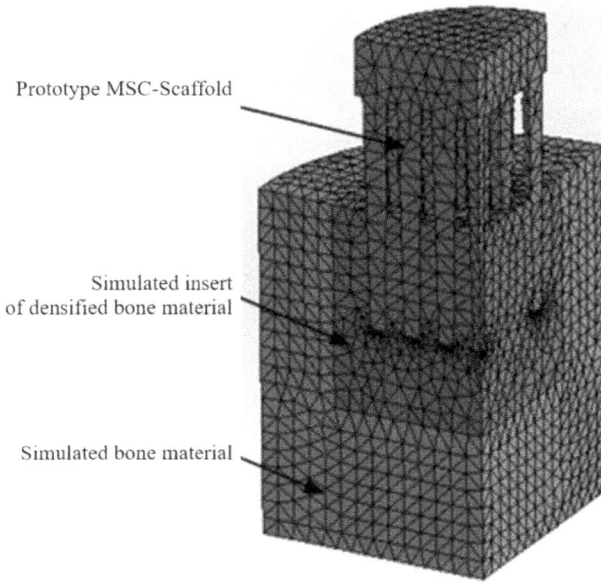

FIGURE 6.14   Modified numerical model of the MSC-Scaffold preprototype embedded in the periarticular bone with an insert that simulates densified bone material.

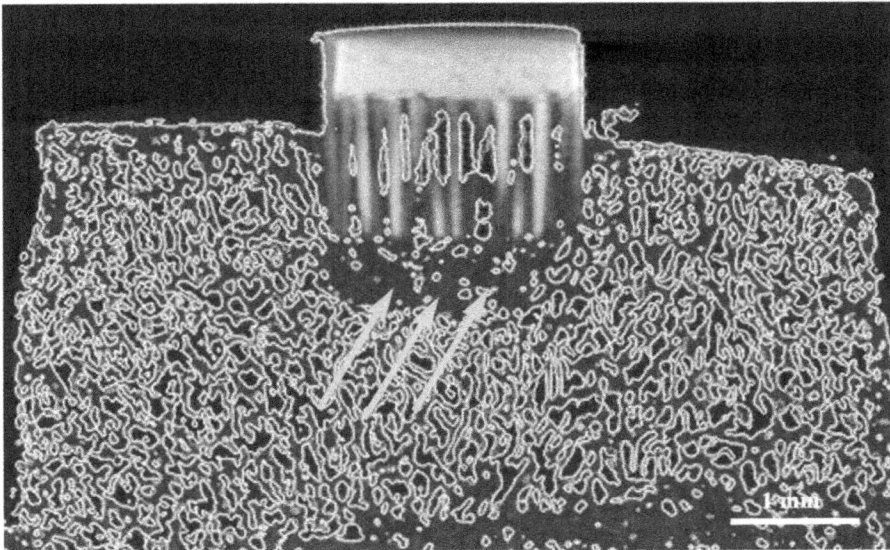

FIGURE 6.15   Reconstructed based on a microtomographic analysis research sample of the preprototype of the MSC-Scaffold mechanically embedded in the periarticular bone; the areas of bone density below the scaffold spikes are indicated by arrows.

densification of the trabecular structure of the periarticular bone located below the tops of the spikes is indicated by arrows.

Figure 6.16 shows the section of the dependence of the embedding force of the MSC-Scaffold in the bone on the displacement (embedment depth) corresponding to phase II of the embedding process of the MSC-Scaffold in the periarticular bone, averaged based on the data obtained from ten measurements performed during experimental tests. This section was juxtaposed with the results of numerical simulations performed based on a modified numerical model, in which an insert that simulates the densified bone material was taken into account. The mechanical properties of this insert, at each embedment level, correspond to the values in Table 6.4. For individual points that reflect the value of the penetration force for a specific embedment depth, representative maps of the HMH reduced stress distributions are presented.

According to the stress distribution presented in the HMH reduced stress maps, the stress gradient between the periapical surface of the MSC-Scaffold spikes and the surrounding periarticular bone area below the MSC-Scaffold spikes decreased.

The change caused by the inclusion in the numerical model of the aforementioned insert caused increased storage of elastic energy in the periarticular bone in the

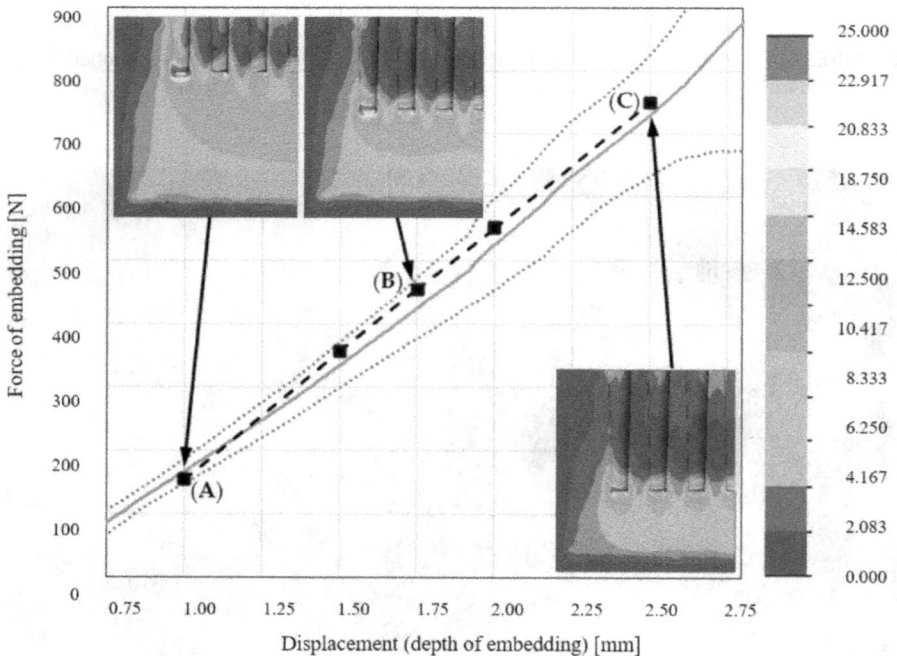

FIGURE 6.16 Phase II of the force-distance curves obtained from experimental measurements (the mean line is presented as the solid grey line, dotted grey lines are ± standard deviations) and the results of re-simulations with FE model modified by the simulated insert of densified bone material (dashed black line) at (A) 1.00 mm embedding displacement and 153 N loading force; (B) 1.75 mm embedding displacement and 453 N loading force; (C) 2.50 mm embedding displacement and 748 N loading force.

interspike spaces and below the spikes, and consequently an increase in the measured embedding force. Comparison of the results of mechanical tests of the embedding of the MSC-Scaffold with the results of numerical simulations of the analogous problem using a modified numerical model taking into account the insert simulating the compaction of bone material gave the value of the statistical index $FVU = 0.02$, which indicates a strong agreement of the experimental and simulation results.

***

The state of quasi-static loading of the MSC-Scaffold partially embedded (i.e. after initial surgical embedded) in the cancellous bone material was researched. For this state, it is important to determine the critical load that does not cause further migration (penetration) of the MSC-Scaffold in periarticular cancellous bone during the physiological controlled loading of the operated limb in the postoperative rehabilitation period.

The bone density assessment by high-resolution computed microtomography was used during the mechanical test of the penetration of the MSC-Scaffold in the periarticular bone to develop a validated numerical model, which allowed to determine the most appropriate geometric structural features of the MSC-Scaffold to the preliminary version of the MSC-Scaffold prototype described in the patents [52–54]. As in other works on numerical modelling of mechanical problems in the implant-bone system [29,31,32], this task combined experimental laboratory study and computational analysis to validate the pre-developed numerical model. As in the study by Cicciù et al. [55,56], microtomographic imaging data were used to adapt the 3D geometric model and the material properties of the subsystems of the finite element model used for the computational simulation of the problem under consideration. Finite element numerical analysis is widely used to study the mechanical stress distribution in the implant and the surrounding bone [57–60]. To ensure the stability of the calculations, solid elements and a hexagonal mesh were used in the constructed numerical model. According to the works [55,61,62], such assumptions allowed the generation of a high-quality model.

One can agree with the opinion of Marangalou et al. [63] that continuum finite element analysis has become the standard computational tool for analysing the mechanical behaviour of bone in orthopaedic biomechanics. In this case, it was assumed that the periarticular bone is a one-phase, transversely isotropic elastic material (cf. [64–66]). Van Rietbergen et al. [64] emphasize that since the trabeculae of the cancellous bone *in vivo* are mainly subjected to bending and compressive loads, the elastic modulus E_2 of the cancellous bone largely determines the mechanical behaviour of this bone. The assumption of transversal isotropy of the cancellous bone can be reasonably considered adequate and it allows for the sufficiently correct analysis of the complex states of load on this bone. The rationale for this may be the work of Krone and Schuster [65] who observed in the experimental analysis and numerical study of the human femur that the transversely isotropic numerical model of the cancellous and cortical bone material gives very similar results to those obtained for the assumed orthotropic model of both these bone materials. Significantly different analysis results were obtained in [66] for the assumed isotropic model of cancellous bone and cortical bone; the isotropic bone model turns out to be too close.

In the experiment carried out, the Huber-von Mises-Hencky criterion was used to determine the submaximal value of the load force applied to the preprototype of the MSC-Scaffold that does not cause further its penetration in bone material. In a comparative study by Keyak and Rossi [67] and Tellache et al. [68], who studied the mechanics of damage resulting from stress and strain state analysis used to predict femoral fractures, it was found that the HMH criterion is robust. This criterion is often used to predict trabecular bone damage – for example, in works by Maknickas et al. [69] or Provatidis et al. [70].

The initial numerical model of the MSC-Scaffold preprototype made of a titanium alloy partially embedded in the elastic transverse isotropic material of the periarticular bone was validated in two steps.

In the first stage, the transfer of mechanical load for different levels of embedding was investigated using this numerical model. The results of the numerical simulations were compared with the results of mechanical tests of the MSC-Scaffold prototype embedded in samples from a swine periarticular bone. The experimental swine model has been used successfully in bone mechanics research [71,72] and is an established animal model for experimental surgical implantation and the mechanical study of implants [73]. Swindle et al. [74] showed that the bones of swine and humans had a similar density and microstructure; moreover, the biostructure of the cartilage of the synovial joint and the ligamentous system is structurally very similar in the joints of swine and humans.

To determine the convergence between the experimental and simulation results obtained, the statistical coefficient FVU was used. In the first step of the validation procedure, it was found that the proposed initial numerical model does not accurately reflect the simulated phenomenon. The value obtained of $FVU = 0.33$ indicated the need to explain the cause of the observed discrepancies and introduce changes to the initial numerical model of the problem.

In the second stage of validation, mechanical tests of the embedding process under microtomographic control were performed to quantify the bone density distribution before and during the quasi-static mechanical embedding of the MSC-Scaffold preprototype. This approach using microtomographic monitoring was also used by other authors [49,55,61]. The microtomographic imaging data were used to modify the initial numerical model by using a simulated insert of densified bone material in the model. This led to a strong convergence between the simulations using the modified model and the experimental results, as evidenced by the reduction of the value of FVU to 0.02.

HMH reduced stress maps showed that load transfer from the MSC-Scaffold to the bone was nearly uniform, as expected based on the biomimetic characteristics of the prototype MSC-Scaffold. In this way, the MSC-Scaffold can provide a close-to-physiological transfer of load into the bone around the implant. As the depth of the embedded spikes increases, the contribution of the lateral surface of the MSC-Scaffold spikes in the load transfer increases, which results in lower stress values in the bone material below the MSC-Scaffold spikes.

Thus, it can be stated that the modified numerical model accurately reflects the mechanical behaviour of the examined implant-bone system in the early postoperative period. The early postoperative period is crucial for the survival of this non-cemented resurfacing arthroplasty endoprosthesis. Controlled loading of such endoprosthesis by the patient in the early postoperative rehabilitation period enables the bone tissue to ingrow into the interspike spaces of the MSC-Scaffold and ensures the final biological fixation of the implant in the bone – provided that the structural accessibility of the MSC-Scaffold for bone ingrowth characterized by its pro-osteoconductive functionality, conditioned by the geometric features of its interspike space (see Chapter 4), is designed appropriately. Therefore, it can be concluded that the early postoperative biomechanical load capacity (loadability) of the articular surface of the non-cemented resurfacing endoprosthesis with the MSC-Scaffold can be considered the crucial design criterion for such endoprostheses.

REFERENCES

1. Patalas, A. Study of the process of embedding in bone of the multi-spiked connecting scaffold for resurfacing arthroplasty endoprosthesis (In Polish: Badanie procesu zagłębiania w kość wieloszpilkowego skafoldu stawowej endoprotezy powierzchniowej). PhD Thesis, Warsaw University of Technology, Warsaw, 2022.
2. Uklejewski, R.; Winiecki, M.; Patalas, A.; Rogala, P. Numerical studies of the influence of various geometrical features of a multi-spiked connecting scaffold prototype on mechanical stresses in peri-implant bone. *Comput Methods Biomech Biomed Engin.* 2018; 21(9): 541–7. doi:10.1080/10255842.2018.1480759
3. Uklejewski, R.; Winiecki, M.; Patalas, A.; Rogala, P. Bone density micro-CT assessment during embedding of the innovative multi-spiked connecting scaffold in periarticular bone to elaborate a validated numerical model for designing biomimetic fixation of resurfacing endoprostheses. *Materials.* 2021; 14(6): 1384. doi:10.3390/ma14061384
4. Huiskes, H.W.J.; Janssen, J.D.; Slooff, T.J.J.H. Finite element analysis for artificial joint fixation problems in orthopaedics, in: Gallagher, R.H.; Simon, B.R.; Johnson, P.C.; Gross, J.F. (Eds.): *Finite Elements in Biomechanics.* John Wiley & Sons, Hoboken, NJ, 1982: 313–343.
5. Cowin, S. *Bone Mechanics Handbook.* CRC Press, Boca Raton, FL, 2001.
6. Long, M.; Rack, H.J. Titanium alloys in total joint replacement—a materials science perspective. *Biomaterials.* 1998; 19(18): 1621–39. doi:10.1016/s0142-9612(97)00146-4
7. Ratner, B.D.; Hoffman, A.S.; Schoen, F.J.; Lemons, J.E. (Eds.): *Biomaterials Science: An Introduction to Materials in Medicine.* 3rd edition, Academic Press, Cambridge, MA, 2012.
8. Geetha, M.; Singh, A.K.; Asokamani, R.; Gogia, A.K. Ti based biomaterials, the ultimate choice for orthopaedic implants – a review. *Prog Mater Sci.* 2009; 54(3): 397–425. doi:10.1016/j.pmatsci.2008.06.004
9. An, Y.; Draughn, R. (Eds.): *Mechanical Testing of Bone and the Bone-Implant Interface.* CRC Press, Boca Raton, FL, 1999.
10. Fields, A.J.; Lee, G.L.; Liu, X.S.; Jekir, M.G.; Guo, X.E.; Keaveny, T.M.; Influence of vertical trabeculae on the compressive strength of the human vertebra. *J Bone Miner Res.* 2011; 26(2): 263–9. doi:10.1002/jbmr.207
11. Tejszerska, D.; Świtoński, E.; Gzik, M. (Eds.): Biomechanika narządu ruchu człowieka. Wydawnictwo Naukowe Instytutu Technologii Eksploatacji – Państwowego Instytutu Badawczego, Radom, 2011.
12. Huiskes, R.; & Verdonschot, N. J. J. Biomechanics of artificial joints: the hip, in: Mow, V. C. & Hayes W. C. (Eds.), *Basic orthopaedic biomechanics.* 2nd edition. Lipincott-Raven Publishers, New York, 1997: 395–460.
13. Rho, J.Y.; Kuhn-Spearing, L.; Zioupos, P. Mechanical properties and the hierarchical structure of bone. *Med Eng Phys.* 1998; 20(2): 92–102. doi:10.1016/s1350-4533(98)00007-1
14. Bankoff, A.D.P. Biomechanical characteristics of the bone, in: Goswami, T.: *Human Musculoskeletal Biomechanics*, IntechOpen, 2012. doi:10.5772/19690

15. Bergmann, G.; Graichen, F.; Rohlmann, A. Hip joint loading during walking and running, measured in two patients. *J Biomech*. 1993; 26(8): 969–90. doi:10.1016/0021-9290(93)90058-m
16. Bergmann, G.; Graichen, F.; Rohlmann, A. Loads acting at the hip joint, in: Sedel, L.; Cabanela, M.E. (Eds): *Hip Surgery: Materials and Developments*, Martin Duntiz, London, 1998, 1–8.
17. Bergmann, G.; Bender, A.; Dymke, J.; Duda, G.; Damm, P. Standardized loads acting in hip implants. *PLoS One*. 2016; 11(5): e0155612. doi:10.1371/journal.pone.0155612
18. Graichen, F.; Bergmann, G.; Rohlmann, A. Hip endoprosthesis for in vivo measurement of joint force and temperature. *J Biomech*. 1999; 32(10): 1113–7. doi:10.1016/s0021-9290(99)00110-4
19. ISO 14242-1:2012 Implants for surgery – Wear of total hip joint prostheses – Part 1: Loading and displacement parameters for wear testing machines and corresponding environmental conditions for test.
20. Hirmand, M.; Vahab, M.; Khoei, A.R. An augmented Lagrangian contact formulation for frictional discontinuities with the extended finite element method. *Finite Elem Anal Des*. 2015; 107: 28–43. doi:10.1016/j.finel.2015.08.003
21. Dos Santos, M.B.F.; Meloto, G.O.; Bacchi, A.; Correr-Sobrinho, L. Stress distribution in cylindrical and conical implants under rotational micromovement with different boundary conditions and bone properties: 3D FEA. *Comput Methods Biomech Biomed Engin*. 2017; 20(8): 893–900. doi:10.1080/10255842.2017.1309394
22. Burkhart, T.A.; Andrews, D.M.; Dunning, C.E. Finite element modeling mesh quality, energy balance and validation methods: a review with recommendations associated with the modeling of bone tissue. *J Biomech*. 2013; 46(9): 1477–88. doi:10.1016/j.jbiomech.2013.03.022
23. Dogru, S.C.; Cansiz, E.; Arslan, Y.Z. A review of finite element applications in oral and maxillofacial biomechanics. *J Mech Med Biol*. 2018; 18: 1830002. doi:10.1142/S0219519418300028
24. Ramos, A.; Simoes, J.A. Tetrahedral versus hexahedral finite elements in numerical modelling of the proximal femur. *Med Eng & Phys*. 2006; 28(9): 916–24. doi:10.1016/j.medengphy.2005.12.006
25. Benzley, S.E.; Perry, E.; Merkley, K.; Clark, B.; Sjaardama, G. A comparison of all hexagonal and all tetrahedral finite element meshes for elastic and elasto-plastic analysis, in: *Proceedings of the 4th International Meshing Roundtable*, Sandia National Laboratories, Albuquerque, NM, 16–17 October 1995, 179–91.
26. Lee, J.S.; Lim, Y.J. Three-dimensional numerical simulation of stress induced by different lengths of osseointegrated implants in the anterior maxilla. *Comput Methods Biomech Biomed Engin*. 2013; 16(11): 1143–9. doi:10.1080/10255842.2012.654780
27. Tsouknidas, A.; Maliaris, G.; Savvakis, S.; Michailidis, N. Anisotropic post-yield response of cancellous bone simulated by stress-strain curves of bulk equivalent structures. *Comput Methods Biomech Biomed Engin*. 2015; 18(8): 839–46. doi:10.1080/10255842.2013.849342
28. Pawlikowski, M.; Skalski, K.; Banczerowski, J.; Makuch, A.; Jankowski, K. Stress-strain characteristic of human trabecular bone based on depth sensing indentation measurements. *Biocybern Biomed Eng*. 2017; 37(2): 272–80. doi:10.1016/j.bbe.2017.01.002
29. Enns-Bray, W.S.; Ariza, O.; Gilchrist, S.; Widmer-Soyka, R.P.; Vogt, P.J.; Palsson, H.; Helgason, B. Morphology based anisotropic finite element models of the proximal femur validated with experimental data. *Med Eng Phys*. 2016; 38(11): 1339–47. doi:10.1016/j.medengphy.2016.08.010
30. Affes, F.; Ketata, H.; Kharrat, M.; Dammak, M. How a pilot hole size affects osteosynthesis at the screw–bone interface under immediate loading. *Med. Eng. Phys*. 2018; 60: 14–22. doi:10.1016/j.medengphy.2018.07.002

31. Huang, H.L.; Hsu, J.T.; Fuh, L.J.; Tu, M.G.; Ko, C.C.; Shen, Y.W. Bone stress and interfacial sliding analysis of implant designs on an immediately loaded maxillary implant: a nonlinear finite element study. *J Dent*. 2008; 36(6): 409–17. doi:10.1016/j.jdent.2008.02.015

32. Du, J.; Lee, J.H.; Jang, A.T.; Gu, A.; Hossaini-Zadeh, M.; Prevost, R.; Curtis, D.A.; Ho, S.P. Biomechanics and strain mapping in bone as related to immediately-loaded dental implants. *J Biomech*. 2015; 48(12): 3486–94. doi:10.1016/j.jbiomech.2015.05.014

33. Wu, D.; Isaksson, P.; Ferguson, S.J.; Persson, C. Young's modulus of trabecular bone at the tissue level: a review. *Acta Biomater*. 2018; 78: 1–12. doi:10.1016/j.actbio.2018.08.001

34. Bailey, S.; Vashishth, D. Mechanical characterization of bone: state of the art in experimental approaches-what types of experiments do people do and how does one interpret the results? *Curr Osteoporos Rep*. 2018; 16(4): 423–33. doi:10.1007/s11914-018-0454-8

35. Liu, S.; Shin, Y.C. Additive manufacturing of Ti6Al4V alloy: a review. *Mater Des*. 2019; 164: 107552. doi:10.1016/j.matdes.2018.107552

36. Zhai, Y.; Galarraga, H.; Lados, D.A. Microstructure, static properties, and fatigue crack growth mechanisms in Ti-6Al-4V fabricated by additive manufacturing: LENS and EBM. *Eng Fail Anal*. 2016; 69: 3–14. doi:10.1016/j.engfailanal.2016.05.036

37. Kerr, A.; Rowe, P. *An Introduction to Human Movement and Biomechanics*, 7th ed.; Elsevier, Amsterdam, The Netherlands, 2019.

38. Uklejewski, R.; Winiecki, M.; Rogala, P.; Patalas, A. Structural-geometric functionalization of the additively manufactured prototype of biomimetic multispiked connecting Ti-Alloy scaffold for entirely noncemented resurfacing arthroplasty endoprostheses. *Appl Bionics Biomech*. 2017; 2017: 5638680. doi:10.1155/2017/5638680

39. An, Y.; Freidman, R. *Animal Models in Orthopaedic Research*, CRC Press, Boca Raton, FL, 1998.

40. Natali, A.N.; Meroi, E.A. A review of the biomechanical properties of bone as a material. *J Biomed Eng*. 1989; 11(4): 266–76. doi:10.1016/0141-5425(89)90058-7

41. Guillén, T.; Zhang, Q.-H.; Tozzi, G.; Ohrndorf, A.; Christ, H.-J.; Tong, J. Compressive behaviour of bovine cancellous bone and bone analogous materials, microCT characterisation and FE analysis. *J Mech Behav Biomed Mater*. 2011; 4(7): 1452–61. doi:10.1016/j.jmbbm.2011.05.015

42. Ozan, F.; Pekedis, M.; Koyuncu, Ş.; Altay, T.; Yıldız, H.; Kayalı, C. Microcomputed tomography and mechanical evaluation of trabecular bone structure in osteopenic and osteoporotic fractures. *J Orthop Surg (Hong Kong)*. 2017; 25(1): 1–6. doi:10.1177/2309499017692718

43. Spiess, A.N.; Neumeyer, N. An evaluation of R^2 as an inadequate measure for nonlinear models in pharmacological and biochemical research: a Monte Carlo approach. *BMC Pharmacol*. 2010; 10: 6. doi:10.1186/1471-2210-10-6

44. Shmueli, G. To explain or to predict? *Statist Sci*. 2010; 25(3): 289–310. doi:10.1214/10-STS330

45. Bruce, A. *Practical Statistics for Data Scientists: 50 Essential Concepts*. Shroff/O'Reilly, Mumbai, India, 2017.

46. Adams, G.J.; Cook, R.B.; Hutchinson, J R.; Zioupos P. Bone apparent and material densities examined by cone beam computed tomography and the Archimedes technique: comparison of the two methods and their results. *Front Mech Eng*. 2018; 3: 23 doi:10.3389/fmech.2017.00023

47. Zioupos, P.; Cook, R.B.; Hutchinson, J.R. Some basic relationships between density values in cancellous and cortical bone. *J Biomech*. 2008; 41(9): 1961–8. doi:10.1016/j.jbiomech.2008.03.025

48. Kaneko, T.S.; Bell, J.S.; Pejcic, M.R.; Tehranzadeh, J.; Keyak, J.H. Mechanical properties, density and quantitative CT scan data of trabecular bone with and without metastases. *J Biomech*. 2004; 37(4): 523–30. doi:10.1016/j.jbiomech.2003.08.010

49. Nobakhti, S.; Shefelbine, S.J. On the relation of bone mineral density and the elastic modulus in healthy and pathologic bone. *Curr Osteoporos Rep.* 2018; 16(4): 404–10. doi:10.1007/s11914-018-0449-5

50. Haba, Y.; Lindner, T.; Fritsche, A.; Schiebenhöfer, A.K.; Souffrant, R.; Kluess, D.; Bader, R. Relationship between mechanical properties and bone mineral density of human femoral bone retrieved from patients with osteoarthritis. *Open Orthop J.* 2012; 6: 458–63. doi:10.2174/1874325001206010458

51. Keenan, M.J.; Hegsted, M.; Jones, K.L.; Delany, J.P.; Kime, J.C.; Melancon, L.E.; Tulley, R.T.; Hong, K.D. Comparison of bone density measurement techniques: DXA and Archimedes' principle. *J Bone Miner Res.* 1997; 12(11): 1903–7. doi:10.1359/jbmr.1997.12.11.1903

52. Rogala, P. Endoprosthesis. EU Patent No. EP072418 B1, 22 December 1999.

53. Rogala, P. Acetabulum Endoprosthesis and Head. U.S. Patent US5,911,759 A, 15 June 1999.

54. Rogala, P. Method and Endoprosthesis to Apply This Implantation. Canadian Patent No. 2,200,064, 1 April 2002.

55. Cicciù, M.; Fiorillo, L.; D'Amico, C.; Gambino, D.; Amantia, E.M.; Laino, L.; Crimi, S.; Campagna, P.; Bianchi, A.; Herford, A.S.; Cervino, G. 3D digital impression systems compared with traditional techniques in dentistry: a recent data systematic review. *Materials.* 2020; 13(8): 1982. doi:10.3390/ma13081982

56. Cicciù, M.; Cervino, G.; Milone, D.; Risitano, G. FEM investigation of the stress distribution over mandibular bone due to screwed over denture positioned on dental implants. *Materials.* 2018; 11(9): 1512. doi:10.3390/ma11091512

57. Bramanti, E.; Cervino, G.; Lauritano, F.; Fiorillo, L.; D'Amico, C.; Sambataro, S.; Denaro, D.; Famà, F.; Ierardo, G.; Polimeni, A.; Cicciù, M. FEM and Von Mises analysis on prosthetic crowns structural elements: evaluation of different applied materials. *Sci World J.* 2017; 2017: 1029574. doi:10.1155/2017/1029574

58. Lauritano, F.; Runci, M.; Cervino, G.; Fiorillo, L.; Bramanti, E.; Cicciù, M. Three-dimensional evaluation of different prosthesis retention systems using finite element analysis and the Von Mises stress test. *Minerva Stomatol.* 2016; 65(6): 353–67.

59. Ramos, A.; Soares dos Santos, M.P.; Mesnard, M. Predictions of Birmingham hip resurfacing implant offset–In vitro and numerical models. *Comput Methods Biomech Biomed Engin.* 2019; 22(4): 352–63. doi:10.1080/10255842.2018.1556973

60. Xu, M.; Yang, J.; Lieberman, I.; Haddas, R. Stress distribution in vertebral bone and pedicle screw and screw-bone load transfers among various fixation methods for lumbar spine surgical alignment: A finite element study. *Med Eng Phys.* 2019; 63: 26–32. doi:10.1016/j.medengphy.2018.10.003

61. Gong, H.; Fan, Q.; Zhou, Y.; Wang, D.; Li, P.; Su, T.; Zhang, H. Simulation of failure processes of as-cast Ti-5Al-5Nb-1Mo-1V-1Fe titanium alloy subjected to quasistatic uniaxial tensile testing. *Mater Des.* 2019; 180: 107962. doi:10.1016/j.matdes.2019.107962

62. Timercan, A.; Brailovski, V.; Petit, Y.; Lussier, B.; Séguin, B. Personalized 3D-printed endoprostheses for limb sparing in dogs: modeling and in vitro testing. *Med Eng Phys.* 2019; 71: 17–29. doi:10.1016/j.medengphy.2019.07.005

63. Hazrati-Marangalou, J.; Ito, K.; van Rietbergen, B. A new approach to determine the accuracy of morphology–elasticity relationships in continuum FE analyses of human proximal femur. *J Biomech.* 2012; 45(16): 2884–92. doi:10.1016/j.jbiomech.2012.08.022

64. Van Rietbergen, B.; Kabel, J.; Odgaard, A.; Huiskes, R. Determination of trabecular bone tissue elastic properties by comparison of experimental and finite element results, in: Sol, H., Oomens, C.W.J. (Eds): *In Material Identification Using Mixed Numerical Experimental Methods*, Springer, Dordrecht, 1997, 183–92. doi:10.1007/978-94-009-1471-1_19

65. Krone, R.; Schuster, P. An Investigation of Importance of Material Anisotropy in Finite-Element Modeling of the Human Femur. SAE Int. 2006; Paper No. 2006-01-0064. doi:10.4271/2006-01-0064

66. Wirtz, D.C.; Schiffers, N.; Pandorf, T.; Radermacher, K.; Weichert, D.; Forst, R. Critical evaluation of known bone material properties to realize anisotropic FE-simulation of the proximal femur. *J Biomech.* 2000; 33(10): 1325–30. doi:10.1016/s0021-9290(00)00069-5

67. Keyak, J.H.; Rossi, S.A. Prediction of femoral fracture load using finite element models: an examination of stress- and strain-based failure theories. *J Biomech.* 2000; 33(2): 209–14. doi:10.1016/s0021-9290(99)00152-9

68. Tellache, M.; Pithioux, M.; Chabrand, P.; Hochard, C. Femoral neck fracture prediction by anisotropic yield criteria. *Eur J Comput Mech.* 2009; 18: 33–41. doi:10.3166/ejcm.18.33-41

69. Maknickas, A.; Alekna, V.; Ardatov, O.; Chabarova, O.; Zabulionis, D.; Tamulaitiene, M.; Kačianauskas, R. FEM-based compression fracture risk assessment in Osteoporotic Lumbar Vertebra L1. *Appl Sci.* 2019; 9: 3013. doi:10.3390/app9153013

70. Provatidis, C.; Vossou, C.; Koukoulis, I.; Balanika, A.; Baltas, C.; Lyritis, G. A pilot finite element study of an osteoporotic L1-vertebra compared to one with normal T-score. *Comput Methods Biomech Biomed Engin.* 2010; 13(2): 185–95. doi:10.1080/10255840903099703

71. Haut, R.C.; Wei, F. Biomechanical studies on patterns of cranial bone fracture using the immature porcine model. *J Biomech Eng.* 2017; 139(2): 021001. doi:10.1115/1.4034430

72. Bowland, P.; Ingham, E.; Fisher, J.; Jennings, L.M. Development of a preclinical natural porcine knee simulation model for the tribological assessment of osteochondral grafts in vitro. *J. Biomech.* 2018; 77: 91–8. doi:10.1016/j.jbiomech.2018.06.014

73. Pilia, M.; Guda, T.; Appleford, M. Development of composite scaffolds for load-bearing segmental bone defects. *Biomed Res Int.* 2013; 2013: 458253. doi:10.1155/2013/458253

74. Swindle, M.M.; Makin, A.; Herron, A.J. Swine as models in biomedical research and toxicology testing. *Vet Pathol.* 2012; 49(2): 344–56. doi:10.1177/0300985811402846

7 Pilot study on the prototype multi-spiked connecting scaffold for non-cemented resurfacing endoprostheses in an animal model

7.1 EXPERIMENTAL DETERMINATION OF THE APPROPRIATE SURGICAL APPROACH TO THE HIP AND KNEE JOINT IN SWINE

Pilot study on an animal model (swine, breed: Polish Large White, approval of the Local Ethics Committee in Poznan) concerning the preprototypes of the MSC-Scaffold and the working prototype of partial resurfacing knee arthroplasty endoprosthesis were carried out in order to:

- determine the appropriate surgical approach to the knee and hip joints of swine,
- gain operational experience in implanting the above-mentioned preprototypes of implants in an experimental animal,
- work out the methodology of postoperative treatment with an experimental animal,
- acquire experience in the field of making bone-implant specimens harvested from experimental implantations,
- conduct initial macroscopic and microscopic evaluation of the bone-implant interface in specimens harvested from experimental animals that had been surgically implanted several weeks earlier with the prototype implants investigated.

The images in Figure 7.1 present photographic documentation of one of the implantations of the MSC-Scaffold preprototypes in the swine knee joint carried out in a veterinary clinic. Figure 7.2 shows the cutting of the bone-implant specimen using

DOI: 10.1201/9781003364498-7

equipment for precise cutting of the bone-metal implant specimens. Figure 7.3 shows an example bone-implant specimen prepared for microscopic evaluation of bone-implant integration.

A lateral approach to the swine hip joint via the gluteal muscles was selected. The animal operated on was placed in the ipsilateral position with the greater trochanter on the edge of the operating table and the gluteal muscles were relaxed. Approach to the head, neck, and acetabulum in swine was difficult. The greater trochanter was hardly felt below the line from the iliac to the ischial tuberosity. A straight lateral

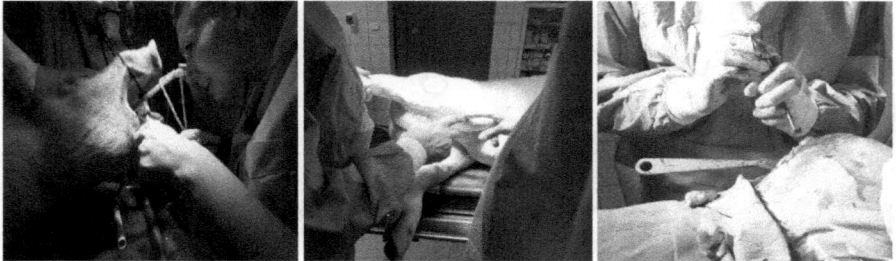

FIGURE 7.1 Photographic documentation of one of the implantations of the prototype MSC-Scaffold in the swine knee joint carried out in a veterinary clinic.

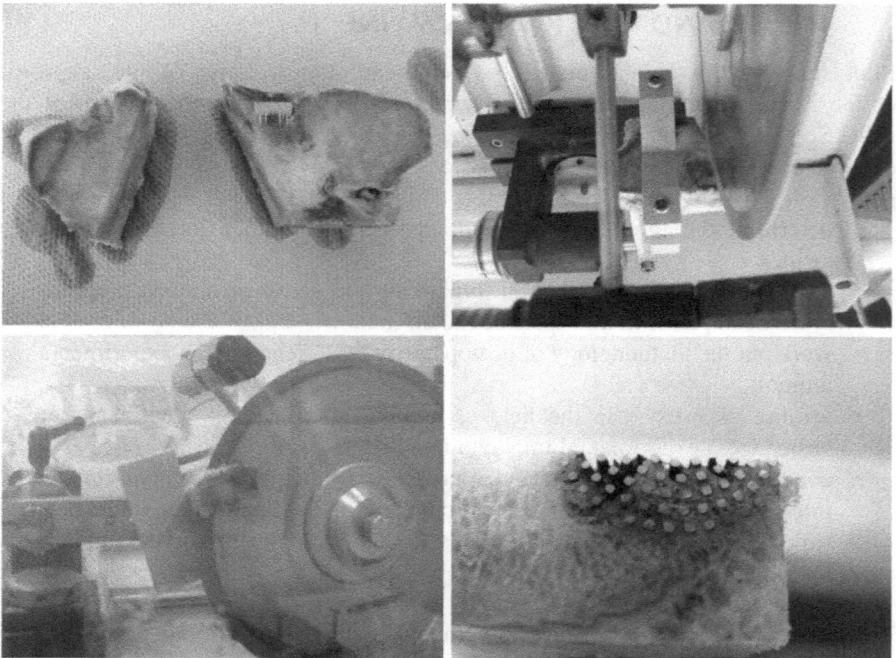

FIGURE 7.2 Cutting the bone-implant specimen.

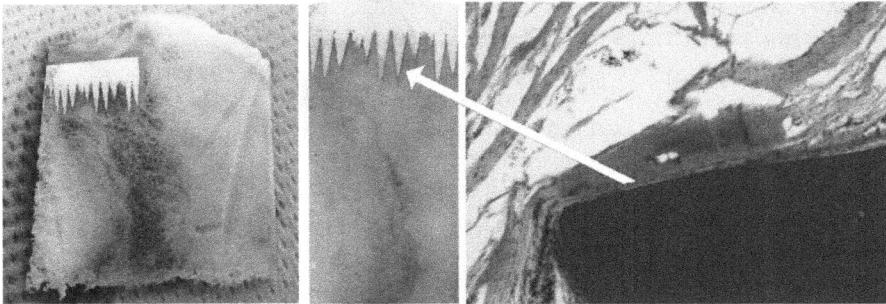

FIGURE 7.3 An example specimen of a bone-implant specimen for the microscopic evaluation of the bone-implant biointegration.

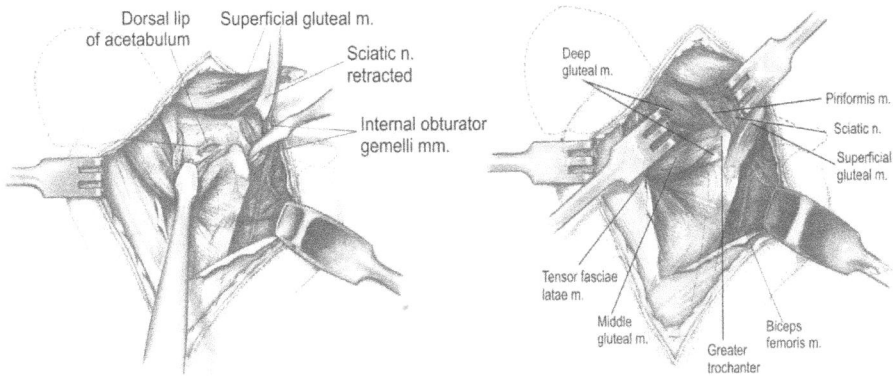

FIGURE 7.4 Sketch of a surgical lateral approach to a swine hip (adapted from the sketches in [1,2]).

skin incision was made along the lateral femoral line, starting from the upper trochanter 8–10 cm above and ending 8–10 cm below the trochanteric area, and then the tensor fasciae latae muscle and the great gluteus muscle were separated along the cut line above the greater trochanter. The broad fascia tensioner was moved anteriorly and the great gluteus muscle posteriorly, revealing the initial attachment of the gluteus maximus and the bone attachment of the gluteus medius. The muscle mass of the gluteus medius and gluteus maximus with its tendon junction was lifted and moved anteriorly. The gluteus medius tendon was incised obliquely along the greater trochanter, leaving its posterior half still attached to the trochanter. An incision was then made proximally along the gluteal median fibres to the junction of the gluteus medius and posterior thirds of the gluteus medius. This gluteal splitting should not extend more than 2–3 cm from the apex of the greater trochanter to avoid damage to the superior gluteal nerve and artery (Figure 7.4). A distal incision was made anteriorly along the broader lateral muscle fibres as far as the bone along the anterolateral surface of the thigh. The gluteus medius tendon is marked. The cut made by this fascia and tendon attachments together with the caudal large lateral and biceps muscle retraction exposed the greater trochanter and the subcranial view of the hip joint. The anterior articular capsule was exposed. A purse incision was needed. Surgical displacement of the femoral head from the acetabulum was performed.

The implantation sites for the two preprototypes of the MSC-Scaffold were prepared in the femoral head using a surgical drill. The first preprototype was implanted near the top of the femoral head and the second preprototype was placed at the equator of the femoral head. The holes in the subchondral bone were gradually milled to their final size with a milling cutter to harbour the implant. During drilling and milling, the bone holes were continuously cooled with a saline solution and then the holes in the femoral head were rinsed with saline to remove bone debris. Placement of the implants in the prepared bone holes was made with a surgical mallet. Two preprototypes of the MSC-Scaffold were embedded in the tissue of the bone openings up to about half the height of their spikes, so that their bases are slightly below the surface of the articular cartilage of the femoral head, as shown in Figure 7.5.

The femoral head was repositioned at the anatomical site. During the operative exit, the gluteus medius tendon was sutured with non-absorbable braided sutures. A layered wound suture is applied. Post-implantation antibiotic regimen was applied: penicillin powder was injected into the subcutaneous layer at the end of the operation.

Figure 7.6 shows the radiograph taken in the fourth week after implantation. Radiographic examination showed no loosening and no migration of the implant in the fourth week after surgery. Figure 7.7 shows a swine hip joint taken eight weeks after implantation with the implanted two preprototypes of the MSC-Scaffold. During resection of the hip joint, macroscopic fragmentation (fracture) of the femoral head

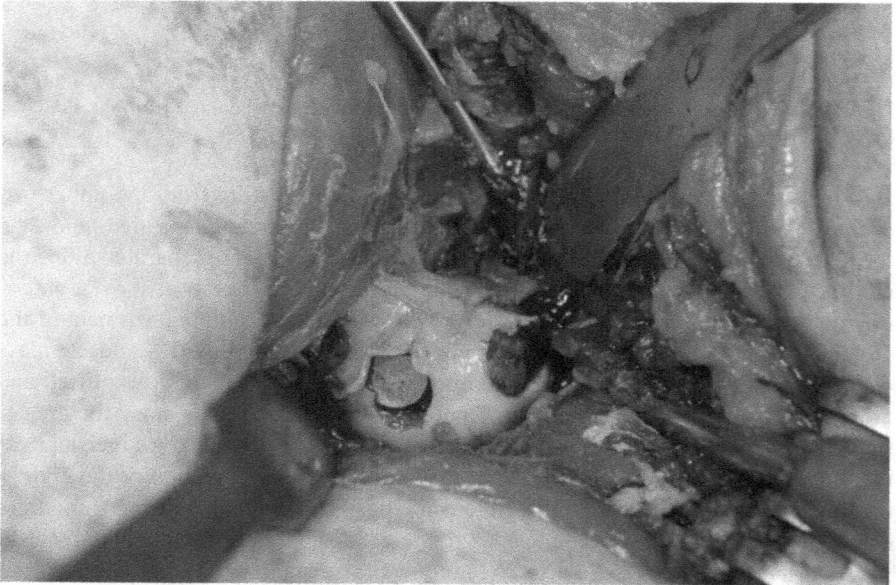

FIGURE 7.5 Intraoperative photo of implantation of two preprototypes of the MSC-Scaffold in the femoral head in a swine.

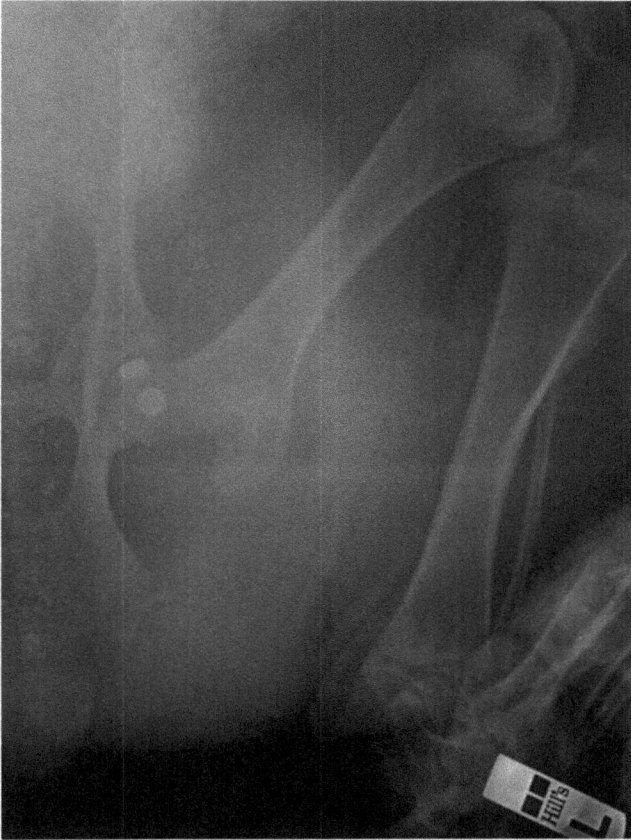

FIGURE 7.6 Radiograph taken fourth week after implantation (X-ray Stenoscop Plus, Mobile C-Arm; GE Medical Systems) in a veterinary clinic.

was found. The implantation of two MSC-Scaffold preprototypes (each of ⌀10 mm) turned out to be too aggravating – the animal had a chronic limp after the procedure and eight weeks after surgical implantation in the excised hip joint after its opening, a fragmented femoral head was found (Figure 7.7).

Thus, it was experimentally found that the swine hip joint is not the right place for further study in an animal model of biointegration of the MSC-Scaffold preprototypes with bone tissue.

Moreover, since the surgical approach to the hip joint in swine and surgical procedures on this joint itself are technically quite difficult, especially due to the lack of specialized instruments dedicated to such surgeries in swine, further experimental studies on the implantation of our prototype implants into the hip joint in these swine were abandoned. For the next research stage, which will be carried out in the next research project, that is, the full standard implantation test of prototypes in an animal model, following the requirements of ISO 10993-2 [3], such specialized instruments

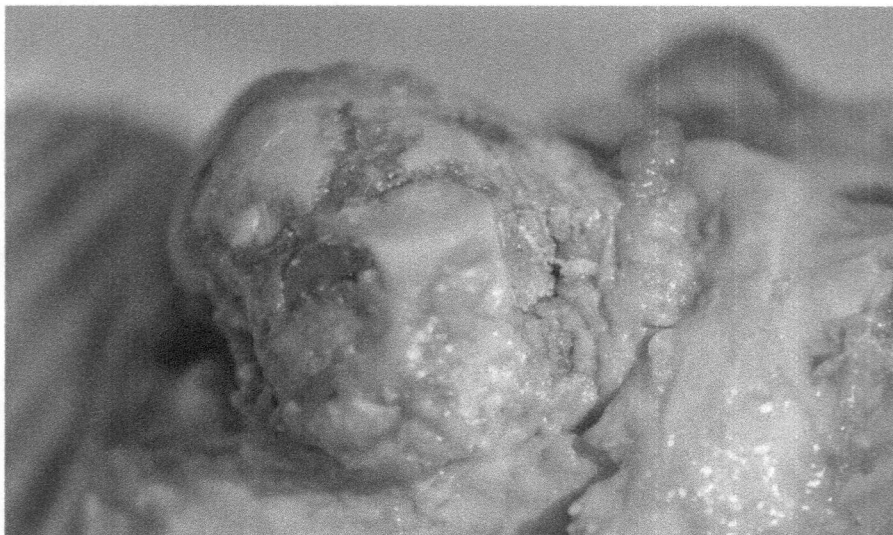

FIGURE 7.7   Fragmented swine femoral head obtained eight weeks after surgical implantation of the MSC-Scaffold preprototypes.

were designed. The patent application was sent to the Patent Office of the Republic of Poland [4].

The need to implant in a comparative study more than one preprototype of the MSC-Scaffold required experimental determination of an appropriate surgical approach to the swine knee joint.

For this purpose, after opening the knee joints in swine, four preprototypes of the MSC-Scaffold were implanted under the surface of the articular cartilage of the medial and lateral femoral condyles.

A lateral parapatellar approach was used to the swine knee due to the normally small abduction in the hip joint and the medial location of the tibial (femoral) nerve, as well as the saphenous artery and vein. An anterolateral skin incision was made over the operated right knee joint, with a length of approximately 8 inches. An approach to the knee joint was used between the lateral edge of the patella and the outer side of the patellar ligament, and then between the vastus lateralis and the rectus femoris muscle. The articular capsule of the knee joint was opened on the lateral edge of the patella, then the patella was dislocated medially, haemostasis was performed, and the patellofemoral area of the knee was exposed (Figure 7.8).

Implantation sites were prepared in both femoral condyles using a surgical drill. The holes in the cancellous bone were gradually milled to their final size with a milling cutter, and an implant (the MSC-Scaffold preprototype) was inserted. During drilling and milling, the bone holes were continuously cooled with a saline solution. The holes in the condyles were rinsed with saline and the bone debris was removed. Four preprototypes of the MSC-Scaffold were placed beneath the surface of the articular cartilage in both femoral condyles in the swine open knee. Implant placement in the drilled bone holes was performed with a surgical mallet. Figure 7.9

presents an intraoperative photogram of the four MSC-Scaffold preprototypes implanted beneath the surface of the articular cartilage in the medial and lateral femoral condyles of the swine knee joint.

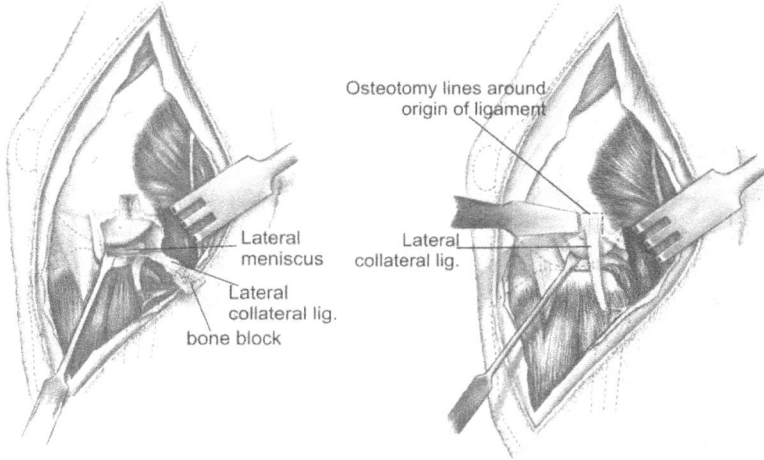

FIGURE 7.8 Sketch of the surgical lateral approach to the swine knee joint (adapted from the sketches in [1,2]).

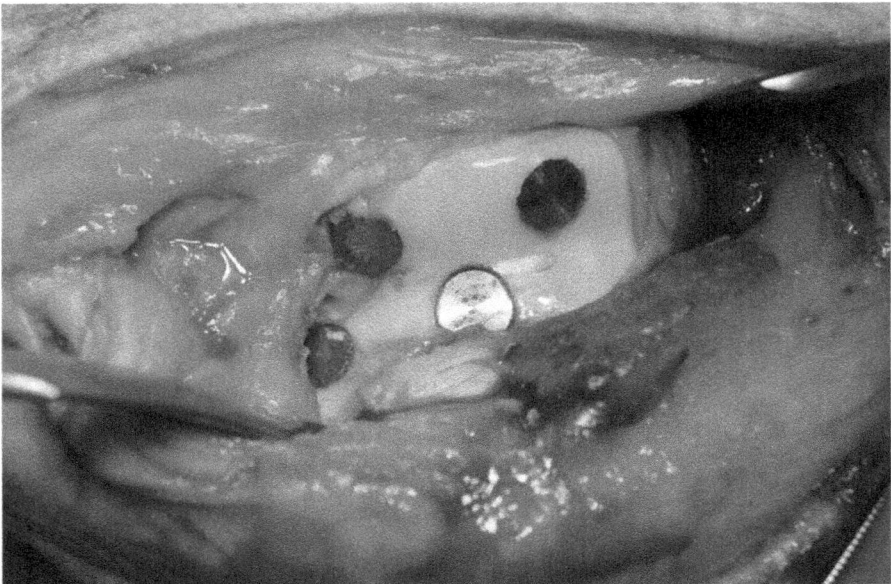

FIGURE 7.9 Intraoperative photo of implantation of four preprototypes of the MSC-Scaffold into the articular subchondral layer of the medial and lateral condyle of the lower epiphysis of the swine femur.

Then the patella was repositioned at the anatomical site. A layered wound suture is applied. After implantation, an antibiotic regimen was applied: at the end of the procedure, penicillin powder was injected into the subcutaneous layer, the wound was covered with a penicillin-soaked mesh, and an antiseptic dressing was applied. After the procedure: Amikacin (Biodacin) 1 g two times a day was administered i.v. (or i.m.) for three days. On the third day after surgery, the swine were allowed to fully load the hind limb.

Eight weeks after implantation of the MSC-Scaffold preprototypes in the operating room of the veterinary clinic (premedication and general anaesthesia as in the case of implantation), surgical removal of the operated joints containing the implants was performed; the procedure was completed with animal sacrifice (Morbital lethal doses of 200 mg/kg b.w., i.v.) according to the protocol approved by the Local Ethics Committee in Poznan.

Figure 7.10 shows a radiograph taken four weeks after implantation. The radiographic examination did not show any loosening or migration of the implant after surgery. Figure 7.11 shows an operated swine knee sample with four preprototypes of the MSC-Scaffold surgically removed eight weeks after implantation. In the resected

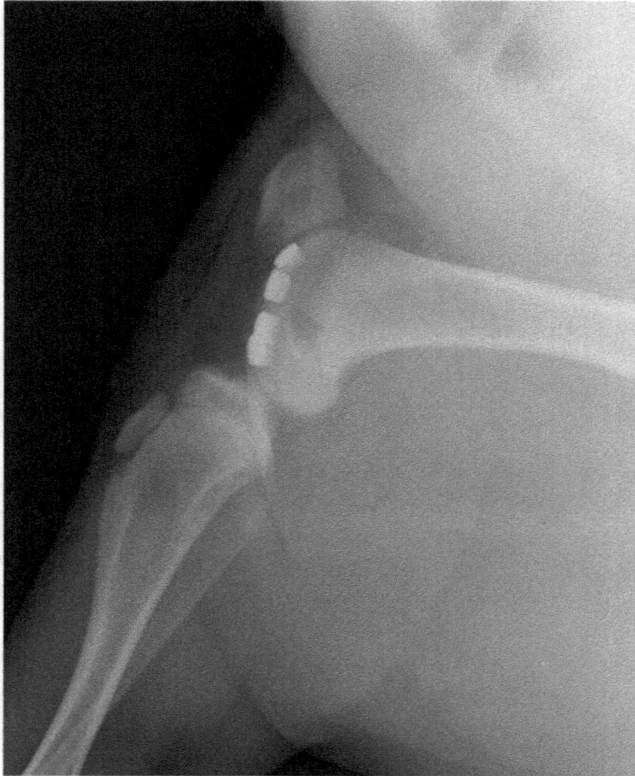

FIGURE 7.10   Radiograph taken at the fourth week after implantation (X-ray Stenoscop Plus, Mobile C-Arm; GE Medical Systems) at a veterinary clinic.

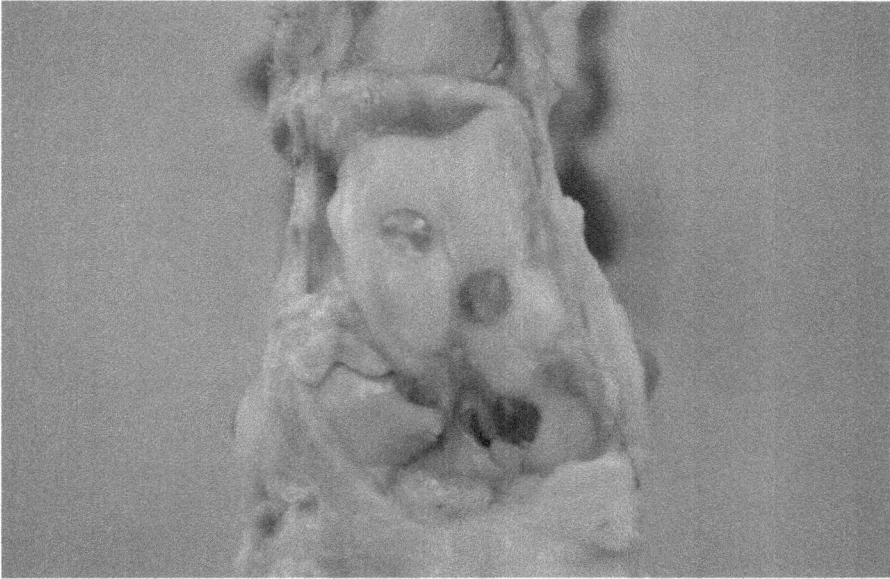

FIGURE 7.11 The knee joint collected eight weeks after the surgical implantation of four preprototypes of the MSC-Scaffold.

knee joint, no damage was observed to the femoral condyles, and the four implanted preprototypes showed good stabilization with no signs of migration.

We concluded that the swine knee joint could be recommended as a suitable site for further research (e.g., comparative research on unmodified and calcium phosphate-coated MSC-Scaffold preprototypes; see Section 5.4).

Based on the results of the surgical study regarding the experimental choice of an adequate surgical technique and the correct implantation site, it can be concluded that the appropriate place for the experimental pilot study in an animal model (swine) of the prototype MSC-Scaffold for the entirely non-cemented resurfacing arthroplasty endoprosthesis, recommended by us, is the swine knee joint (with the lateral approach).

7.2 VERIFICATION OF THE WORKING PROTOTYPE OF PARTIAL RESURFACING KNEE ARTHROPLASTY ENDOPROSTHESIS IN TEN EXPERIMENTAL ANIMALS

Initially, two working prototypes of partial resurfacing knee arthroplasty endoprosthesis were implanted in two animals (swine, Polish Large White breed) to experimentally determine the correct surgical technique for implanting the working prototype of partial resurfacing knee arthroplasty endoprosthesis with the biomimetic MSC-Scaffold. Implantation procedures were performed in the operating room of a veterinary clinic with the consent of the Local Ethics Committee in Poznan.

The selection of an appropriate animal model to experimentally implant a prototype resurfacing endoprosthesis is essential for the transfer of the results of the experimental study to clinical applications [5–10]. It is known that the swine model is used successfully in the preclinical study of surgical treatment of bone defects with various biosubstitutes. The density and microstructure of the swine bone were confirmed to be similar to those of human bone. A certain limitation in the study carried out in this animal model appears to be the large weight of the animals, and accelerated bone growth makes it difficult to distinguish early and late remodelling [5,6,9]. Swines have well-developed Havers systems in growing and mature bone [5] and blood circulation, metabolism, and bone remodelling largely correspond to these processes in humans [11]. The structure of the swine synovial joint is structurally a system of cartilage and ligaments very similar to the human joint [9,10]. Therefore, swine is recognized as the experimental animal of choice in a preclinical surgical study involving, inter alia, surgical techniques of implantation [11–13].

During surgical implantation of the working prototype of partial resurfacing knee arthroplasty endoprosthesis, general inhalation anaesthesia with endotracheal intubation [14–16] and monitoring of anaesthesia with a pulse oximeter (swine ear sensor) and cardio monitor (Dräger AT-1 anaesthesia machine, Drägerwerk AG & Co. KGaA, Lubeck, Germany) were done; anaesthesia was maintained with isoflurane inhalation anaesthetic; premedication was administered intramuscularly in one syringe of Cepetor/Medetomidine hydrochloride (0.02–0.04 mg/kg b.w., i.m.) and Levomethadone (0.25–0.5 mg/kg b.w., i.m.).

The first operation (swine, breed: Polish Large White, weight 87 kg) was performed by cutting the attachment of the collateral ligament of the lateral knee joint together with a thin bone fragment. The articular surface was prepared with a surgical chisel to obtain the geometry of the bone base that corresponds to the implant. The implant was embedded in the bone with a surgical mallet; the MSC-Scaffold spikes were embedded in the subchondral trabecular bone to a depth approximately half its height, allowing the limb to be loaded on the third day after surgery. Two screws were used to reattach the severed lateral collateral ligament.

In the second animal (swine, breed: Polish Large White, weight 80 kg), the surgical approach to the lateral femoral condyle was preceded by cutting off only one-third of the anterior collateral ligament attachment of the knee joint. Following implantation, this third of the anterior ligament attachment was reattached by positioning the bone suture.

The characteristics of the swine used in the study are presented in Table 7.1.

Figure 7.12a presents the working prototype of partial resurfacing knee arthroplasty endoprosthesis implanted into the lateral femoral condyle of the first animal, while Figure 7.12b shows the working prototype of partial resurfacing knee arthroplasty endoprosthesis implanted into the lateral femoral condyle of the knee joint in the second swine.

A layered wound suture was applied. Following implantation, an antibiotic regimen was introduced: at the end of the procedure, penicillin powder was applied to the subcutaneous layer, the wound was covered with a penicillin-soaked mesh, and an antiseptic dressing was applied. After the procedure: Amikacin (Biodacin) 1 g two times a day was administered i.v. (or i.m.) for three days.

TABLE 7.1

Summary of data on operations performed to determine the appropriate surgical technique to implant the working prototype of partial resurfacing knee arthroplasty endoprosthesis with the MSC-Scaffold

No of Swine	Weight (kg)	Knee	Bone Screws Used to Reattach the Severed Lateral Ligament Attachment	Stability in Radiological Examination	Stability of Operated Joint in Clinical Examination (Likert Scale)	Destruction of Femoral Condyle
1	87	Left	Yes	Very good	5	None
2	80	Right	No	Migration	2	None

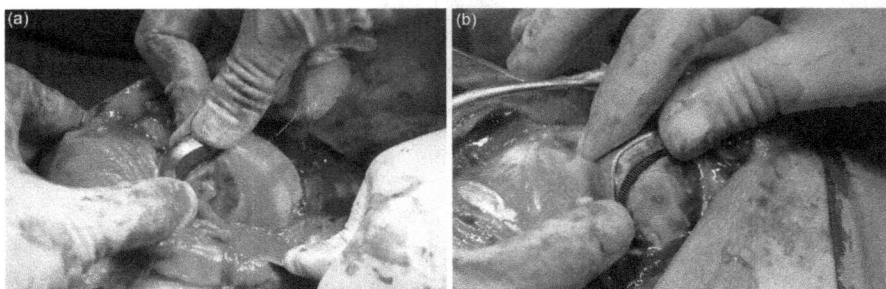

FIGURE 7.12 Intraoperative image of implantation in the swine knee joint of the working prototype of partial resurfacing knee arthroplasty endoprosthesis with partial resurfacing with the MSC-Scaffold: the first experimental animal (a), the second experimental animal (b).

On the third day after surgery, the swine were allowed to fully load the operated hindlimb. Four weeks after implantation, a premedicated postoperative X-ray examination of the animals was performed in a veterinary clinic, as in the case of implantation, using the Stenoscop Plus X-ray machine, Mobile C-Arm (GE Medical Systems, Japan). Eight weeks after implantation of the working prototype of partial resurfacing knee arthroplasty endoprosthesis in a veterinary clinic (premedication and general anaesthesia as during implantation), the implants were harvested together with the surrounding bone tissue. The procedure was completed with euthanasia of the animals (Morbital lethal dose of 200 mg/kg b.w., i.v.) according to a protocol approved by the Local Ethics Committee in Poznan. The extracted knee joints were examined by digital radiography (XPERT 40, Kubtec, USA).

Figures 7.13–7.15 present the results of the initial implantation of two working prototypes of partial resurfacing knee arthroplasty endoprosthesis into the lateral femoral condyle of two experimental animals. The results of a radiological examination performed four weeks after implantation (X-ray Stenoscop Plus, Mobile C-Arm,

GE Medical Systems, Japan) in a veterinary clinic are presented in Figure 7.13, where Figure 7.13a concerns the first of the animals, while Figure 7.13b is for the second animal. Similarly, Figures 7.14a and 7.14b present the surgically removed knee joint eight weeks after the implantation of the first and second animals, respectively. Similarly, Figures 7.15a and 7.15b present digital radiographs of knee joints resected after eight weeks.

The operative procedure used in the first animal provided surgical access to the entire femoral condyle for the embedding of the working prototype of partial resurfacing knee arthroplasty endoprosthesis and allows it to be firmly anchored. Clinical and radiological examination confirmed the very good stability of the knee joint

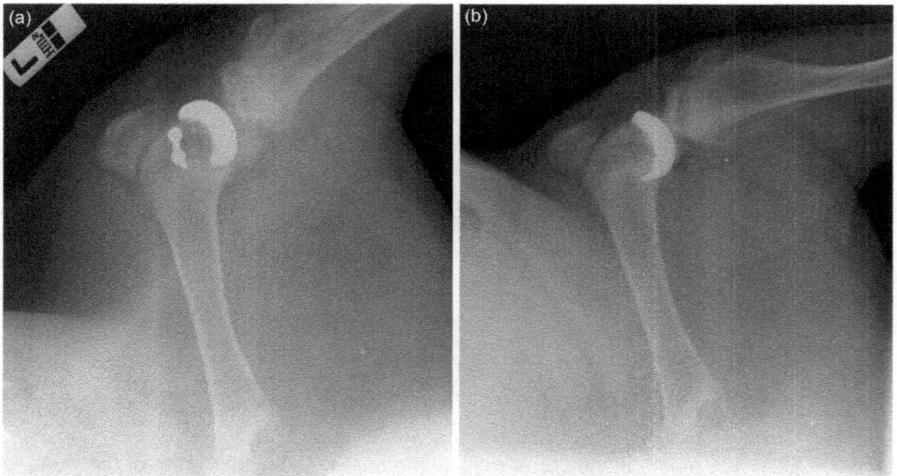

FIGURE 7.13 Radiograph of knee joints with the working prototype implanted of the partial knee resurfacing arthroplasty endoprosthesis performed in the veterinary clinic on the first (a) and second (b) animal four weeks after implantation.

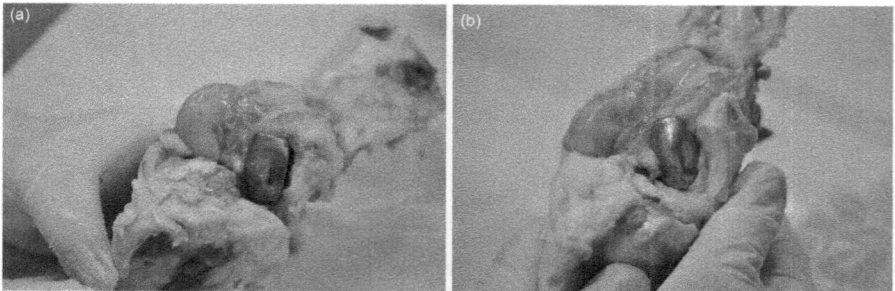

FIGURE 7.14 Knee joints harvested eight weeks after surgical implantation in the first experimental animal (a) and the second experimental animal (b).

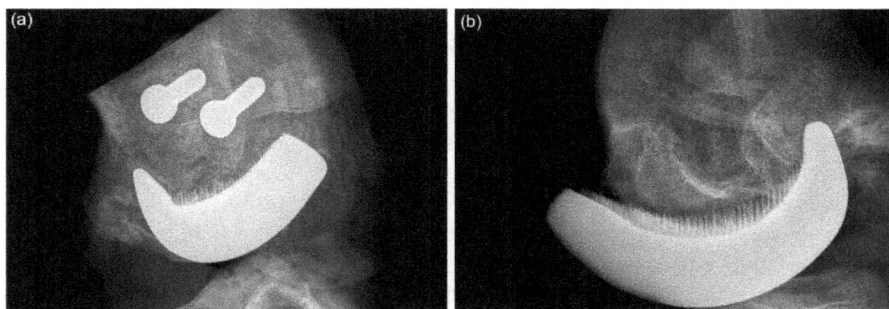

FIGURE 7.15   Digital radiograph of the knee joints resected after eight weeks (XPERT 40, Kubtec, USA) showing: the MSC-Scaffold interspike space occupied with remodelled bone tissue and two bone screws with which the excised lateral ligament attachment of the knee joint was reattached to the bone along with a thin bone fragment (a); slight implant migration in the area of the anterior surface of the lateral condyle and the interspike space partially occupied with the ingrown bone tissue (b).

and the absence of implant migration. No destruction of the femoral condyles was observed in the resected knee joint. A good seating of the implanted prototype of a working surface of partial knee endoprosthesis with the MSC-Scaffold was observed without any signs of migration. The digital radiograph of the resected knee joint shows the interspike space of the MSC-Scaffold occupied with the ingrown bone tissue and the two bone screws used to reattach the severed lateral ligament attachment of the swine lateral knee joint to the bone along with a thin bone fragment.

The operating procedure applied to the second test animal allows easy access to the anterior part of the lateral femoral condyle in the knee joint and limited access to the posterior part of this condyle. Clinical and radiological examination confirmed sufficient stability of the operated knee joint. In the resected knee joint, no destruction of the condyles was observed, but the working prototype of the partial resurfacing knee arthroplasty endoprosthesis with the MSC-Scaffold had minimal migration in the anterior part of the lateral femoral condyle. The digital radiograph of the knee joint resected after eight weeks can confirm a slight migration of the implant in the anterior part of the lateral femoral condyle and the interspike space of the MSC-Scaffold partially occupied with rebuilt peri-implant bone tissue.

In our opinion, the limited surgical approach to the posterior femoral condyle due to bone separation of only one-third of the anterior part of the fibular collateral ligament results in inadequate implant seating and leads to observed implant migration.

The tests of the working prototype of partial resurfacing knee arthroplasty endoprosthesis with partial resurfacing with the MSC-Scaffold were carried out on a group of ten swine of the Polish Large White breed, using the surgical technique selected experimentally during the preliminary study as more favourable. Before implantation, the bone-contacting surface of spikes of the MSC-Scaffold were modified with the calcium phosphate coating. This modification was made by electrochemical cathodic deposition under experimentally determined conditions (see Section 5.2).

Figure 7.16 shows an SEM image of the surface of the spikes of the MSC-Scaffold subjected to the modification mentioned above. The arrows show the lamellar calcium phosphate crystals on the lateral surface of the MSC-Scaffold spikes.

Clinical evaluation of joint stability after the implantation of the working prototype of partial resurfacing knee arthroplasty endoprosthesis of partial resurfacing was carried out according to [17] with the modification: total/medial stability of the joint was measured. The assessment of radiological stability (component loosening) was assessed on a 4-point scale. Radiolucency around the element was assessed in terms of thickness and position [18]. Statistica 12.0 (StatSoft, Tulsa, USA) was used for the statistical analysis of the results. Descriptive values of the variables are expressed as mean ± standard deviation or median (minimum–maximum).

A summary of the data on the operations performed is included in Table 7.2. In nine cases, good (30%) and very good (60%) stability of the operated knee joints was found, except for the one case where a septic complication occurred (Table 7.3). In the case of the remaining nine animals, no destruction of the femoral condyles was recorded in the knee joints harvested eight weeks after implantation of the working prototype of partial resurfacing knee arthroplasty endoprosthesis with the MSC-Scaffold. Joint stability was determined in a clinical trial using the 5-point Likert scale (Table 7.2). The mean body weight of the experimental animals was 82.0 ± 7.6 kg (Table 7.4).

Histological evaluation and microtomographic examination of the resected knee joints were performed.

Bone-implant specimens were fixed in 10% formalin solution (formaldehyde in phosphate buffer) for a week, and then dehydrated in ethanol at a concentration of 70%, 80%, 90%, 99%, and 100% after 48 h at each concentration and embedded in resin. Fragments of bone-implant specimens with a thickness of 200 μm were cut using the IsoMet™ 4000 Linear Precision Saw (Buehler, Esslingen am Neckar, Germany) and then ground to a thickness of 20 μm using the MetaServ 250 grinder

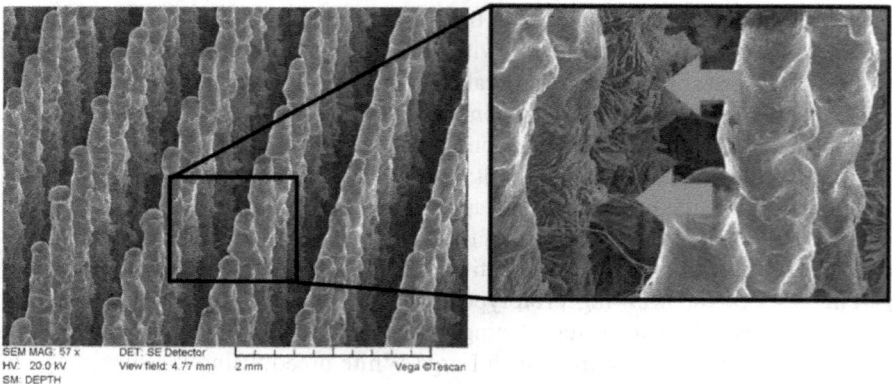

SEM MAG: 57 x   DET: SE Detector
HV: 20.0 kV   View field: 4.77 mm   2 mm   Vega ©Tescan
SM: DEPTH

FIGURE 7.16   SEM image of the surface of the MSC-Scaffold spikes connecting the working prototype of partial resurfacing knee arthroplasty endoprosthesis subjected to electrochemical modification of Ca-P, the arrows show lamellar calcium phosphate crystals on the lateral surface of the spikes.

TABLE 7.2
Summary of data on the performed surgeries of implantation of the working prototype of partial resurfacing knee arthroplasty endoprosthesis with the MSC-Scaffold

No of Swine	Weight (kg)	Sex	Age (Months)	Knee	Stability in Radiological Examination	Stability of Operated Joint in Clinical Examination (Likert Scale)	Destruction of Femoral Condyle
1	76	M	8	Left	Good	4	None
2	91	F	9	Right	Good	4	None
3	77	F	7	Left	Very good	5	None
4	69	M	8	Left	Very good	5	None
5	94	F	9	Right	Migration	2	None
6	78	M	8	Left	Very good	5	None
7	91	F	9	Left	Good	3	None
8	86	M	8	Right	Very good	4	None
9	81	M	9	Right	Very good	5	None
10	74	F	7	Right	Very good	4	None

TABLE 7.3
Stability characteristics of the implanted working prototype of working prototype of partial resurfacing knee arthroplasty endoprosthesis with the MSC-Scaffold, determined on radiological examination ($N = 10$)

Stability in Radiological Examination	Number (%)
Migration	1 (10)
Good	3 (30)
Very good	6 (60)

TABLE 7.4
Characterization of body weight and stability determined in a clinical study in ten animals implanted with the working prototype of partial resurfacing knee arthroplasty endoprosthesis with the MSC-Scaffold

Parameters	Mean ± SD	Median (min–max)
Weight (kg)	82.0 ± 7.6	80.5 (69–94)
Age (months)	8.2 ± 0.8	
Stability scale in clinical examination		4 (2–5)

polisher (Buehler, Esslingen am Neckar, Germany). Thin sections (20 μm) of bone-implant specimens were stained with haematoxylin and eosin and then examined with the Olympus CX41 light microscope (Olympus, Tokyo, Japan).

Figure 7.17 presents thin sections and stained histological sections (H&E) made of macro-specimens harvested eight weeks after the implantation of the prototype knee endoprostheses. Demonstrated are sections in the longitudinal (Figure 7.17a) and crosswise (Figure 7.17b) directions to the spike axis.

Histological section specimens show the interspike space occupied with peri-implant cancellous tissue and bone trabeculae in contact with the MSC-Scaffold spikes. In the eighth week following the procedure, no morphological exponents of inflammation were found in bone tissue from the stained histological samples. Almost all of the MSC-Scaffold spikes in the longitudinal and transverse sections are surrounded by mature bone tissue. There were no morphological markers of the osteogenesis

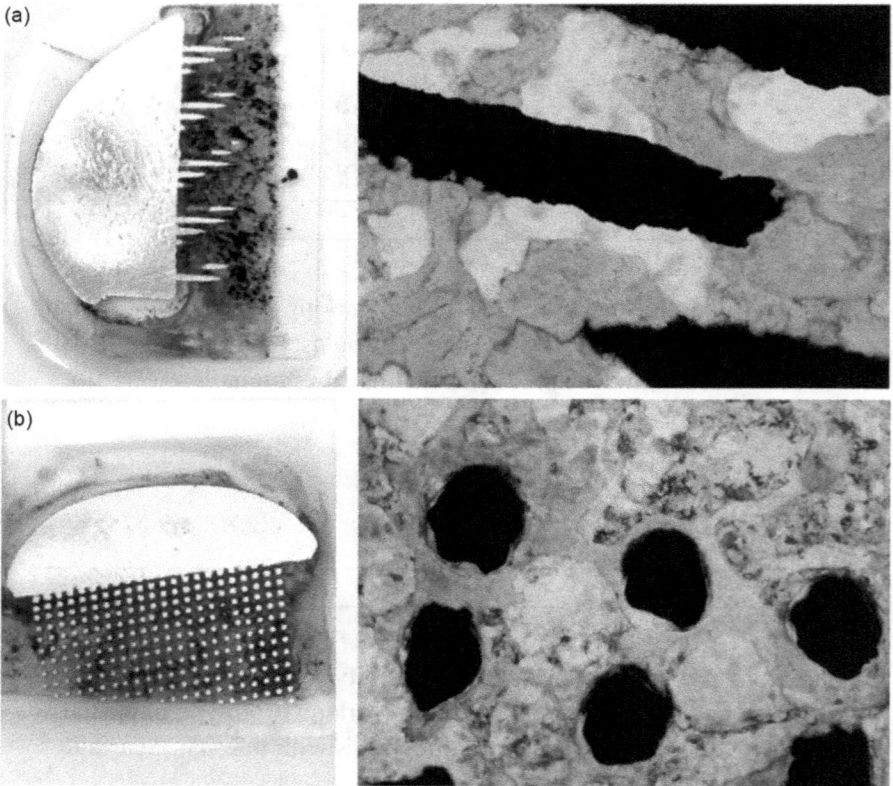

FIGURE 7.17 Microscopic and histopathological samples of the bone-implant section (H&E) made from bone-implant specimens harvested eight weeks after implantation, containing the working prototype of the knee arthroplasty endoprosthesis with the MSC-Scaffold: parallel (a) and perpendicular (b) in relation to the axis of the MSC-Scaffold spikes.

process. It can be concluded that the periscaffold trabecular bone is of similar age and maturity in these histological sections.

Microtomographic examination of knee joint specimens collected eight weeks post-implantation was performed using the SkyScan 1173 microtomographic X-ray scanner (Bruker, Kontich, Belgium). During the test, the samples were immersed in formalin and mounted on the turntable in the microtomography measurement chamber so that the axis of the spikes was parallel to the rotation axis of the table. The following scanning parameters were used: source energy 130 keV, source intensity 61 μA, resolution 9.92 μm, filter 0.25 mm brass filter, irradiation time 4,000 ms, rotation 360°, every 0.2°, scanning time approximately 6 h. 3D reconstruction of the bone-implant specimen scanned post-operatively from experimental animals after eight weeks and 2D quantitative analysis were performed using the SkyScan CT-Analyzer software (Bruker, Kontich, Belgium).

In 3D reconstructions of bone implants, cuboid-shaped fragments were virtually extracted for further quantitative and qualitative analysis. Based on the differences in radiological density, the radiological phases for the MSC-Scaffold, trabecular bone, and soft tissues, including bone marrow, were distinguished. In each of the virtually separated subareas of the micro-CT scan of the bone-implant specimen, six reference levels, spaced every 0.5 mm from each other, were determined, crossing the axes of the MSC-Scaffold spikes at right angles below their tops. The percentage of radiologically separated phases was measured at each of the scanning levels. The cube-shaped fragments were virtually separated for further quantitative and qualitative analysis. Figure 7.18 shows an example 2D micro-CT scan image of a periarticular bone specimen with the working prototype of partial resurfacing knee arthroplasty endo-prosthesis with the MSC-Scaffold, taken eight weeks after implantation. Figure 7.19 presents a microtomographic visualization of the bone-implant specimen, where a fragment was virtually isolated using dedicated software, showing the biointegration of the MSC-Scaffold with periarticular bone tissue.

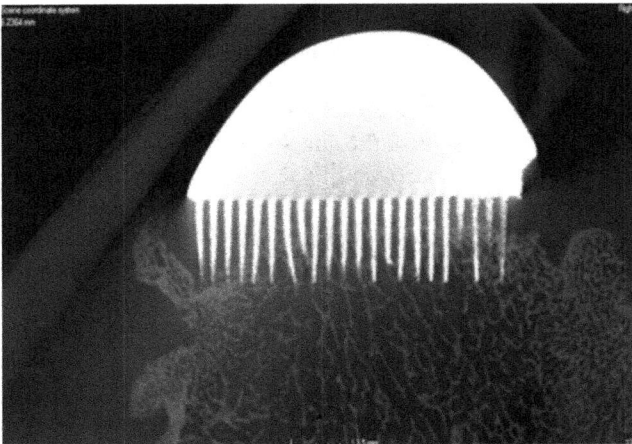

FIGURE 7.18   An example of a digital micro-CT scan of a swine knee joint sample with the working prototype of the partial resurfacing knee arthroplasty endoprosthesis with the MSC-Scaffold, taken eight weeks after implantation.

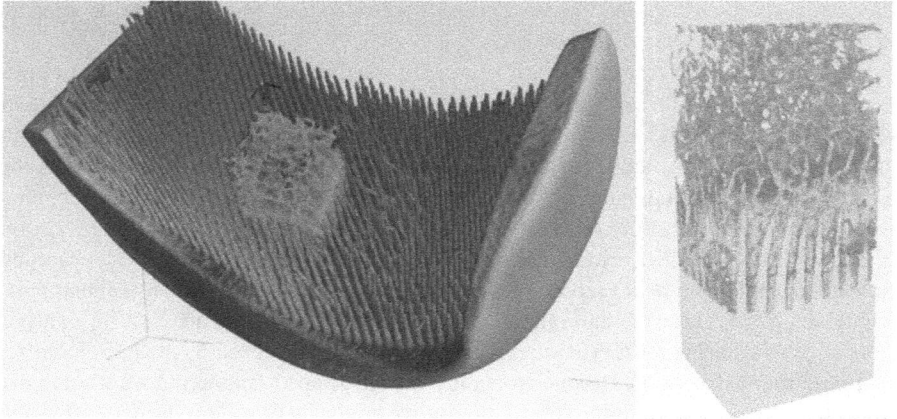

FIGURE 7.19 Microtomographic visualization of the periarticular bone specimen with the working prototype of partial resurfacing knee arthroplasty endoprosthesis with the MSC-Scaffold collected eight weeks after implantation; in the image of this specimen, using dedicated software, the fragment was virtually isolated, visualizing the biointegration of the MSC-Scaffold with periarticular bone tissue.

Figure 7.20 presents an example series of six images representing the determined reference levels, where based on radiological density, individual subareas (phases) such as the implant, trabecular bone, and soft tissues, including bone marrow, were distinguished, and the percentage of radiologically distinguished phases was measured.

Qualitative analysis of the radiological microstructure of the trabecular bone phase in the interspike space of the MSC-Scaffold reveals that at the reference levels closer to the tops of the spikes (Figures 7.20a–c) there is a bone-like trabecular structure near the MSC-Scaffold. At the reference levels closer to the base of the spikes (Figures 7.20d–f), we can see an initial stage of bone tissue ingrowth in the form of its creeping substitution on the lateral surface of the spikes. This initial stage is followed by an appositional growth of bone tissue gradually filling the interspike space of the MSC-Scaffold. The results of the quantitative analysis of the biointegration of the MSC-Scaffold with the periarticular bone tissue in the apical area of the MSC-Scaffold are presented in Figure 7.21; the graph shows the changes in the percentage share of the identified radiological phases (the MSC-Scaffold of titanium alloy, trabecular bone, and soft tissues) as a function of the distance from the base of the spikes at individual reference levels.

The percentage of the trabecular bone increases with the distance from the bases of the spikes from 44 ± 4% (female) and 41 ± 4% (male) to a maximum value of 66 ± 5% (female) and 70 ± 4% (male) in a distance of 2.5–3 mm from the bases of the spikes, while the percentage of soft tissues decreases from a value of 38 ± 4% approximately similar for both genders to a minimum value of 23% ± 5% (female) and 22% ± 4% (male) at a distance of 2.5 mm from the base of the spikes. The percentage of the material phase of the spikes decreases linearly with the increase of the distance from the spikes' bases – which is in line with the expectations resulting

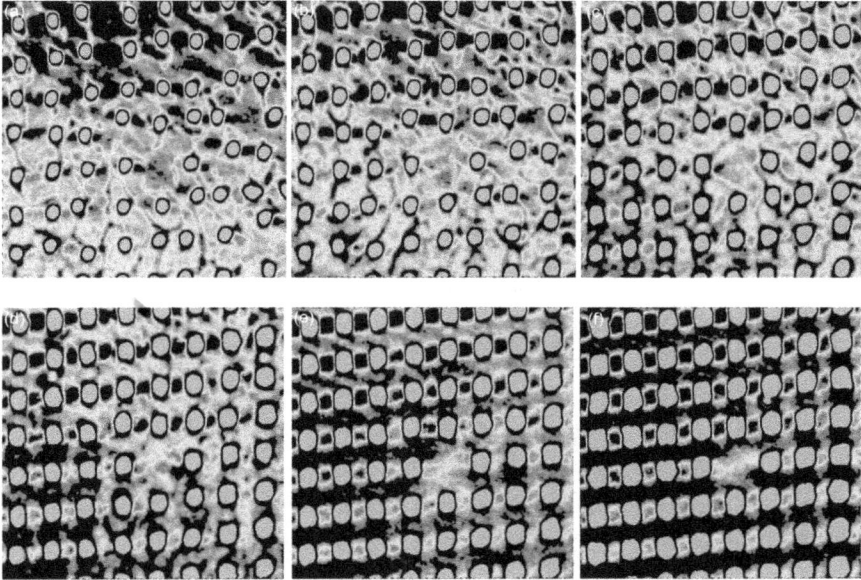

FIGURE 7.20   Series of six exemplary micro-CT scan slices of the explanted bone-implant specimen established at six reference levels at distances of (a) 3.5 mm, (b) 3.0 mm, (c) 2.5 mm, (d) 2.0 mm, (e) 1.5 mm, and (f) 1.0 mm from the spike bases of the MSC-Scaffold.

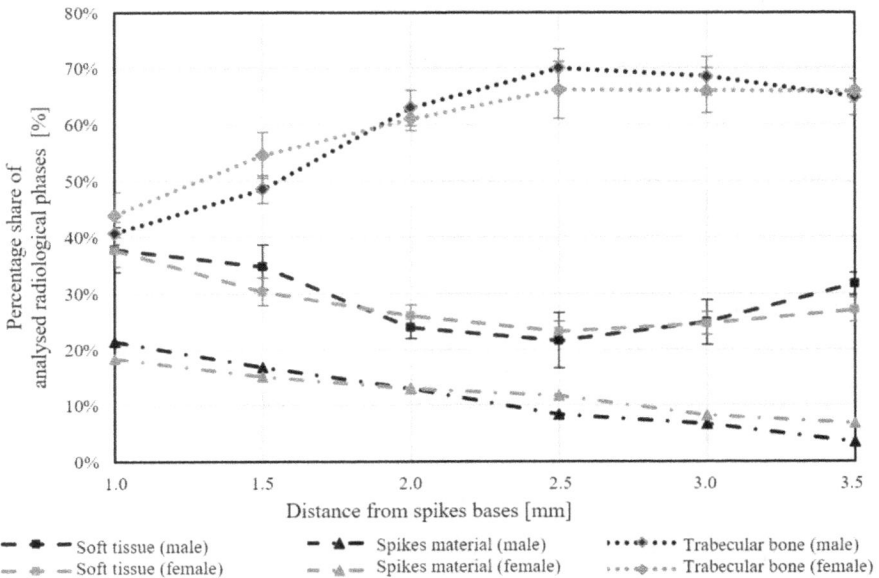

FIGURE 7.21   The percentage share of the radiological phases analysed: trabecular bone, spike material, and soft tissue of the explanted bone-implant specimen as a function of the distance from the spike bases.

from the geometric shape of the spikes and, at the same time, is the correctness of the results of the microtomographic quantitative analysis.

The distance from the bases of the reference level increases where the share of the peri-implant trabecular bone reaches the maximum (2.5 to 3 mm) corresponding to the initial depth of surgical embedding of the MSC-Scaffold in the periarticular bone. At this level, the maximum loads are transferred from the MSC-Scaffold to the surrounding trabecular bone, resulting in a relatively higher percentage of the ingrown bone relative to the percentage of soft tissues visible at that location.

The qualitative results obtained here may provide some insight into the course of the mechanical phenomena that accompany the intraoperative embedding of the MSC-Scaffold in the periarticular trabecular bone up to about half the height of its spikes, which is carried out by a surgeon implanting a prototype non-cemented resurfacing endoprosthesis.

***

Preliminary results of the experimental surgical determination of the appropriate surgical technique for implanting the working prototype of the partial resurfacing knee arthroplasty endoprosthesis with the biomimetic MSC-Scaffold show that the preferred surgical technique in the planned preclinical study of the first biomimetic method of fixation resurfacing joint endoprostheses using the working prototype of the partial resurfacing knee arthroplasty endoprosthesis should include: first cutting off the entire collateral ligament attachment of the lateral knee joint together with a thin bone fragment, and then reattaching this ligament to the bone with two bone screws.

The results of the pilot radiological, histological, and microtomographic study of biomimetic fixation of the working prototype of partial resurfacing knee arthroplasty endoprosthesis, carried out on bone-implant specimens from ten experimental animals (swine, breed: Polish Large White), eight weeks after the implantation of these implants, showed that:

- part of the interspike space of the MSC-Scaffold was occupied with newly formed and rebuilt mature bone tissue, proving that there was an initial biointegration of the prototype MSC-Scaffold with the periarticular trabecular bone;
- in the reconstruction of the 3D scanned bone-implant specimen obtained postoperatively from experimental animals, eight weeks after implantation in the deeper areas, near to the spikes bases of the MSC-Scaffold, the early stage of the osseointegration process was identified in the form of creeping substitution of the peri-implant bone tissue onto the lateral surface of the spikes;
- micro-CT study also enabled detailed measurements of the percentage changes in the proportion of each radiologically different phase (identified as a titanium MSC-Scaffold, peri-implant trabecular bone, and soft tissues) as a function of the distance from the bases of the spikes. Microtomographic examinations have been practically verified as a very useful tool in future planned research on the qualitative and quantitative evaluation of bone biointegration in the MSC-Scaffold spike region.

These results show that the biomimetic method of fixation of the working prototype of partial resurfacing knee arthroplasty endoprosthesis via the MSC-Scaffold ensures entirely non-cemented fixation (anchoring) of the resurfacing endoprosthesis component in the trabecular bone of the periarticular bone [19].

REFERENCES

1. Johnson, K.A. *Piermattei's Atlas of Surgical Approaches to the Bones and Joints of the Dog and Cat*, 5th edition. Elsevier/Saunders, St. Louis, Missouri, 2014.
2. Popesko, P. *Atlas of Topographical Anatomy of Domestic Animals Book*, 4th edition. Vydavatelstvo Priroda, s.r.o. Slovakia, 2012.
3. ISO 10993-2:2006 Biological evaluation of medical devices – Part 2: Animal welfare requirements.
4. Rogala, P.; Rogala, J.; Rogala, S.; Zawadzki P. A unit for the reaming of the surface of joint cartilage and of periarticular bone of an acetabulum and femoral head. PCT/PL2020/000006, WO2021112698A1, 29 January 2020.
5. An, Y.; Freidman, R. *Animal Models in Orthopaedic Research*, CRC Press, Boca Raton, FL, 1998.
6. Pilia, M.; Guda, T.; Appleford, M. Development of composite scaffolds for load-bearing segmental bone defects. *Biomed Res Int*. 2013; 2013: 458253. doi:10.1155/2013/458253
7. Schlegel, K.A.; Rupprecht, S.; Petrovic, L.; Honert, C.; Srour, S.; von Wilmowsky, C.; Felszegy, E.; Nkenke, E.; Lutz, R. Preclinical animal model for de novo bone formation in human maxillary sinus. *Oral Surg Oral Med Oral Pathol Oral Radiol Endod*. 2009; 108(3): e37–44. doi:10.1016/j.tripleo.2009.05.037
8. Helke, K.L. Ezel, P.C.; Duran-Struuck, R.; Swindle, M.M. Biology and diseases of swine; in: Fox, J.G.; Anderson, L.C.; Otto, G.; Pritchett-Corning, K.R.; Whary, M.T.; (Eds.): *Laboratory Animal Medicine*, 3rd ed. Academic Press, Cambridge, MA, 2015: 695–769.
9. Swindle, M.M.; Makin, A.; Herron, A.J. Swine as models in biomedical research and toxicology testing. *Vet Pathol*. 2012; 49(2): 344–56. doi:10.1177/0300985811402846
10. Swindle, M.M. *Swine in the Laboratory: Surgery, Anesthesia, Imaging, and Experimental Techniques*, 2nd ed. CRC Press: Boca Raton, FL, 2007.
11. Moran, C.J.; Ramesh, A.; Brama, P.A.; O'Byrne, J.M.; O'Brien, F.J.; Levingstone, T.J. The benefits and limitations of animal models for translational research in cartilage repair. *J Exp Orthop*. 2016; 3(1): 1. doi:10.1186/s40634-015-0037-x
12. Pearce, A.I.; Richards, R.G.; Milz, S.; Schneider, E.; Pearce, S.G. Animal models for implant biomaterial research in bone: a review. *Eur Cell Mater*. 2007; 13: 1–10. doi:10.22203/ecm.v013a01
13. Botchwey, E.A.; Pollack, S.R.; El-Amin, S.; Levine, E.M.; Tuan, R.S.; Laurencin, C.T. Human osteoblast-like cells in three-dimensional culture with fluid flow. *Biorheology*. 2003; 40(1–3): 299–306.
14. Søndergaard, L.V.; Dagnæs-Hansen, F.; Herskin, M.S. Welfare assessment in porcine biomedical research – suggestion for an operational tool. *Res Vet Sci*. 2011; 91(3): e1–9. doi:10.1016/j.rvsc.2011.02.008
15. Kaiser, G.M.; Heuer, M.M.; Frühauf, N.R.; Kühne, C.A.; Broelsch, C.E. General handling and anesthesia for experimental surgery in pigs. *J Surg Res*. 2006; 130(1): 73–9. doi:10.1016/j.jss.2005.07.012
16. Golriz, M.; Fonouni, H.; Nickkholgh, A.; Hafezi, M.; Garoussi, C.; Mehrabi, A. Pig kidney transplantation: an up-to-date guideline. *Eur Surg Res*. 2012; 49(3–4): 121–9. doi:10.1159/000343132

17. Scuderi, G.R.; Bourne, R.B.; Noble, P.C.; Benjamin, J.B.; Lonner, J.H.; Scott, W.N. The new knee society knee scoring system. *Clin Orthop Relat Res.* 2012; 470(1): 3–19. doi:10.1007/s11999-011-2135-0

18. Mercier, N.; Wimsey, S.; Saragaglia, D. Long-term clinical results of the Oxford medial unicompartmental knee arthroplasty. *Int Orthop.* 2010; 34(8): 1137–43. doi:10.1007/s00264-009-0869-z

19. Rogala, P.; Uklejewski, R.; Winiecki, M.; Dąbrowski, M.; Gołańczyk, J.; Patalas, A. First Biomimetic Fixation for Resurfacing Arthroplasty: Investigation in Swine of a Prototype Partial Knee Endoprosthesis. *Biomed Res Int.* 2019; 2019: 6952649. doi:10.1155/2019/6952649

8 Pilot micro-CT study of the impact of embedding the multi-spiked connecting scaffold on the density and compressive strength of the subchondral trabecular bone of femoral heads from patients with osteoarthritis

Osteoarthritis (OA) is a common disease that primarily involves cartilage destruction, synovial inflammation, osteophyte formation, and subchondral trabecular bone sclerosis with progressive functional disability and reduced quality of life [1]. For OA of the hip, the main treatment option is total hip arthroplasty (THA), which is widely used, and there are many methods of fixation of implants and bearing surfaces [1,2]. Total hip resurfacing arthroplasty (THRA) has several potential advantages over traditional long-stem THA arthroplasty, such as preservation of the bone stock and close-to-physiological bone and joint biomechanics, better stability, and an excellent functional outcome [3–5]. For the appropriate bioengineering design of the innovative prototype MSC-Scaffold for resurfacing endoprostheses components with the periarticular bone, which could be used in the surgical treatment of patients with OA, it is necessary to examine using microcomputed tomography (micro-CT) the subchondral trabecular bone in the heads of the femurs of OA patients treated with THA, before and after mechanical embedding of the prototype MSC-Scaffold in these heads, including determination of the relative area of the subchondral trabecular bone (bone area/total area

DOI: 10.1201/9781003364498-8

ratio, BA/TA) and the density of subchondral trabecular bone in the examined femoral heads and the compressive strength of that bone.

Quantitative computed tomography (QCT) of the microstructure of subchondral trabecular bone in the medial proximal tibia and femoral head in patients with OA was the subject of works by Shiraishi et al., Okazaki et al., and Li et al. [6–9]. The changes in the microstructure of the trabecular bone that were analysed the most frequently in patients with osteoarthritis affecting the medial part of the knee joint were to investigate the relationship between the microstructure of this bone and the stage of the disease and the position of the lower extremities [6]. Changes in microarchitecture and reconstruction of subchondral trabecular bone in patients with osteoarthritis were also analysed in terms of age and gender [8].

Evaluation of the density of the subchondral trabecular bone, carried out by micro-CT in fresh bones of experimental animal heads (swine, Polish Large White breed), published in [10], revealed that the embedding of the MSC-Scaffold prototype in the periarticular bone of femoral heads causes bone material densification under the embedded MSC-Scaffold that affects its mechanical properties. Therefore, it can be hypothesized that the densification of the subchondral trabecular bone microarchitecture on the femoral heads of OA patients treated with THA surgery due to the embedding of the MSC-Scaffold in the specimens of these femoral heads may depend on the initial bone density in these femoral heads.

The main objective of the study was micro-CT assessment of the relative area and density of the subchondral trabecular bone in the femoral heads removed during THA from OA patients carried out before and after mechanical embedding of the innovative MSC-Scaffold prototype for THRA endoprostheses in these heads. The specific aim of the study was to evaluate the influence of the initial surgical embedding of the MSC-Scaffold prototype for THRA endoprostheses on the change in the microstructure of the trabecular microarchitecture of the subchondral trabecular bone of femoral heads from OA patients, as possible, depending on the initial value of the subchondral trabecular bone relative area in these heads.

The pilot microtomography study used femoral heads from four patients, all of whom had advanced stages of primary osteoarthritis of the hip and underwent total hip arthroplasty. Exclusion criteria were secondary degenerative changes and hip fractures, a history of cancer, and liver or kidney failure. The study, approved by the Bioethics Committee of the Poznan University of Medical Sciences (consent No. 146/2018), was carried out as part of a research grant from the Poznan University of Medical Sciences.

All subjects included in this study were undergoing bilateral anteroposterior radiography of the hip. The orthopaedist assessed the radiographs by using the Kellgren-Lawrence (KL) radiographic scale. Stage 2 is described as definite osteophyte formation with possible joint space narrowing, stage 3 – multiple osteophytes, definite joint space narrowing, sclerosis, and possible bony deformity, and stage 4 – large osteophytes, marked joint space narrowing, severe sclerosis, and definite bone deformity. The visual analogue scale (VAS) score is used to measure the pain intensity of the hip joint. It has a range of 0–10, and 0 is no pain while 10 is extreme pain.

All femoral heads were collected intraoperatively from patients undergoing THA for hip OA. The shape of the examined femoral epiphyses was changed by a degenerative process. Bone tissue was densified in the upper lateral part of the femoral head and cysts were found in the head and neck of the femoral. The articular surface showed damage, which was emphasized in the loading area. The articular cartilage was pathologically altered, softened, and disintegrated, with areas of local destruction caused by subchondral congestion and blood vessel infiltration.

To prevent their drying, the femoral heads after surgical resection were covered with a dressing soaked in 0.9% saline solution (NaCl) and placed in a sealed heat-insulating container. Subsequently, bone specimens were transported to the test site in a portable refrigerator, processed with a cutter to remove a piece of cartilage around the top of the femoral head with continuous cooling of the head and femoral neck area with water, and immediately scanned with the GE Phoenix Vltomelx s240 microtomography scanner (Waygate Technologies, Wunstorf, Germany) with the following parameters: radiation source energy 130 keV, source current: 125 mA, resolution: 17.5 μm, filter: brass 1.5 mm, exposure time: 300 ms, rotation: 180°, every 0.5°, scan time: 20 min. The total time between the surgical resection of the femoral heads and the completion of their scanning did not exceed 6 h.

After micro-CT scanning of every femoral head sample, the titanium MSC-Scaffold prototype was placed on the top of the sample and, applying the specialized device, the MSC-Scaffold embedding in the femoral head sample was carried out with a speed of 0.1 mm/s to halfway up the spikes. The embedding process was controlled radiologically to achieve the appropriate depth of embedding. Afterwards, the micro-CT scanning of the femoral head specimen was done again with the same scanning parameters.

To accurately reconstruct the trabecular microarchitecture of subchondral trabecular bone in femoral head specimens, before and after the mechanical embedding of the MSC-Scaffold prototype to perform the qualitative and quantitative micro-CT analyses of this microarchitecture, the following image processing steps (necessary for the acquired projection data sets) were performed: 3D image reconstruction of femoral head specimens, elimination of imaging artefacts, segmentation of images.

Based on the radiological density criterion, the following elements (the so-called radiological phases) in the reconstructed 3D images were identified as an implant (MSC-Scaffold made of a titanium alloy) and mineralized trabecular bone (trabeculae) and soft tissues between the trabeculae (including bone marrow).

An additional correction by the thresholding method was applied; the above method assigns different greyscale voxels to a specific phase based on a selected threshold, which increases control over the determination of the discriminant boundaries. Such an approach is widely used in the case of microtomographic images of porous materials [11–14]. The same approach and identification procedure was used for the femoral head specimens before the MSC-Scaffold preprototype embedding, using the same criteria for identifying only two radiological phases: mineralized trabecular bone and soft tissue between the trabeculae.

The same coordinate systems have been established for digitally reconstructed femoral head specimens before and after mechanical embedding of the MSC-Scaffold preprototype and the data sets were compared using professional software (Volume Graphics 2.2, Heidelberg, Germany). Cylindrical fragments of the femoral head reconstruction located in the region of the MSC-Scaffold preprototype embedment site were digitally extracted. The axis of the bone cylinder was consistent with the direction of the resultant compressive force acting on the femoral head during physiological loading of the lower limb [15,16]. An example of a 3D reconstruction of a microtomographic image of the femoral head is shown in Figure 8.1. Example cross sections of the reconstructed microtomographic images of the femoral head specimens obtained before and after embedding the MSC-Scaffold preprototype are presented in Figure 8.2.

Subsequently, cross sections for quantitative analysis of micro-CT have been determined in each digitally extracted reconstruction of a cylinder-shaped sample. The plane tangent to the tops of the spikes of the recessed prototype MSC-Scaffold was established as the reference level (reference cross section), and the following cross sections were spaced 0.5 mm apart. In the case of digital reconstruction of a cylindrical sample of the femoral head before the embedding of the preprototype MSC-Scaffold, the reference level was set at the same level concerning the upper part of the cylinder. In each micro-CT reconstructed cross section, the radiological compartments representing bone trabeculae and intertrabecular regions (pore space) with soft tissues were identified.

The relative area of the subchondral trabecular bone was determined as the ratio of the subchondral trabecular bone area to the total area (BA/TA). Measurements were made on binarized images (cf. [17]). As is generally known, for trabecular bone (considered a porous material) [18, 19], the mean value of the surface share of the mineralized bone phase (BA/TA mean) is equal to the relative value of the volume share of the mineralized bone phase (BV/TV).

The volume density of the trabecular bone (ρ_b) was determined based on the formula (6.2) – see Section 6.2. Then, to determine the changes in the mechanical

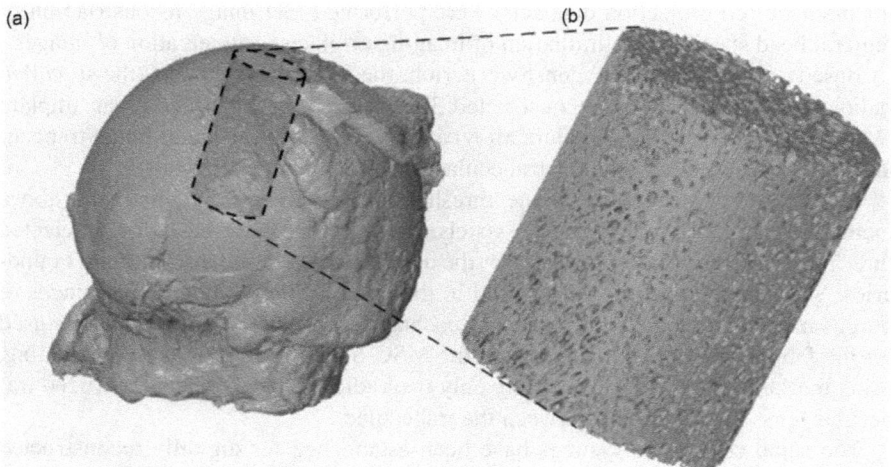

FIGURE 8.1 Micro-CT reconstruction of the femoral head sample (a) and digitally extracted cylinder-shaped bone sample (b) for further micro-CT evaluation of the bone trabecular microarchitecture and density.

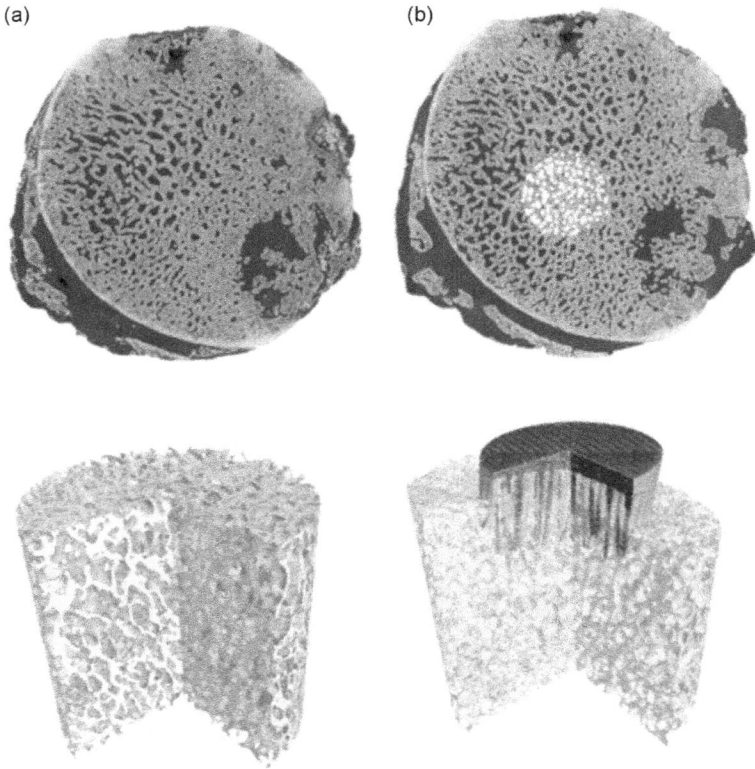

FIGURE 8.2 Micro-CT 3D reconstruction of femoral head bone specimens: (a) before and (b) after embedding of the MSC-Scaffold prototype.

strength of the bone caused by the embedding of the prototype MSC-Scaffold, the values of the compressive strength S of the subchondral bone of the examined femoral heads were calculated in designated elements, before and after the embedding, using the empirical formula [20,21]:

$$S = 25 \cdot (\rho_A)^{1.8}, \qquad\qquad (8.1)$$

where: ρ_A – apparent density of the trabecular bone(= $\alpha \cdot \rho_T$) [g/cm^3], α– fraction of the mineralized bone phase = BV/TV = mean BA/TA, ρ_T – bone trabecular density (comparable to cortical bone density, assumed to be 1.85 g/cm^3).

Detailed medical characteristics of the patients are presented in Table 8.1. The study involved two women and two men in the advanced stages of primary OA. Examples of preoperative anterior-posterior X-rays of the right hip joints of two patients are presented in Figure 8.3. The mean age of the patients at the time of surgery was 61.2 years (age range 51–72 years). The mean pain intensity of the patients on the VAS was 7.0. The preoperative X-ray examination of the hip indicated grade 4 hip osteoarthritis (KL4) in two patients and grade 3 (KL3) in two patients. Patients

TABLE 8.1
Characteristics of the patients

Patient No.	Age	Sex	BMI	Opposite Side OA	Duration of Pain (Years)	Orthopaedic Supports	KL	VAS
1	72	M	27.5		5	Orthopaedic walker	3	6
2	54	F	24.0		1	Without orthopaedic supports	4	7
3	68	F	28.8		2	Elbow crutches	3	7
4	51	M	33.2		2	Elbow crutches	4	8

KL, Kellgren-Lawrence radiographic stage of OA; VAS, Visual Analogue Scale.

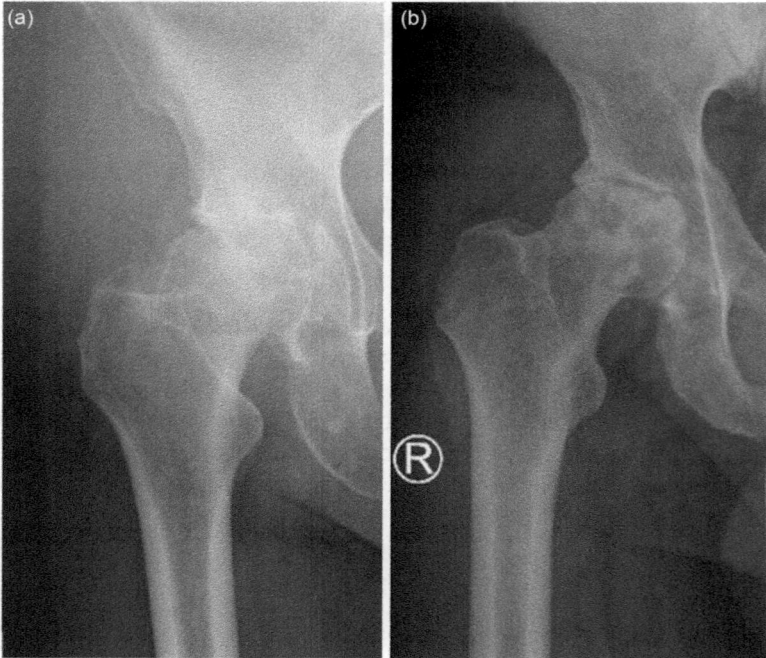

FIGURE 8.3 Preoperative anteroposterior X-ray of the right hip joints of two patients: (a) patient 2; (b) patient 4.

had hip flexion contracture with limited flexion up to 80°–90° and internal rotation up to 5°, accompanied by pain. The patient walked with a limp on the right lower limb. It was the first THA for all of these patients. Men had high blood pressure and diabetes, and women had no comorbidities.

Examples of binarized images of cross sections of a digitally extracted reconstruction of a bone sample (patient 1) in the shape of a cylinder, determined for the quantitative analysis of micro-CT, have been presented in Figure 8.4. For comparison, cross sections from a similar location were compiled before and after embedding the spikes of the prototype MSC-Scaffold.

Comparison of binarized images of cross sections of the bone sample analysed before (Figures 8.4a–f) and after (Figures 8.4g–l) the mechanical embedding of the MSC-Scaffold prototype reveals changes in the microarchitecture of the subchondral trabecular bone caused by the embedding of the MSC-Scaffold spikes. For binarized images of the cross sections of the bone sample after mechanical embedding of the MSC-Scaffold spikes, making a comparison of the cross sections located at successive levels representing the elements of the trabecular bone spaced successively every 0.5 mm from the reference level (Figures 8.4g–l), a decrease in the extent of the densified area of the subchondral trabecular bone can be observed with an increase in the distance from the reference level.

Figures 8.5–8.8 show, respectively: subchondral trabecular bone relative area BA/ TA, subchondral trabecular bone in the heads of the femur of patients with osteoarthritis, determined based on microtomographic imaging before and after the MSC-Scaffold embedding, expressed as percentage points of change in BA/TA value caused by embedding the MSC-Scaffold spikes into the bone, corresponding to these changes, calculated values of the density, and compressive strength of the subchondral trabecular bone (before and after embedding of the MSC-Scaffold). The values of all measured and calculated values are given in Table 8.2.

The BA/TA values of the subchondral trabecular bone in micro-CT analysed femoral head specimens before the MSC-Scaffold embedding varied from 38.7% for patient 3 to 58.4% for patient 1, but did not change significantly within the volume of each analysed sample (the changes in BA/TA values did not exceed 1.5% in each

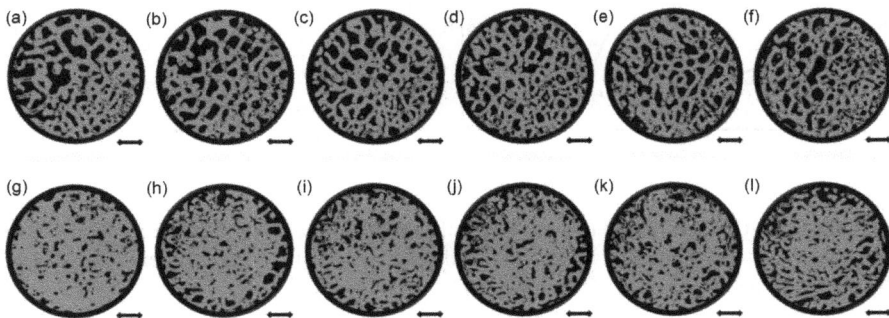

FIGURE 8.4 Quantitative micro-CT analysis of the microarchitecture of femoral head bone specimens before and after mechanical embedding of the MSC-Scaffold prototype. Views of cross sections of bone specimens below the reference plane: before the MSC-Scaffold embedding: (a) 0 mm, (b) 0.5 mm, (c) 1 mm, (d) 1.5 mm, (e) 2 mm, (f) 2.5 mm; and after the MSC-Scaffold embedding: (g) 0 mm, (h) 0.5 mm, (i) 1 mm, (j) 1.5 mm, (k) 2 mm, (l) 2.5 mm; bar = 2 mm.

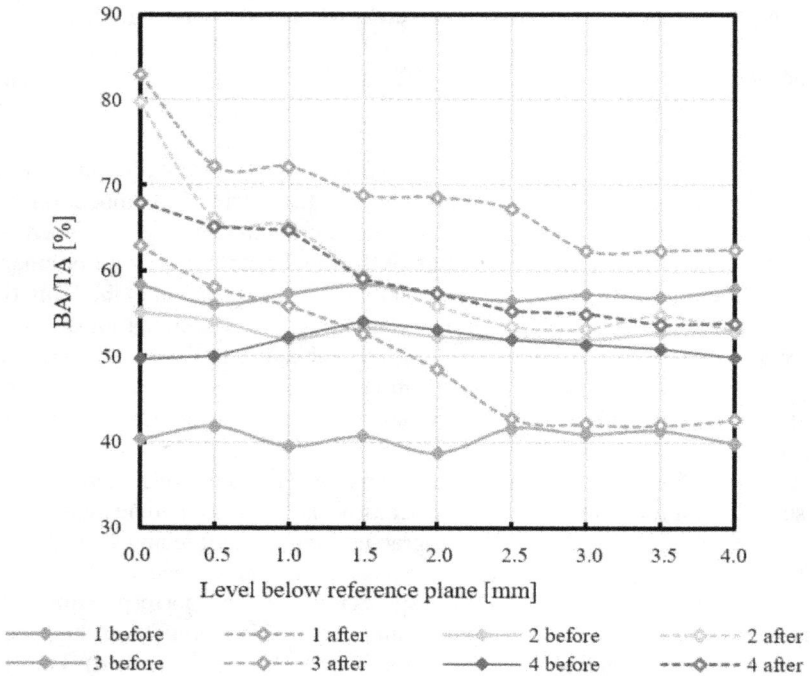

FIGURE 8.5   Subchondral trabecular bone relative area (BA/TA, bone area/total area ratio) values in micro-CT analysed femoral head specimens removed during THA from patients with OA before and after the embedding of the MSC-Scaffold prototype, at various levels of the section below the reference plane.

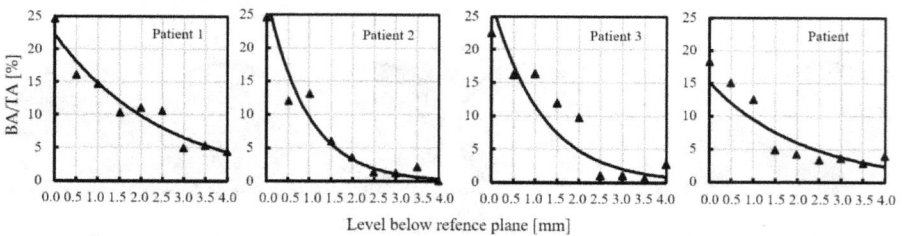

FIGURE 8.6   Changes in the relative area values of the subchondral trabecular bone (BA/TA, bone area/total area ratio) in femoral head specimens analysed at different levels below the reference plane.

sample). The calculated mean subchondral trabecular bone density ρ_b and the mean compressive strength of the subchondral trabecular bone S before MSC-Scaffold embedding varied from 1.34 ± 0.01 g/cm^3 and 14.9 ± 0.7 MPa for patient 3, respectively, to 1.49 ± 0.01 g/cm^3 and 27.8 ± 0.7 MPa for patient 1.

After the MSC-Scaffold embedding, BA/TA values were significantly higher and varied from 62.4% for patient 3 to 83.0% for patient 1 at the level just below the reference

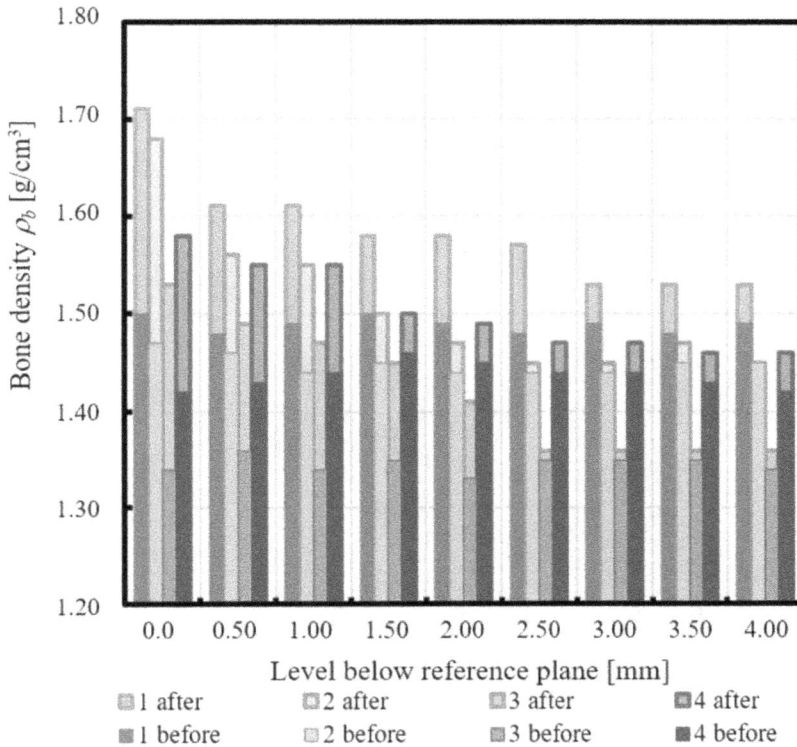

FIGURE 8.7 Changes in subchondral trabecular bone volumetric density ρ_b values in femoral head specimens analysed at different levels below the reference plane.

plane, while the corresponding calculated subchondral trabecular bone density ρ_b for the reference plane ranged from 1.53 to 1.71 g/cm^3, and the predicted compressive strength of the subchondral trabecular bone ranged from 32.8 to 54.1 MPa.

The subchondral trabecular bone density ρ_b relative change at the level below the reference plane was from 11.1% to 14.4%, while the subchondral trabecular bone compressive strength S relative change at the level below the reference plane was from 75.3% to 88.6%.

The BA/TA values then decreased at the next levels and the decrease rate varied from 4.2 p.p. to 18.3 p.p. per 1 mm, while the subchondral trabecular bone density ρ_b relative change and the subchondral trabecular bone compressive strength S relative change varied from 6.1% to 10.0% and from 34.3% to 86.2%, respectively. Such a decrease rate can be observed on average up to 2.0 mm depth below the reference plane. The BA/TA values decrease rates are different in each analysed femoral head sample and the curves of best fit were estimated for each patient individually (Figure 8.6). As can be seen in Figure 8.6, the particular best-fit curves of the BA/TA decrease reach a plateau at the level of 1.5 to 3.0 mm below the reference plane. Below these levels, the changes in subchondral trabecular bone BA/TA, the relative change in subchondral trabecular bone density ρ_b relative change, and compressive

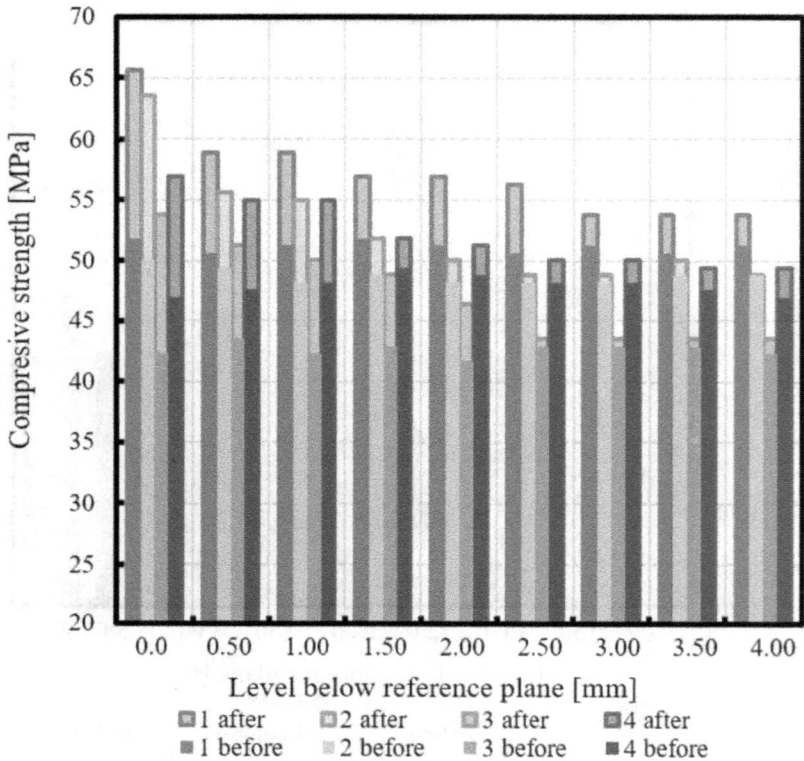

FIGURE 8.8 Changes in the compressive strength S values of the subchondral trabecular bone in analysed femoral head specimens due to the initial embedding of the MSC-Scaffold at different levels below the reference plane.

strength of subchondral trabecular bone S are minor (below 5 p.p.), up to 3.1% and up to 17.8%, respectively.

Based on this, the spatial extent of subchondral trabecular bone densification due to the initial embedding of the MSC-Scaffold prototype was established and it is marked with an asterisk in Table 8.2.

It should be underlined that the BA/TA values of the subchondral trabecular bone of the femoral head specimens presented in Table 8.2 are mean values, calculated from the three BA/TA measurements: the (middle) cross section at a given level below the reference plane and the two adjacent slices (located above and below 0.5 mm from this median section); these BA/TA values are, as it is known [19,22], equal to the bone relative volume BV/TV values (at a given level below the reference plane). The values assessed here with micro-CT subchondral trabecular bone relative area (BA/TA) in femoral head specimens removed during THA from patients with OA are between 38.7% and 58.4% and correspond to the data provided by other researchers' research reported in the literature, e.g.: 60.2% [8,9], 32.7% to 59.7% [23]. The

TABLE 8.2

Subchondral trabecular bone relative area (BA/TA) values in femoral heads of patients with OA measured in micro-CT before and after MSC-Scaffold (MSCS) embedding, percentage point changes in BA/TA values, calculated corresponding subchondral trabecular bone densities ρ_b, and compressive strength of subchondral trabecular bone S, before and after MSC-Scaffold embedding, and changes in subchondral trabecular bone densities ρ_b and subchondral trabecular bone S

Patient No.		0.0	0.5	1.0	1.5	2.0	2.5	3.0	3.5	4.0	Mean ± SD
					Levels Below Reference Plane (mm)						
1	BA/TA before MSCS embedding (%)	58.4	56.1	57.3	58.4	57.3	56.5	57.2	56.9	57.9	57.3 ± 0.8
	BA/TA after MSCS embedding (%)	83.0	72.2	72.1	68.8	68.5	67.1	62.3	62.3	62.4	
	Change in BA/TA (%)	24.7	16.1	14.8	10.4	11.2	10.6	5.0*	5.4	4.5	
	ρ_b before MSCS embedding (g/cm³)	1.50	1.48	1.49	1.50	1.49	1.48	1.49	1.48	1.49	1.49 ± 0.01
	ρ_b after MSCS embedding (g/cm³)	1.71	1.61	1.61	1.58	1.58	1.57	1.53	1.53	1.53	
	ρ_b relative change (%)	14.3	9.0	8.3	5.6	6.3	6.1	2.9	3.1	2.5	
	S before MSCS embedding (MPa)	28.7	26.7	27.8	28.7	27.8	27.1	27.7	27.4	28.3	27.8 ± 0.7
	S after MSCS embedding (MPa)	54.1	42.0	41.9	38.5	38.3	36.9	32.2	32.3	32.4	
	S relative change (%)	88.6	57.5	51.0	34.3	37.7	36.3	16.3	17.8	14.3	
2	BA/TA before MSCS embedding (%)	55.1	54.1	52.0	53.2	52.2	52.0	51.9	52.7	52.8	52.9 ± 1.1
	BA/TA after MSCS embedding (%)	79.7	66.1	65.2	59.3	55.9	53.5	53.2	54.8	52.9	
	Change in BA/TA (%)	24.6	12.0	13.2	6.0	3.7*	1.4	1.3	2.1	0.1	
	ρ_b before MSCS embedding (g/cm³)	1.47	1.46	1.44	1.45	1.44	1.44	1.44	1.45	1.45	1.45 ± 0.01
	ρ_b after MSCS embedding (g/cm³)	1.68	1.56	1.55	1.50	1.47	1.45	1.45	1.47	1.45	
	ρ_b relative change (%)	14.4	6.9	7.5	3.3	1.8	0.6	0.6	1.5	0.1	
	S before MSCS embedding (MPa)	25.9	25.0	23.3	24.3	23.5	23.3	23.2	23.8	23.9	24.0 ± 0.9
	S after MSCS embedding (MPa)	50.3	35.9	35.0	29.5	26.5	24.5	24.3	25.6	24.1	
	S relative change (%)	94.3	43.2	50.1	21.3	12.9	5.0	4.5	7.3	0.5	

(Continued)

TABLE 8.2 (CONTINUED)

Patient No.		Levels Below Reference Plane (mm)									
		0.0	0.5	1.0	1.5	2.0	2.5	3.0	3.5	4.0	Mean ± SD
3	BA/TA before MSCS embedding (%)	40.3	41.9	39.6	40.7	38.7	41.7	41.0	41.4	39.9	40.6 ± 1.0
	BA/TA after MSCS embedding (%)	62.9	58.1	55.9	52.6	48.5	42.8	42.1	42.0	42.6	
	Change in BA/TA (%)	22.6	16.2	16.3	11.9	9.8*	1.1	1.1	0.6	2.8	
	ρ_b before MSCS embedding (g/cm^3)	1.34	1.36	1.34	1.35	1.33	1.35	1.35	1.35	1.34	1.34 ± 0.01
	ρ_b after MSCS embedding (g/cm^3)	1.53	1.49	1.47	1.45	1.41	1.36	1.36	1.36	1.36	
	ρ_b relative change (%)	14.0	9.9	10.0	7.7	6.1	0.4	0.9	0.6	1.6	
	S before MSCS embedding (MPa)	14.7	15.8	14.2	15.0	13.7	15.7	15.2	15.4	14.5	14.9 ± 0.7
	S after MSCS embedding (MPa)	32.8	28.5	26.5	23.8	20.6	16.4	15.9	15.9	16.3	
	S relative change (%)	122.7	80.2	86.2	58.9	49.9	4.8	4.8	4.8	12.8	
4	BA/TA before MSCS embedding (%)	49.7	50.0	52.2	54.0	53.1	51.9	51.4	50.9	49.9	51.4 ± 1.5
	BA/TA after MSCS embedding (%)	67.9	65.0	64.7	59.0	57.4	55.3	55.0	53.7	53.9	
	Change in BA/TA (%)	18.2	15.0	12.5	4.9*	4.3	3.4	3.6	2.8	4.0	
	ρ_b before MSCS embedding (g/cm^3)	1.42	1.43	1.44	1.46	1.45	1.44	1.44	1.43	1.42	1.44 ± 0.01
	ρ_b after MSCS embedding (g/cm^3)	1.58	1.55	1.55	1.50	1.49	1.47	1.47	1.46	1.46	
	ρ_b relative change (%)	11.1	8.8	7.4	2.8	2.7	2.0	2.3	1.9	2.5	
	S before MSCS embedding (MPa)	21.5	21.8	23.5	25.0	24.2	23.2	22.8	22.4	21.6	22.9 ± 1.2
	S after MSCS embedding (MPa)	37.7	34.9	34.5	29.2	27.8	26.0	25.8	24.7	24.8	
	S relative change (%)	75.3	60.3	47.1	17.1	15.1	12.0	13.0	10.2	14.9	

* Spatial extent of subchondral trabecular bone densification due to initial embedding of the MSC-Scaffold prototype (mm).

values of the mean calculated subchondral trabecular bone density ρ_b also correspond to data provided by other authors [24,25].

Since the value of bone strength cannot be measured in patients *in vivo*, therefore, the empirical relationships linking bone density with its biomechanical properties (such as bone strength or Young's elastic modulus) have been determined in laboratory biomechanical examinations carried out on bone preparations from different anatomical locations in the skeleton. A review of published scientific papers on this issue is included in the work by Fleps et al. [21]. It is known that the volumetric density of subchondral trabecular bone can be treated as the key parameter because its values can be assessed in humans *in vivo* in various localizations in the skeleton, for example, utilizing quantitative computed tomography (QCT, pQCT).

Due to these laboratory biomechanical studies and the published results of these studies, one can now use these known empirical relationships and calculate (with acceptable accuracy) the values of specific bone biomechanical parameters based on the values of bone density measured at various anatomical locations in the skeleton in a given patient. Therefore, we have used the empirical formula (8.1) established in [20,21] to determine the values of subchondral trabecular bone strength S based on the assessed values of subchondral trabecular bone density ρ_b in examined femoral heads.

The changes in the subchondral trabecular bone relative area BA/TA values before and after embedding of the MSC-Scaffold prototype differed between analysed femoral head specimens from OA patients. Detailed medical characteristics of each patient have been included in the study [26].

Based on the results of the study in individual patients, it can be concluded that the highest (approximately 14%) density of subchondral trabecular bone directly under the MSC-Scaffold was obtained in patients (patient 1 and patient 2) with higher baseline BA/TA and the calculated bone density. The high baseline bone quality in these patients is probably due to a normal baseline bone density compared to other authors with OA [9]. Differences in the spatial extent of subchondral trabecular bone densification due to the initial embedding of the MSC-Scaffold prototype between these cases can be noticed, with a definite advantage in the male patient 1 (2.5 mm vs. 1.5–2 mm).

In all patients, the change in BA/TA 1 mm below baseline was similar and ranged from 12.5 to 16.3 p.p. Interestingly, the highest change in density was obtained at the level of 1 mm in the patient with the lowest initial density (patient 3).

The performed pilot study of the micro-CT assessment and analyses of the MSC-Scaffold embedding in the human femoral subchondral heads of patients with OA determined the range of effect of the subchondral trabecular bone densification, taking into account different initial bone densities. Densification of the subchondral trabecular bone in the examined femoral heads caused by embedding of the MSC-Scaffold spikes results in an increase in the mechanical strength of the bone. In the case of surgical treatment using the innovative entirely non-cemented resurfacing endoprosthesis with the MSC-Scaffold, based on the results presented here, it can be expected that the improvement in the mechanical properties of the subchondral trabecular bone located below the surgically inserted MSC-Scaffold will determine the initial stability of the femoral component of the resurfacing endoprosthesis. The limitation of this study was the small sample size (four femoral heads of patients with OA treated with THA) and the lack of a control group due to the difficulty in finding patients of the appropriate age and sex categories with healthy bone within the femoral head. More research is needed in this area to verify the results of the pilot study.

***

The embedding of the MSC-Scaffold in subchondral trabecular bone causes the change in its relative area (BA/TA) ranging from 18.2% to 24.7% (translating to the calculated density ρ_b relative change from 11.1% to 14.4%, and the predicted compressive strength S relative change from 75.3% to 122.7%) regardless of its initial density (before the embedding).

The densification of the subchondral trabecular bone due to the initial embedding of the MSC-Scaffold gradually decreases with the increasing distance from the apexes of the MSC-Scaffold spikes, while the spatial extent of the densification of the subchondral trabecular bone ranged from 1.5 to 2.5 mm.

It may be suggested (despite the limited number of examined cylindrical bone specimens from femoral heads) that the impact magnitude of the initial surgical embedding of the MSC-Scaffold in the trabecular bone of the femoral head may be a factor determining the long-term maintenance of this innovative MSC-Scaffold in the bone, and thus the joint resurfacing endoprosthesis embedded in the periarticular bone through the MSC-Scaffold. The results indicate that the greater the extent of the subchondral trabecular bone biostructure densification, the greater the bone mechanical strength, thus resulting in better conditions for the postoperative functioning of the MSC-Scaffold fixation in the periarticular bone. Increased mechanical strength of the subchondral trabecular bone prevent the possible implant migration during postoperative limb loading.

It can be suggested (despite the limited number of examined femoral head specimens) that the size of the influence of the MSC-Scaffold's initial embedding on subchondral trabecular bone may be a factor in its maintenance. It seems that the deeper this effect of subchondral trabecular bone densification, the better the strength of subchondral trabecular bone and, consequently, the better postoperative embedding of the MSC-Scaffold in the bone should be expected. The increased strength of the subchondral trabecular bone can prevent the undesirable migration of implant during the postoperative limb loading.

The team received approval from the Bioethics Committee of the Poznan University of Medical Sciences to conduct (by 2024) an extended programme of clinical diagnostic tests and quantitative microtomographic tests on the heads of human femurs of patients with osteoarthritis (OA) of the hip qualified for surgical treatment using the THA method using long-stem hip endoprostheses.

REFERENCES

1. Agarwal, N.; To, K.; Khan, W. Cost-effectiveness analyses of total hip arthroplasty for hip osteoarthritis: a PRISMA systematic review. *Int J Clin Pract.* 2021; 75: e13806. doi:10.1111/ijcp.13806

2. Suárez, J.C.; Forero, A.; Llinás, A.; Bonilla, G.; Rodríguez, H.; Amado, O. Bearing surfaces in primary hip arthroplasty. Is there any difference? *Acta Ortop Mex.* 2020; 34: 22–66. doi:10.35366/94619

3. Daniel, J.; Pradhan, C.; Ziaee, H.; Pynsent, P.B.; McMinn, D.J. Results of Birmingham hip resurfacing at 12 to 15 years: a single-surgeon series. *Bone Jt J.* 2014; 96: 1298–306. doi:10.1302/0301-620X.96B10.33695

4. Ford, M.C.; Hellman, M.D.; Kazarian, G.S.; Clohisy, J.C.; Nunley, R.M.; Barrack, R.L. Five to ten-year results of the Birmingham hip resurfacing implant in the US: a single institution's experience. *J Bone Jt Surg Am.* 2018; 100: 1879–87. doi:10.2106/JBJS.17.01525

5. Hellman, M.D.; Ford, M.C.; Barrack, R.L. Is there evidence to support an indication for surface replacement arthroplasty?: a systematic review. *Bone Jt J.* 2019; 101: 32–40. doi:10.1302/0301-620X.101B1.BJJ-2018-0508.R1

6. Shiraishi, K.; Chiba, K.; Okazaki, N.; Yokota, K.; Nakazoe, Y.; Kidera, K.; Yonekura, A.; Tomita, M.; Osaki, M. In vivo analysis of subchondral trabecular bone in patients with osteoarthritis of the knee using second-generation high-resolution peripheral quantitative computed tomography (HR-pQCT). *Bone.* 2020; 132: 115155. doi:10.1016/j.bone.2019.115155

7. Okazaki, N.; Chiba, K.; Motoi, M.; Osaki, M. Analysis of subchondral bone microstructure by HR-PQCT: relationship with the severity of knee osteoarthritis and alignments of lower extremities. *Osteoarthr Cartil.* 2017; 25: S263. doi:10.1016/j.joca.2017.02.442

8. Li, G.; Zheng. Q.; Landao-Bassonga, E.; Cheng, T.S.; Pavlos, N.J.; Ma, Y.; Zhang, C.; Zheng, M.H. Influence of age and gender on microarchitecture and bone remodeling in subchondral bone of the osteoarthritic femoral head. *Bone.* 2015; 77: 91–7. doi:10.1016/j.bone.2015.04.019

9. Li, G.; Chen, L.; Zheng, Q.; Ma, Y.; Zhang, C.; Zheng, M.H. Subchondral bone deterioration in femoral heads in patients with osteoarthritis secondary to hip dysplasia: a case-control study. *J Orthop Transl.* 2019; 24: 190–7. doi:10.1016/j.jot.2019.10.014

10. Uklejewski, R.; Winiecki, M.; Patalas, A.; Rogala, P. Bone density Micro-CT assessment during embedding of the innovative multi-spiked connecting scaffold in periarticular bone to elaborate a validated numerical model for designing biomimetic fixation of resurfacing endoprostheses. *Materials.* 2021; 14(6): 1384. doi:10.3390/ma14061384

11. Shah, S.M.; Gray, F.; Crawshaw, J.P.; Boek, E.S. Microcomputed tomography pore-scale study of flow in porous media: effect of voxel resolution. *Adv Water Resour.* 2016; 95: 276–87. doi:10.1016/j.advwatres.2015.07.012

12. Tuller, M.; Kulkarni, R.; Fink, W. Segmentation of X-ray CT data of porous materials: a review of global and locally adaptive algorithms, in: Anderson, S.H.; Hopmans, J.W.; (Eds.): *Soil–Water–Root Processes: Advances in Tomography and Imaging.* Soil Science Society of America Special Publications, Madison, WI, 2013; 61: 157–82. doi:10.2136/sssaspecpub61.c8

13. Akhter, M.P.; Recker, R.R. High-resolution imaging in bone tissue research-review. *Bone.* 2021; 143: 115620. doi:10.1016/j.bone.2020.115620

14. Buccino, F.; Colombo, C.; Vergani, L.M. A Review on multiscale bone damage: from the clinical to the research perspective. *Materials.* 2021; 14: 1240. doi:10.3390/ma14051240

15. Gregory, J.; Stewart, A.; Undrill, P.; Reid, D.; Aspden, R. Bone shape, structure, and density as determinants of osteoporotic hip fracture: a pilot study investigating the combination of risk factors. *Invest Radiol.* 2005; 40: 591–7. doi:10.1097/01.rli.0000174475.41342.42

16. San Antonio, T.; Ciaccia, M.; Müller-Karger, C.; Casanova, E. Orientation of orthotropic material properties in a femur FE model: a method based on the principal stresses directions. *Med Eng Phys.* 2012; 34: 914–9. doi:10.1016/j.medengphy.2011.10.008

17. Chappard, D.; Retailleau-Gaborit, N.; Legrand, E.; Baslé, M.F.; Audran, M. Comparison insight bone measurements by histomorphometry and microCT. *J Bone Miner Res.* 2005; 20: 1177–84. doi:10.1359/JBMR.050205

18. Vandeweghe, S.; Coelho, P.G.; Vanhove, C.; Wennerberg, A.; Jimbo, R. Utilizing microcomputed tomography to evaluate bone structure surrounding dental im-plants: a comparison with histomorphometry. *J Biomed Mater Res Part B Appl Biomater.* 2013; 101: 1259–66. doi:10.1002/jbm.b.32938

19. Martin, R.B. Porosity and specific surface of bone. *Crit Rev Biomed Eng.* 1984; 10: 179–222.

20. Lotz, J.C.; Gerhart, T.N.; Hayes, W.C. Mechanical properties of trabecular bone from the proximal femur: a quantitative CT study. *J Comput Assist Tomogr.* 1990; 14: 107–14. doi:10.1097/00004728-199001000-00020

21. Fleps, I.; Bahaloo, H.; Zysset, P.K.; Ferguson, S.J.; Pálsson, H.; Helgason, B. Empirical relationships between bone density and ultimate strength: a literature review. *J Mech Behav Biomed Mater.* 2020; 110: 103866. doi:10.1016/j.jmbbm.2020.103866

22. Ito, M.; Nakamura, T.; Matsumoto, T.; Tsurusaki, K.; Hayashi, K. Analysis of trabecu-lar microarchitecture of human iliac bone using microcomputed tomography in patients with hip arthrosis with or without vertebral fracture. *Bone.* 1998; 23: 163–9. doi:10.1016/s8756-3282(98)00083-0

23. Ryan, M.; Barnet, L.; Rochester, J.; Wilkinson, J.M.; Dall'Ara, E. A new approach to comprehensively evaluate the morphological properties of the human femoral head: Example of application to osteoarthritic joint. *Sci Rep.* 2020; 10: 5538. doi:10.1038/s41598-020-62614-7

24. Adams, G.J.; Cook, R.B.; Hutchinson, J R.; Zioupos P. Bone apparent and material densities examined by cone beam computed tomography and the Archimedes tech-nique: comparison of the two methods and their results. Front Mech Eng. 2018; 3: 23. doi:10.3389/fmech.2017.00023

25. Zioupos, P.; Cook, R.B.; Hutchinson, J.R. Some basic relationships between density values in cancellous and cortical bone. J Biomech. 2008; 41(9): 1961–8. doi:10.1016/j.jbiomech.2008.03.025

26. Dąbrowski, M.; Rogala, P.; Uklejewski, R.; Patalas, A.; Winiecki, M.; Gapiński, B. Subchondral bone relative area and density in human osteoarthritic femoral heads assessed with micro-CT before and after mechanical embedding of the innovative multi-spiked connecting scaffold for resurfacing THA endoprostheses: a pilot study. *J Clin Med.* 2021; 10(13): 2937. doi:10.3390/jcm10132937

9 Summary, conclusions, and final remarks

Initial research tasks within the planned research schedule included: (1) identification and experimental selection of appropriate technology for the manufacturing of the prototype MSC-Scaffold, ensuring biomimetic, completely cement-free fixation (anchoring) of components of joint resurfacing endoprostheses in the periarticular bone; (2) the development of initial design and the technological guidelines for the manufacturing of the first prototype of a biomimetic resurfacing endoprosthesis intended for experimental surgical treatment of osteoarthritis, along with (3) the design and manufacturing of preprototypes of such MSC-Scaffold and prototypes of such endoprostheses, intended for further stages of bioengineering research and *in vivo* pilot study in experimental animals.

During the surgical implantation of a prototype resurfacing arthroplasty endoprosthesis implanted in the bone in an entirely non-cemented way using the MSC-Scaffold, the spikes of the MSC-Scaffold are inserted into the intertrabecular space of the periarticular trabecular bone (it is the initial surgical fixation of a resurfacing endoprosthesis component in bone); therefore, it was crucial to adjust the geometric structural features of this scaffold to the characteristic dimensions of the intertrabecular microstructure of the pore space of the periarticular trabecular bone constituting the interconnected system of marrow cavities.

Design guidelines for the manufacturing of the MSC-Scaffold have been developed based on the analysis of the so-called structural compatibility of the tested design variants of the MSC-Scaffold with the periarticular trabecular bone of the animal femoral head. To this end, parameters such as the implant-bone contact area increase factor and the trabecular bone marrow lacunae and the spikes' coincidence index were defined, and based on the microscopic study of the trabecular bone tissue taken from the swine femoral heads and for various shapes and arrangements of the MSC-Scaffold spikes, we have analysed the changes in the values of the proposed parameters. Based on these studies, we have proposed to use in the prototype MSC-Scaffold for resurfacing arthroplasty endoprostheses the concentrically arranged pyramid-shaped spikes with a square base of a side length of 0.50 mm.

CAD models of the MSC-Scaffold preprototypes have been developed in the form of their representative fragments related to the target shape of the femoral component of the hip resurfacing arthroplasty endoprosthesis, as well as CAD models of the prototypes of a hip endoprosthesis for total hip arthroplasty and the working prototype of partial resurfacing knee arthroplasty endoprosthesis for implantation in experimental animals.

To evaluate the possibility of manufacturing the MSC-Scaffold that ensures non-cemented fixation of the components of resurfacing endoprostheses in the

DOI: 10.1201/9781003364498-9

periarticular bone, we have made preprototypes of this scaffold and prototypes of endoprostheses using various methods:

- by stereolithography (from Accura SI 10 resin on the Viper Si2 SLA printer by 3D Systems),
- by the method of precision wire-cut electrical discharge machining and die-sinker electrical discharge machining (made of 40H steel hardened to 45 HRC, on the Robofil 290 EDM machine manufactured by the Swiss company Charmilles),
- by selective laser melting (powders of Ti-6Al-7Nb and Ti-6Al-4V alloys on ReaLizer SLM 100 and ReaLizer SLM 250 machines by MTT Technologies Group, Germany),
- in addition, in other related and commercially available additive technologies such as selective laser sintering and electron beam melting.

Based on the analysis of the technological possibilities of that time (the mid-2000s), we have acknowledged and confirmed, based on the prototyping, that the manufacturing of the MSC-Scaffold for fixation in the periarticular bone of components of joint resurfacing endoprostheses, and being an integral part of those endoprostheses, is not possible without the use of additive manufacturing technologies. Further prototyping within these technologies revealed several unacceptable defects in the preprototypes manufactured. The requirements for the manufacturing of elements with uniform density and with mechanical properties comparable to those made of homogeneous materials directed our attention to the technology of selective laser melting (SLM). Based on our experimental comparative research and the data available in the literature, SLM technology was found to be suitable for the manufacturing components of prototype biomimetic resurfacing endoprostheses with the MSC-Scaffold.

We have developed design guidelines for the most favourable geometric features of the MSC-Scaffold for resurfacing endoprostheses, taking into account the SLM technological guidelines, as well as the shaping and finishing machining guidelines. We have prepared CAD documentation for the design of the prototypes of the resurfacing endoprosthesis, which included technological handles and technological allowances for shaping and finishing (grinding and lapping) of both components of the prototype hip joint endoprosthesis.

We have also analysed the issues of post-production processing (using abrasive blasting technology) of the bone-contacting surface of the prototype MSC-Scaffold for entirely non-cemented resurfacing endoprostheses manufactured using SLM technology. We have identified difficulties in removing the micro-residues adhering to the surface of the MSC-Scaffold in the form of not fully melted particles of the alloy powder, and variously shaped splatted forms. It required the development of nonstandard technological tasks for their removal, especially from the hard-to-reach areas around the base of the MSC-Scaffold spikes. As a result of the carried out tests, we have developed an effective variant of post-production treatment with a developed abrasive mixture and we have identified the appropriate parameters of such treatment of the prototype MSC-Scaffold of innovative resurfacing endoprostheses manufactured in the SLM technology.

We have evaluated the possibility of the formation of the structural and pro-osteoconductive potential of the interspike space of the prototype MSC-Scaffold. The research aimed to determine the technologically achievable conditions for bio-mimetic structural-osteoconductive functionalization of its microgeometric structural features, which ultimately allowed for the improvement of the conditions for the subsequent osseointegration of the prototype MSC-Scaffold with periarticular trabecular bone tissue. The analysis was carried out based on a proposed set of parameters for evaluation of the pro-osteoconductive functionality of the MSC-Scaffold manufactured prototype.

We have compared the microgeometric features of the CAD models for the prototype MSC-Scaffold and the prototypes manufactured on that basis using SLM technology, which allowed for a precise correction of the technological limitations thus identified. The study was carried out on a prototype of an entirely non-cemented hip resurfacing arthroplasty endoprosthesis with the MSC-Scaffold by measuring the effective height of its spikes using a confocal microscope and by structurally assessing samples representing different geometric variants of the prototype MSC-Scaffold fragments for both components of the prototype resurfacing endoprosthesis. In the CAD model samples of two series of modelled prototype MSC-Scaffold fragments, the nominal height of the MSC-Scaffold spikes and the shape of the spikes were alternatively and independently altered, thus verifying the changes of the MSC-Scaffold geometric features as assumed in CAD models on the prototypes produced based on the said CAD models using SLM technology.

The results of the investigation led to the conclusion that the values of the effective height of the MSC-Scaffold spikes of the prototype hip endoprosthesis manufactured using SLM technology based on CAD models designed according to the technological guidelines of the research project No. 4T07C05629 were significantly lower than the effective height value of the spikes in above-mentioned CAD models (by $48 \pm 9\%$ in the case of the femoral component of the prototype of an entirely non-cemented hip resurfacing endoprosthesis and by $51 \pm 9\%$ for the acetabular component of the prototype of the same endoprosthesis), which significantly reduces the structural and osteoconductive potential of the interspike space of the manufactured prototype MSC-Scaffold.

Based on the structural evaluation of the samples representing different geometric variants of the fragments of the prototype MSC-Scaffold for both components of the prototype resurfacing endoprosthesis, it was found that altering the shape of the MSC-Scaffold spikes in the CAD model, and leaving the nominal height of the spikes unchanged, allows for having some control over the structural and osteoconductive potential of its interspike space by increasing (by approximately 20%) the effective height of these spikes in the SLM prototypes. The most beneficial effect of influencing the structural and osteoconductive potential of the interspike space of the MSC-Scaffold can be achieved by modifying the geometric features of the spike structure, including both the change of their nominal height and their shape in the CAD model.

The obtained results allowed for revising the constructional assumptions of the primary prototype of the MSC-Scaffold and provided key information on the need to compensate for the identified technological limitations of selective laser melting when establishing design directives, i.e. a method of improving structural pro-osteoconductive functionality to properly design subsequent prototypes of the knee and hip joint resurfacing endoprostheses (partial and total) with the MSC-Scaffold.

Initial biological evaluation under the conditions of a ten-day human osteoblasts culture on preprototypes of the MSC-Scaffold carried out after structural-osteoconductive functionalization of their interspike space confirmed that the adjacent spikes of the MSC-Scaffold constitute an osteoconductive surface for osteoblasts. Fluorescent microscopic images taken after ten days of culturing human osteoblasts on the MSC-Scaffold preprototype showed the formation of interconnected cytoplasmic processes of osteoblasts on the surface of the MSC-Scaffold preprototypes, indicating a tendency to create a three-dimensional intercellular network that is a characteristic element of the biostructure of the lamellar bone tissue of which the trabeculae of the trabecular bone are built. The MSC-Scaffold spikes provide an osteoconductive surface for proliferating and spreading osteoblasts.

Pilot surgical implantation in an animal model (swines of the Polish Large White breed) of structurally functionalized MSC-Scaffold preprototypes did not show postoperative implant loosening, migration, or other possible early complications. Histopathological evaluation of the peri-spike bone tissue revealed that: (1) most of the interspike space of the MSC-Scaffold preprototype was occupied with newly formed and remodelled (mineralized) bone tissue, ensuring the primary biological fixation of the MSC-Scaffold preprototypes in the periarticular trabecular bone and (2) to improve contact with bone, the surface of the MSC-Scaffold should be physicochemically modified with calcium phosphates to obtain a surface that is to some extent biochemically mimetic with respect to the native bone biomineral (hydroxyapatite).

Therefore, the study of the calcium phosphate (CaP) modification of the bone-contacting surface of the MSC-Scaffold preprototypes by electrochemical cathodic deposition of calcium phosphates was undertaken – suitable for the geometrically complex bone-contacting surface. Attempts to modify this method, initially carried out at constant current densities, were satisfactory, i.e. it was confirmed that the deposition of the calcium phosphate coating on the bone-contacting surface of the MSC-Scaffold preprototypes can be controlled by regulating the current density. The increase in the osteoinductive potential of the bone-contacting surface of the CaP-modified prototype MSC-Scaffold was confirmed in an experimental pilot study of this scaffold in an animal model (in swine of the Polish Large White breed) and osteoblasts cultures. After the structural-geometric functionalization of the MSC-Scaffold, it was observed that the results of the calcium phosphate modification of the bone-contacting surface of the MSC-Scaffold prototypes performed during the potentiostatic cathodic deposition process showed a much higher reproducibility compared to the results of the CaP modification performed during the galvanostatic electrochemical cathodic deposition process. In the further study on the CaP modification of the bone-contacting surface of the MSC-Scaffold preprototypes carried out during the potentiostatic electrochemical cathodic deposition process, the task was to determine the most appropriate range of conditions for this process. The tests were carried out for electric potential values ranging from -9 to -3 V. It was found that the appropriate conditions for this process were largely influenced by the geometric features of the MSC-Scaffold prototype, i.e. mainly by the distance between the spikes. In the case of insufficient space between the

MSC-Scaffold spikes, it has been observed that the calcium phosphate deposits were located between the spikes and not on their lateral surface.

Based on the characteristics of the physicochemical properties of the coating manufactured on lateral surface of spikes of the MSC-Scaffold preprototypes – in terms of structural (EDS) and morphological (SEM) properties and the study of mass growth of the preprototypes caused by the deposition of the calcium phosphate coating on the surface – it was found that the electric potential range of the process from −5.25 to −4.75 V ensures a good quality CaP modification of the bone-contacting surface of a variant of the MSC-Scaffold preprototype characterized by an interspike distance of 350 μm. In addition, the effect of preceding acid-alkali treatment was investigated using a range of electric potential values determined to allow the coatings on the lateral surface of the MSC-Scaffold spikes to achieve a Ca/P molar ratio corresponding to the Ca/P values in native bone hydroxyapatite. The characterization of the CaP coating properties was extended to include surface EDS mapping and quantitative crystal phase analysis (XRD). For variants of the MSC-Scaffold preprototypes subjected to acid-alkali treatment, an increase in the degree of coverage of the lateral surface of the spikes and greater uniformity of surface coverage were found. This treatment also prevents the formation of microcracks on the surface in contact with the bone of the MSC-Scaffold and increases the degree of coverage of the lateral surface of the spikes. The Ca/P molar ratios of the deposits on the lateral surface of the spikes in all these modified preprototypes were consistent with the value of the Ca/P molar ratio in native bone hydroxyapatite, and on the bone-contacting surface of the prototype MSC-Scaffold subjected to acid-alkali treatment, there were lamellar and needle crystals of calcium phosphate deposited.

The relatively best results of CaP modification on the bone-contacting surface of the MSC-Scaffold preprototypes have been obtained in the potentiostatic process of electrochemical cathodic deposition carried out at an electric potential of −5.00 V, that is, biomineral coverage was obtained with values of the Ca/P molar ratio of deposits similar to this value of the ratio of native bone hydroxyapatite and the highest mean mass growth of the coating and the highest degree of coating of the lateral surface of the spikes (even for prototypes modified without the preceding acid-alkali treatment). The numerous microcracks observed in the MSC-Scaffold preprototypes modified in the electrochemical cathodic deposition process conducted at an electric potential of −5.00 V without acid-alkali treatment were eliminated by the applying of this preceding treatment. It finally guaranteed the relatively highest homogeneity compared to the preprototypes modified at other values the electric potential of the electrochemical cathodic deposition process, falling within a predetermined range of this potential.

Evaluation of the results of a ten-day culture of human osteoblasts in preprototypes of the MSC-Scaffold – unmodified and with a calcium phosphate-modified surface – shows that the factors which have a significant impact on the enzymatic activity of alkaline phosphatase (and thus on mineralization) are the distance between the prototype MSC-Scaffold spikes and applying modification with a layer of calcium phosphate on the bone-contacting surface of the MSC-Scaffold spikes.

Evaluation of the biointegration of these prototypes of the MSC-Scaffold implanted into the knee joint of swine carried out eight weeks post-implantation indicated that most of the interspike space of the MSC-Scaffold was occupied with newly formed and rebuilt mature bone tissue, and in the 3D images of the bone-implant specimens reconstructed using computed microtomography and taken eight weeks post-implantation, we have detected an approximately 12% increase in bone trabeculae in the interspike spaces for the calcium phosphate surface-modified pre-prototypes as compared to preprototypes with a non-modified surface.

Based on the numerical simulations of the influence of the geometric features of the MSC-Scaffold on the distribution of mechanical stress in the periprosthetic bone, where the MSC-Scaffold partially embedded in the periarticular bone was mechanically loaded, we have determined the most important geometric features of the MSC-Scaffold, ensuring a physiological load transfer from the MSC-Scaffold to the peri-implant bone. The results indicated that the following geometric structural features of the MSC-Scaffold had an impact on the stress level in the bone around the MSC-Scaffold spikes: (a) the distance between the bases of adjacent spikes a, (b) the vertical angle of spikes β, and (c) the height of the spikes' spherical cap h. Distribution of Huber-von Mises-Hencky reduced stress in the area around the implant, it was found that the vertical angle of spikes β and the distance between the bases of the adjacent spikes a are the key geometric features that determine the correct design of a suitable prototype of the MSC-Scaffold for innovative non-cemented resurfacing endoprostheses. The influence of the height of the spherical cap h of the spikes of the MSC-Scaffold is of secondary importance.

Further research aimed to develop and validate a numerical model that allows for the design of the prototype MSC-Scaffold that ensures biomimetic fixation of components of the new generation of non-cemented resurfacing endoprosthesis of the hip joint (and other joints). The quantitative micro-CT evaluation of bone biostructure carried out during the laboratory study of the mechanical embedding of the prototype MSC-Scaffold in the heads of swine femurs allowed analysis of the changes observed in bone density that occur directly under the embedded MSC-Scaffold. Following the analysis, we have made the initial numerical model of the subject of the study more realistic by introducing an insert simulating the densified bone material under the embedded MSC-Scaffold. This modification of the initial numerical model of the studied mechanical process led to a significant improvement in convergence between the results of the laboratory and simulation tests: the calculated value of the fraction of variance unexplained (FVU) index for the compared studies increased significantly to 0.02, indicating a very good convergence; thus, the experimental validation of the modified numerical model of the problem studied was carried out (i.e. mechanical loading of the prototype biomimetic MSC-Scaffold initially and partially embedded in the periarticular bone).

The structural biomimetism of the prototype MSC-Scaffold ensures physiological, uniform surface transfer of the mechanical load from the spikes of the MSC-Scaffold to the trabeculae of the periarticular trabecular bone – it was confirmed based on the analysis of HMH reduced stress maps obtained based on a simulation study of the embedding process using a modified and validated numerical model of the subject of the study. Since we have used a well-known and widely recognized method of validating numerical problems that is applied to many problems in the mechanics of intraosseous implants (the method combines experimental research and numerical analyses), the results obtained from a numerical simulation analysis of the distribution of stress in the periarticular bone around the mechanically loaded partially embedded prototype MSC-Scaffold, performed using a validated numerical model, can be considered as reliable. Thus, it can be stated that the modified numerical model accurately reflects the mechanical behaviour of the examined implant-bone system in the early postoperative period. Controlled loading of the innovative non-cemented resurfacing arthroplasty endoprosthesis with the MSC-Scaffold by the patient in the early postoperative rehabilitation period enables the bone tissue to ingrow into the interspike spaces of the MSC-Scaffold and ensures the final biological fixation of the implant in the bone (which is achieved by bone tissue ingrow and osseointegration with CaP-modified MSC-Scaffold surface).

So, it can be concluded that: (1) the resulting validated numerical model of the considered problem can be used in the bioengineering design of a new type of entirely non-cemented biomimetic fixation of the components of resurfacing arthroplasty endoprostheses in the periarticular bone, replacing degenerative or traumatically damaged synovial joints, and (2) the early postoperative biomechanical load capacity (loadability) of the articular surface of the non-cemented resurfacing endoprosthesis with MSC-Scaffold can be considered the crucial design criterion for such innovative endoprostheses.

To demonstrate in a pilot experiment on an animal model that the innovative MSC-Scaffold allows for an entirely non-cemented and biomimetic fixation of the components of resurfacing arthroplasty endoprostheses in the periarticular trabecular bone, the CAD model of the working prototype of partial resurfacing knee arthroplasty endoprosthesis for swine was developed using reverse engineering methods. The working prototypes of partial resurfacing knee arthroplasty endoprosthesis were manufactured in SLM technology according to the developed CAD model, and the bone-contacting surface of the MSC-Scaffold spikes was modified by depositing a calcium phosphate coating, and then the endoprostheses were implanted in the knee joints of ten swine of the Polish Large White breed. Radiological, histopathological, and microtomographic examinations were performed on bone-implant specimens harvested after eight weeks. In the postoperative clinical examination of the operated knee joints of the above animals, the clinical stability of these joints was good and very good (mean score of 4 on the 5-point Likert scale). Postoperative radiological examinations have indicated good implant fixation (radiolucency less than 2 mm) with no signs of implant migration. The interspike spaces in the MSC-Scaffold of the implanted prototype implants were occupied with the ingrown bone tissue. Histological specimens obtained from bone-implant samples harvested from operated animals eight weeks after implantation (according to the protocol approved by the Local Ethics Committee in Poznan) indicated the presence of newly formed trabecular bone tissue in the spaces between the MSC-Scaffold spikes, with the trabeculae in contact with the spikes. According to the quantitative microtomographic analysis, it was found that the highest percentage of bone tissue ingrowth in the space between the spikes occurs at a distance of 2.5–3.0 mm from the base of the spikes. The experimental pilot implantations in ten swine of the working prototype of partial resurfacing knee arthroplasty endoprosthesis have indicated that it was possible successfully and without the use of cement to anchor the components of resurfacing arthroplasty endoprostheses in the periarticular bone using the innovative biomimetic MSC-Scaffold.

Pilot studies have also been carried out on human femoral heads (with the approval of the Bioethics Committee of the Poznan University of Medical Sciences), including a quantitative microtomographic evaluation of the impact of the mechanical embedding of the MSC-Scaffold concerning the density and compressive strength of the subchondral trabecular bone of femoral heads from four patients with osteoarthritis treated surgically using long-stem hip endoprostheses. Using microcomputed tomography, the microarchitecture of the subchondral trabecular bone was analysed before and after the mechanical embedding of the MSC-Scaffold in the heads of the human femoral bone. There were differences in bone volume density in the heads of the femurs of individual patients with osteoarthritis who underwent surgery. The embedding of the MSC-Scaffold in the subchondral trabecular bone allowed the observation, using microtomographic digital reconstructions of the examined bone, of a change in the ratio of the subchondral trabecular bone area to the total area (BA/TA) ranging from 18.2% to 24.7% (translating to the relative change of the calculated density ρ_b relative change from 11.1% to 14.4%, and the relative change of the predicted compressive strength S from 75.3% to 122.7%) regardless of its initial density (before the embedding). Due to the mechanical embedding of the MSC-Scaffold, the density of the subchondral trabecular bone gradually decreases with increasing distance from the tops of its spikes, while the spatial extent of the densification of the subchondral trabecular bone ranged from 1.5 to 2.5 mm (which is about half the height of the spikes of the MSC-Scaffold). Therefore, we can conclude, despite the limited number of human femoral heads subject to study, that: (1) the magnitude of the impact of the initial surgical embedding of the MSC-Scaffold on the subchondral trabecular bone of the femoral head appears to be a factor determining the long-term maintenance of this innovative MSC-Scaffold (and of the resurfacing endoprosthesis fixed in the periarticular bone via this MSC-Scaffold) also in the case of reduced bone volume density of the femoral head; (2) the greater the extent of the subchondral trabecular bone densification, the greater the mechanical strength of the bone, thus resulting in better conditions for the postoperative functioning of the fixation of the MSC-Scaffold in the periarticular bone. The suggestions formulated here obviously require verification in a larger sample of human femoral heads obtained from postoperative material from patients with hip osteoarthritis treated with THA using long-stem hip endoprostheses (the team received approval from the Bioethics Committee of the Poznan University of Medical Sciences to carry out such extended research by 2024).

CONCLUSIONS AND FINAL REMARKS

- the prototype of the hip joint resurfacing arthroplasty endoprosthesis with the MSC-Scaffold, designed and manufactured using SLM technology of titanium alloy powder, fixed in the periarticular bone without the use of cement via the MSC-Scaffold (Figure 3.31) constitutes fundamental bioengineering progress as compared to the early demonstration prototype of the hip joint resurfacing arthroplasty endoprosthesis manufactured of chromium steel by die-sinker electrical discharge machining (Figure 3.15) for the patent held by the author of the concept of this endoprosthesis (P. Rogala) before starting the above-mentioned research projects;

- the structural biomimetism of the developed prototype of the MSC-Scaffold for fixation in periarticular bone of the components of the new-generation non-cemented hip and knee endoprostheses causes the biomechanical loads acting on the articular surface of the innovative endoprosthesis to be transferred as stresses almost uniformly to the trabeculae of the periarticular trabecular bone – so we can expect that the occurrence of the undesirable effect of the so-called *stress shielding* around intraosseous implants will be significantly reduced in these innovative endoprostheses;
- a pilot experimental study carried out on an animal model (hip joints and knee joints of swines of Polish Large White breed) has proven the effectiveness of entirely non-cemented fixation in the periarticular bone of components of resurfacing arthroplasty endoprostheses via a biomimetic prototype of the MSC-Scaffold developed by our team; the evaluation of the MSC-Scaffold biointegration with the periarticular bone, carried out eight weeks post-implantation, has shown that the majority of the interspike space of the MSC-Scaffold was occupied with the ingrown, newly formed, and mineralized bone tissue, i.e. it was demonstrated that the MSC-Scaffold allows for the so-called *biological fixation* of the components of resurfacing endoprostheses in the periarticular bone;
- the resulting validated numerical model of the considered problem (partially embedded in bone prototype MSC-Scaffold mechanically loaded) can be used in the bioengineering design of a new type of entirely non-cemented biomimetic fixation in the periarticular bone of the components of resurfacing arthroplasty endoprostheses replacing degenerative or traumatically damaged synovial joints;
- the early postoperative biomechanical load capacity (loadability) of the articular surface of the non-cemented resurfacing arthroplasty endoprosthesis with MSC-Scaffold can be considered the crucial design criterion for such innovative endoprostheses (because controlled loading of the innovative non-cemented resurfacing arthroplasty endoprosthesis by the patient in the early postoperative rehabilitation period enables the bone tissue to ingrow into the interspike spaces of the MSC-Scaffold and ensures the final biological fixation of the implant in the bone);
- we have completed bioengineering preclinical research for the development of a biomimetic prototype of the MSC-Scaffold for a new generation of entirely non-cemented resurfacing arthroplasty endoprostheses, and thus it was prepared the next stage of clinical surgical research in humans was prepared, including experimental surgical treatment of damaged knee and hip joints using prototype resurfacing endoprostheses with the biomimetic MSC-Scaffold.

***

In our opinion, the new generation of entirely non-cemented resurfacing arthroplasty endoprostheses for the hip and other joints, whose components are fixed in the periarticular bone via the biomimetic prototype MSC-Scaffold, developed by the bioengineering and clinical research team in Poznan, Poland, is going to be the first generation of biomimetic resurfacing arthroplasty endoprostheses and biomimetic endoprostheses at all.

Appendix 1
Patents front pages scans (US, Canada, Europe)

The Commissioner of
Patents and Trademarks

The
United
States
of
America

Has received an application for a patent for a new and useful invention. The title and description of the invention are enclosed. The requirements of law have been complied with, and it has been determined that a patent on the invention shall be granted under the law.

Therefore, this

United States Patent

Grants to the person(s) having title to this patent the right to exclude others from making, using, offering for sale, or selling the invention throughout the United States of America or importing the invention into the United States of America for the term set forth below, subject to the payment of maintenance fees as provided by law.

If this application was filed prior to June 8, 1995, the term of this patent is the longer of seventeen years from the date of grant of this patent or twenty years from the earliest effective U.S. filing date of the application, subject to any statutory extension.

If this application was filed on or after June 8, 1995, the term of this patent is twenty years from the U.S. filing date, subject to any statutory extension. If the application contains a specific reference to an earlier filed application or applications under 35 U.S.C. 120, 121 or 365(c), the term of the patent is twenty years from the date on which the earliest application was filed, subject to any statutory extension.

Acting Commissioner of Patents and Trademarks

Attest

US005911759A

United States Patent [19]

Rogala

[11]	Patent Number:	5,911,759
[45]	Date of Patent:	Jun. 15, 1999

[54] **ACETABULUM ENDOPROSTHESIS AND HEAD**

[76] Inventor: **Piotr Rogala**, Podolska 6, PL-60-615 Poznan, Poland

[21] Appl. No.: **08/809,117**

[22] PCT Filed: **Sep. 14, 1995**

[86] PCT No.: **PCT/PL95/00020**

§ 371 Date: **May 14, 1997**

§ 102(e) Date: **May 14, 1997**

[87] PCT Pub. No.: **WO96/08214**

PCT Pub. Date: **Mar. 21, 1996**

[30] **Foreign Application Priority Data**

Sep. 16, 1994 [PL] Poland 305060

[51] **Int. Cl.⁶** **A61F 2/32**
[52] **U.S. Cl.** **623/22**; 623/19; 623/18
[58] **Field of Search** 623/22, 23, 20, 623/19, 18, 16

[56] **References Cited**

U.S. PATENT DOCUMENTS

2,910,978	11/1959	Urist .	
3,840,904	10/1974	Tronzo .	
4,659,331	4/1987	Matthews et al.	623/22
4,919,677	4/1990	Stuhmer et al.	623/22
5,108,448	4/1992	Gautier	623/22
5,358,532	10/1994	Evans et al.	623/22
5,609,646	3/1997	Field et al.	623/22

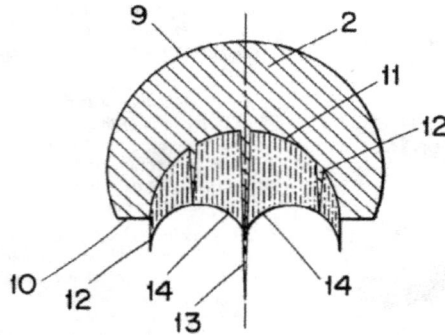

FOREIGN PATENT DOCUMENTS

009 148	4/1980	European Pat. Off. .
013 863	8/1980	European Pat. Off. .
2 598 908	5/1986	France .
2 519 545	1/1992	France .
2 686 503	1/1992	France .
2 150 441	7/1985	United Kingdom .

Primary Examiner—Michael J. Milano
Assistant Examiner—Tram A. Nguyen
Attorney, Agent, or Firm—Burns, Doane, Swecker & Mathis, L.L.P.

[57] **ABSTRACT**

An implantation method is described which involves the successive introduction of projecting multilateral needles into the spongy bone of a joint. The needles are symmetrically spaced on the terminal surfaces of the endoprosthesis up to a resistance edge on one portion of an endoprosthesis and up to a resistance surface on a second portion of the endoprosthesis. The remaining free area between the projecting multilateral needles is filled up to the terminal surfaces in the "biological silence" by osteoblasts. The endoprosthesis also includes a glenoid cavity and a head which have round terminal surfaces with the projecting multilateral needles placed thereon. The projecting multilateral needles have different lengths and mutually parallel axes which are perpendicular to the planes in which the round resistance edge of the glenoid cavity and the resistance plane of the head are located.

20 Claims, 1 Drawing Sheet

Office de la propriété intellectuelle du Canada

Un organisme d'Industrie Canada

Canadian Intellectual Property Office

An Agency of Industry Canada

Brevet canadien / Canadian Patent

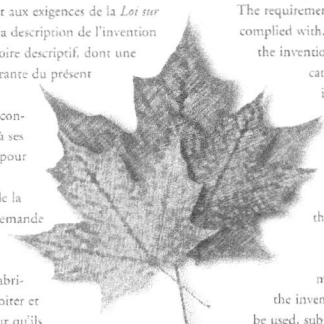

✤ Le commissaire aux brevets a reçu une demande de délivrance de brevet visant une invention. Ladite requête satisfait aux exigences de la *Loi sur les brevets*. Le titre et la description de l'invention figurent dans le mémoire descriptif, dont une copie fait partie intégrante du présent document.

Le présent brevet confère à son titulaire et à ses représentants légaux, pour une période expirant vingt ans à compter de la date du dépôt de la demande au Canada, le droit, la faculté et le privilège exclusif de fabriquer, construire, exploiter et vendre à d'autres, pour qu'ils l'exploitent, l'objet de l'invention, sauf jugement en l'espèce rendu par un tribunal compétent, et sous réserve du paiement des taxes périodiques.

✤ The Commissioner of Patents has received a petition for the grant of a patent for an invention. The requirements of the *Patent Act* have been complied with. The title and a description of the invention are contained in the specification, a copy of which forms an integral part of this document.

The present patent grants to its owner and to the legal representatives of its owner, for a term which expires twenty years from the filing date of the application in Canada, the exclusive right, privilege and liberty of making, constructing and using the invention and selling it to others to be used, subject to adjudication before any court of competent jurisdiction, and subject to the payment of maintenance fees.

BREVET CANADIEN   **2,200,064**   CANADIAN PATENT

Date à laquelle le brevet a été accordé et délivré	**2003/04/01**	Date on which the patent was granted and issued
Date du dépôt de la demande	**1995/09/14**	Filing date of the application
Date à laquelle la demande est devenue accessible au public pour consultation	**1996/03/21**	Date on which the application was made available for public inspection

Commissaire aux brevets / Commissioner of Patents

Canadä

3258 (CIPO 91/02-2

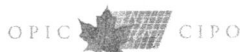

OPIC   CIPO

Office de la Propriété   Canadian   CA 2200064 C 2003/04/01
Intellectuelle   Intellectual Property
du Canada   Office   (11)(21) 2 200 064

Un organisme   An agency of   (12) BREVET CANADIEN
d'Industrie Canada   Industry Canada   CANADIEN PATENT
                                                                          (13) C

(86) Date de dépôt PCT/PCT Filing Date: 1995/09/14   (51) Cl.Int.^{6}/Int.Cl.^{6} A61F 2/34, A61F 2/36, A61F 2/32
(87) Date publication PCT/PCT Publication Date: 1996/03/21 (72) Inventeur/Inventor:
(45) Date de délivrance/Issue Date: 2003/04/01   ROGALA, PIOTR, PL
(85) Entrée phase nationale/National Entry: 1997/03/14   (73) Propriétaire/Owner:
(86) N° demande PCT/PCT Application No.: PL 1995/000020   ROGALA, PIOTR, PL
(87) N° publication PCT/PCT Publication No.: 1996/008214   (74) Agent: RICHES, MCKENZIE & HERBERT LLP
(30) Priorité/Priority: 1994/09/16 (P.305060) PL

(54) Titre : ENDOPROTHESE
(54) Title: ENDOPROSTHESIS

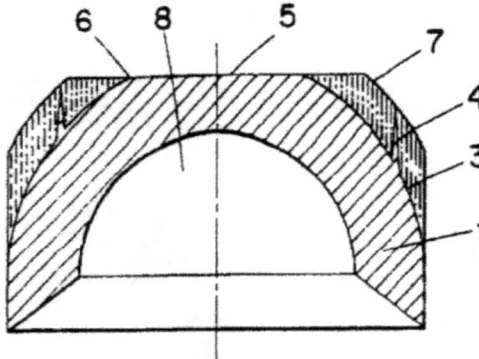

(57) Abrégé/Abstract:
An implantation method is described which involves the successive introduction of projecting multilateral needles into the spongy bone of a joint. The needles are symmetrically spaced on the terminal surfaces of the endoprosthesis up to a resistance edge on one portion of an endoprosthesis and up to a resistance surface on a second portion of the endoprosthesis. The remaining free area between the projecting multilateral needles is filled up to the terminal surfaces in the "biological silence" by osteoblasts. The endoprosthesis also includes a glenoid cavity and a head which have round terminal surfaces with the projecting multilateral needles placed thereon. The projecting multilateral needles have different lengths and mutually parallel axes which are perpendicular to the planes in which the round resistance edge of the glenoid cavity and the resistance plane of the head are located.

‖‖‖‖‖‖‖‖‖‖‖‖‖‖‖‖‖‖‖‖‖‖‖‖‖‖‖‖

(19) **BUNDESREPUBLIK DEUTSCHLAND**

(12) **Übersetzung der europäischen Patentschrift**

(97) EP 0 782 418 B 1

(10) **DE 695 14 110 T 2**

(51) Int. Cl.⁷:
A 61 F 2/32
A 61 F 2/34
A 61 F 2/36

DE 695 14 110 T 2

DEUTSCHES PATENT- UND MARKENAMT

(21) Deutsches Aktenzeichen:	695 14 110.4	
(86) PCT-Aktenzeichen:	PCT/PL95/00020	
(96) Europäisches Aktenzeichen:	95 930 745.5	
(87) PCT-Veröffentlichungs-Nr.:	WO 96/08214	
(86) PCT-Anmeldetag:	14. 9. 1995	
(87) Veröffentlichungstag der PCT-Anmeldung:	21. 3. 1996	
(97) Erstveröffentlichung durch das EPA:	9. 7. 1997	
(97) Veröffentlichungstag der Patenterteilung beim EPA:	22. 12. 1999	
(47) Veröffentlichungstag im Patentblatt:	27. 4. 2000	

EP 13367

(30) Unionspriorität:

30506094   16. 09. 1994   PL

(73) Patentinhaber:

Rogala, Piotr, Poznan, PL

(74) Vertreter:

Grünecker, Kinkeldey, Stockmair & Schwanhäusser, 80538 München

(84) Benannte Vertragsstaaten:

AT, CH, DE, ES, FR, GB, IT, LI, SE

(72) Erfinder:

gleich Anmelder

(54) ENDOPROTHESE

DE 695 14 110 T 2

BUNDESDRUCKEREI 03.00 002 317/379/3G   1

Appendix 2
Letter of thanks from the Rector of the Poznan University of Technology, Poland

A letter of thanks from the Rector of the Poznan University of Technology and the Dean for the bioengineering team for many years of research and teaching activities in the field of biomedical engineering at the Poznan University of Technology (addressed to the head of the team).

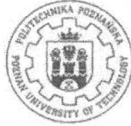

POZNAN UNIVERSITY OF TECHNOLOGY

Prof. Teofil Jesionowski
Rector

Poznan, 16th of June 2022

Professor

Dr hab. Eng. MD, PhD Ryszard UKLEJEWSKI

Dear Professor,

please accept sincere thanks for your active and constructive research and teaching cooperation in the field of biomedical engineering with the Faculty of Mechanical Engineering (previously Faculty of Mechanical Engineering and Management) and the Faculty of Chemical Technology of the Poznan University of Technology.

Initiated by you, Professor, since 2005 together with a bioengineering and clinical-orthopaedic scientific team, active research and teaching activities, connected an academic centers: Poznan University of Technology, Poznan University of Medical Sciences and the Kazimierz Wielki University in Bydgoszcz. Research cooperation in the field of biomedical engineering has resulted in numerous research projects, published research articles, patents and doctorates, conducted in cooperation with, among others, employees of the Poznan University of Technology. Today's very important achievement of the team's work is the latest research monograph "Prototype of a biomimetric scaffold connecting with the bone the components of a new generation of cementless surface joint endoprostheses - design, bioengineering research and pilot experiments on animal model" by Ryszard Uklejewski, Piotr Rogala, and Mariusz Winiecki.

You have also promoted four doctors in the field of engineering sciences, and a lot of masters and engineers. Of particular importance for the Poznan University of Technology, especially for strengthening the academic staff of the Faculty of Mechanical Engineering PUT in the field of biomedical engineering, is the public defense of the distinguished doctoral thesis by M. Sc. Adam Patalas (an assistant at the Faculty of Mechanical Engineering PUT) carried out under your, Professor, guidance in the Warsaw University of Technology in the field of biomedical engineering, in June 2022.

Let us emphasize the participation of the Professor in creating the field of *Biomedical engineering* at the Faculty of Mechanical Engineering PUT as one of the first in Poland.

Dear Professor,

thank you for your and your team cooperation as well as research and teaching work. We are deeply convinced that it will be continued in the coming years on many other different levels.

Yours faithfully

Dean
of Faculty of Mechanical Engineering

Rector
of Poznan University of Technology

5 M. Skłodowska-Curie Square, 60-965 Poznan, Poland, tel.: +48 61 665 3537, 61 833 3881, fax: +48 61 665 3770
e-mail: rektor@put.poznan.pl, www.put.poznan.pl

Index

For Product Safety Concerns and Information please contact our EU
representative GPSR@taylorandfrancis.com
Taylor & Francis Verlag GmbH, Kaufingerstraße 24, 80331 München, Germany

www.ingramcontent.com/pod-product-compliance
Lightning Source LLC
Chambersburg PA
CBHW070712220326
41598CB00024BA/3121